T0263022

Challenges After Treatment for Childhood Cancer

Editors

MAX J. COPPES
LEONTINEN C.M. KREMER

PEDIATRIC CLINICS
OF NORTH AMERICA

www.pediatric.theclinics.com

Consulting Editor
BONITA F. STANTON

December 2020 • Volume 67 • Number 6

ELSEVIER

1600 John F. Kennedy Boulevard • Suite 1800 • Philadelphia, Pennsylvania, 19103-2899

http://www.theclinics.com

THE PEDIATRIC CLINICS OF NORTH AMERICA Volume 67, Number 6
December 2020 ISSN 0031-3955, ISBN-13: 978-0-323-71078-7

Editor: Kerry Holland
Developmental Editor: Casey Potter

The Pediatric Clinics of North America (ISSN 0031-3955) is published bimonthly by Elsevier Inc., 360 Park Avenue South, New York, NY 10010-1710. Months of issue are February, April, June, August, October, and December. Periodicals postage paid at New York, NY and additional mailing offices. Subscription prices are $240.00 per year (US individuals), $695.00 per year (US institutions), $315.00 per year (Canadian individuals), $924.00 per year (Canadian institutions), $362.00 per year (international individuals), $924.00 per year (international institutions), $100.00 per year (US students and residents), $100.00 per year (Canadian students and residents), and $165.00 per year (international residents and students). To receive students/resident rare, orders must be accompanied by name of affiliated institution, date of term, and the signature of program/residency coordinator on institution letterhead. Orders will be billed at individual rate until proof of status is received. Foreign air speed delivery is included in all *Clinics* subscription prices. All prices are subject to change without notice. **POSTMASTER:** Send address changes to *The Pediatric Clinics of North America*, Elsevier Health Sciences Division, Subscription Customer Service, 3251 Riverport Lane, Maryland Heights, MO 63043. **Customer Service: 1-800-654-2452 (US and Canada). From outside of the US and Canada: 1-314-447-8871. Fax: 1-314-447-8029. For print support, E-mail: JournalsCustomerService-usa@elsevier.com. For online support, E-mail: JournalsOnlineSupport-usa@elsevier.com.**

Reprints. For copies of 100 or more, of articles in this publication, please contact the Commercial Reprints Department, Elsevier Inc., 360 Park Avenue South, New York, NY 10010-1710. Tel.: 212-633-3874; Fax: 212-633-3820; E-mail: reprints@elsevier.com.

The Pediatric Clinics of North America is also published in Spanish by McGraw-Hill Inter-americana Editores S.A., Mexico City, Mexico; in Portuguese by Riechmann and Affonso Editores, Rua Comandante Coelho 1085, CEP 21250, Rio de Janeiro, Brazil; and in Greek by Althayia SA, Athens, Greece.

The Pediatric Clinics of North America is covered in *MEDLINE/PubMed (Index Medicus)*, *Excerpta Medica*, *Current Contents*, *Current Contents/Clinical Medicine*, *Science Citation Index*, *ASCA*, *ISI/BIOMED*, and *BIOSIS*.

PROGRAM OBJECTIVE

The goal of the *Pediatric Clinics of North America* is to keep practicing physicians and residents up to date with current clinical practice in pediatrics by providing timely articles reviewing the state-of-the-art in patient care.

TARGET AUDIENCE

All practicing pediatricians, physicians and healthcare professionals who provide patient care to pediatric patients.

LEARNING OBJECTIVES

Upon completion of this activity, participants will be able to:
1. Review the impact of late effects of childhood cancer treatment.
2. Discuss the critical role of Clinical Practice Guidelines (CPGs) for long-term follow up, and how these have been and continue to be developed.
3. Recognize how lessons learned early on from cancer treatment influenced a new and still evolving field of medicine.

ACCREDITATIONS

Physician Credit

The Elsevier Office of Continuing Medical Education (EOCME) is accredited by the Accreditation Council for Continuing Medical Education (ACCME) to provide continuing medical education for physicians.

The EOCME designates this journal-based activity for a maximum of 15 *AMA PRA Category 1 Credit*(s)™. Physicians should claim only the credit commensurate with the extent of their participation in the activity.

All other healthcare professionals requesting continuing education credit for this this journal-based activity will be issued a certificate of participation.

ABP Maintenance of Certification Credit

Successful completion of this CME activity, which includes participation in the activity and individual assessment of and feedback to the learner, enables the learner to earn up to 15 MOC points in the American Board of Pediatrics' (ABP) Maintenance of Certification (MOC) program. It is the CME activity provider's responsibility to submit learner completion information to ACCME for the purpose of granting ABP MOC credit.

DISCLOSURE OF CONFLICTS OF INTEREST

The EOCME assesses conflict of interest with its instructors, faculty, planners, and other individuals who are in a position to control the content of CME activities. All relevant conflicts of interest that are identified are thoroughly vetted by EOCME for fair balance, scientific objectivity, and patient care recommendations. EOCME is committed to providing its learners with CME activities that promote improvements or quality in healthcare and not a specific proprietary business or a commercial interest.

The planning committee, staff, authors and editors listed below have identified no financial relationships or relationships to products or devices they or their spouse/life partner have with commercial interest related to the content of this CME activity:

Gregory T. Armstrong, MD, MSCE; Julie Berbis, MD; Smita Bhatia, MD, MPH; Annelies M.E. Bos, MD, PhD; Tara M. Brinkman, PhD; Sharon M. Castellino, MD, MSc; Regina Chavous-Gibson, MSN, RN; Wassim Chemaitilly, MD, PhD; Eric J. Chow, MD, MPH; Richard J. Cohn, MBBCh, FCP (SA), FRACP; Louis S. Constine, MD; Max J. Coppes, MD, PhD, MBA; Florent de Vathaire, PhD; Jaap den Hartogh, MA; Stephanie B. Dixon, MD, MPH; Matthew J. Ehrhardt, MD, MS; E.A.M. (Lieke) Feijen, PhD; Caitlin Forbes, MA; Martha Grootenhuis, PhD; Matthew D. Hall, MD, MBA; Riccardo Haupt, MD; Michael Magnus Hawkins, BSc, MSc, Dphil; Tara Henderson; Lars Hjorth, MD; Kerry Holland; Melissa M. Hudson, MD; J. Martin Johnston, MD; David M. Johnstone; Line Kenborg, MSc, PhD; Anita Kienesberger, MA; Chrysoula Kosmeri, MD, PhD; Leontien C.M. Kremer, MD, PhD; Kevin Krull, PhD; Claudia E. Kuehni, MD, MSc; Wendy Landier, PhD, CRNP; Anita Mahajan, MD; Alexandros Makis, MD, PhD; Rajkumar Mayakrishnann; Mary L. McBride, MSc; Lillian R. Meacham, MD, PhD; Gisela Michel, PhD; Lindsay M. Morton, PhD; Sogol Mostoufi-Moab, MD, PhD; Renée L. Mulder, PhD; Paul C. Nathan, MD, MSc; Kirsten K. Ness, PhD; Filippa Nyboe Norsker, PhD; Kevin C. Oeffinger, MD; Maria Otth, MD; Michaela Patton, BA; Arnold C. Paulino, MD; Camilla Pedersen, PhD; Saskia Pluijm, PhD; Leslie L. Robison, PhD; Brooke Russell, MSc; Carina Schneider; Fiona Schulte, PhD; Ekaterini Siomou, MD, PhD; Roderick Skinner, MB ChB, PhD, FRCPCH; Jop C. Teepen, PhD; Zuzana Tomášiková,

MSc; Emily S. Tonorezos, MD, PhD; Sophia Tsabouri, MD, PhD; Marianne D. van de Wetering, MD, PhD; Marry M. van den Heuvel-Eibrink, MD, PhD; Helena J. van der Pal, MD, PhD; Rebecca J. van Kalsbeek, MD; Henk Visscher, MD, PhD; Claire E. Wakefield, PhD; W. Hamish Wallace, MD, PhD; Jeanette Falck Winther, MD, DMSc; Suzanne Wolden, MD; Amanda Wurz, PhD; Adam Yan, MD

The planning committee, staff, authors and editors listed below have identified financial relationships or relationships to products or devices they or their spouse/life partner have with commercial interest related to the content of this CME activity:

Joshua D. Palmer, MD: research support from Varian Medical Systems, Inc and speaker's fees from DePuy Synthes

Hanneke M. van Santen, MD, PhD: speaker's fees from Pfizer Inc and Ferring B.V.

UNAPPROVED/OFF-LABEL USE DISCLOSURE
The EOCME requires CME faculty to disclose to the participants:
1. When products or procedures being discussed are off-label, unlabelled, experimental, and/or investigational (not US Food and Drug Administration [FDA] approved); and
2. Any limitations on the information presented, such as data that are preliminary or that represent ongoing research, interim analyses, and/or unsupported opinions. Faculty may discuss information about pharmaceutical agents that is outside of FDA-approved labelling. This information is intended solely for CME and is not intended to promote off-label use of these medications. If you have any questions, contact the medical affairs department of the manufacturer for the most recent prescribing information.

TO ENROLL
To enroll in the *Pediatric Clinics of North America* Continuing Medical Education program, call customer service at 1-800-654-2452 or sign up online at http://www.theclinics.com/home/cme. The CME program is available to subscribers for an additional annual fee of USD 300.00.

METHOD OF PARTICIPATION
In order to claim credit, participants must complete the following:
1. Complete enrolment as indicated above.
2. Read the activity.
3. Complete the CME Test and Evaluation. Participants must achieve a score of 70% on the test. All CME Tests and Evaluations must be completed online.

In order to claim MOC points, participants must complete the following:
1. Complete steps listed above for claiming CME credit
2. Provide your specialty board ID#, birth date (MM/DD), and attestation.
3. Online MOC submission is only available for the American Board of pediatrics' (ABP) Maintenance of Certification (MOC) program

CME INQUIRIES/SPECIAL NEEDS
For all CME inquiries or special needs, please contact elsevierCME@elsevier.com.

Contributors

CONSULTING EDITOR

BONITA F. STANTON, MD
Founding Dean, and Robert C. and Laura C. Garrett Endowed Chair, Hackensack Meridian School of Medicine, President, Academic Enterprise, Hackensack Meridian Health, Nutley, New Jersey

EDITORS

MAX J. COPPES, MD, PhD, MBA
Professor and Nell J. Redfield Chair of Pediatrics, University of Nevada Reno School of Medicine, Physician-in-Chief, Renown Children's Hospital, Reno, Nevada, USA

LEONTINE C.M. KREMER, MD, PhD
Principle Investigator Survivorship Research, Princess Máxima Center for Pediatric Oncology, Utrecht, The Netherlands; Professor of Pediatrics, University of Amsterdam, Amsterdam, The Netherlands

AUTHORS

GREGORY T. ARMSTRONG, MD, MSCE
Member, Department of Epidemiology and Cancer Control, St. Jude Children's Research Hospital, Memphis, Tennessee, USA

JULIE BERBIS, PhD
Assistance Publique Hôpitaux de Marseille, Aix-Marseille University, EA 3279 CEReSS, Health Service Research and Quality of Life Center, Marseille, France

SMITA BHATIA, MD, MPH
Director, Institute for Cancer Outcomes and Survivorship, Professor, Department of Pediatrics, School of Medicine, University of Alabama at Birmingham, Birmingham, Alabama, USA

ANNELIES M.E. BOS, MD, PhD
Associate Professor, Gynecologist, Subspecialist, Reproductive Medicine, Fertility Specialist, Department of Reproductive Medicine and Gynecology, University Medical Centre, Utrecht, Utrecht, The Netherlands

TARA M. BRINKMAN, PhD
Associate Member, Departments of Epidemiology and Cancer Control and Psychology, St. Jude Children's Research Hospital, Memphis, Tennessee, USA

SHARON M. CASTELLINO, MD, MSc
Department of Pediatrics, Hematology-Oncology, Emory University School of Medicine, Aflac Cancer and Blood Disorders Center, Children's Healthcare of Atlanta, Atlanta, Georgia, USA

WASSIM CHEMAITILLY, MD, PhD
Pediatric Endocrinologist, Division of Endocrinology, St. Jude Children's Research Hospital, Memphis, Tennessee, USA

ERIC J. CHOW, MD, MPH
Associate Professor, Fred Hutchinson Cancer Research Center, University of Washington, Seattle, Washington, USA

RICHARD J. COHN, MBBCh, FCP (SA), FRACP
Conjoint Professor, School of Women's and Children's Health, UNSW Sydney and Clinical Program Director, Medicine, Head, Clinical Oncology, Kids Cancer Centre, Sydney Children's Hospital, Sydney, New South Wales, Australia

LOUIS S. CONSTINE, MD
Departments of Radiation Oncology and Pediatrics, University of Rochester, The Philip Rubin Professor of Radiation Oncology and Pediatrics, Vice Chair, Department of Radiation Oncology, Director, The Judy DiMarzo Cancer Survivorship Program, James P. Wilmot Cancer Institute, University of Rochester Medical Center, Rochester, New York, USA

FLORENT DE VATHAIRE, PhD
Research Director, Institut Gustave Roussy, Villejuif, France

JAAP DEN HARTOGH, MA
Vereniging Ouders, Kinderen en Kanker, Childhood Cancer International Europe, Nieuwegein, The Netherlands

STEPHANIE B. DIXON, MD, MPH
Instructor, Division of Cancer Survivorship, Department of Oncology, St. Jude Children's Research Hospital, Memphis, Tennessee, USA

MATTHEW J. EHRHARDT, MD, MS
Department of Oncology, St. Jude Children's Research Hospital, Department of Epidemiology and Cancer Control, St. Jude Children's Research Hospital, Memphis, Tennessee, USA

E.A.M. (LIEKE) FEIJEN, PhD
Post doc, Princess Máxima Center for Pediatric Oncology, Utrecht, The Netherlands

CAITLIN FORBES, MSc
University of Calgary, Alberta Children's Hospital, Calgary, Alberta, Canada

MARTHA GROOTENHUIS, PhD
Professor, Princess Máxima Center for Pediatric Oncology, Utrecht, the Netherlands

MATTHEW D. HALL, MD, MBA
Department of Radiation Oncology, Miami Cancer Institute and Nicklaus Children's Hospital, Miami, Florida, USA

RICCARDO HAUPT, MD
IRCCS Istituto Giannina Gaslini, Genova, Italy

MICHAEL HAWKINS, DPhil
Chair in Epidemiology & Director of Centre, Centre for Childhood Cancer Survivor Studies, Institute of Applied Health Research, Professor, University of Birmingham, Birmingham, United Kingdom

TARA O. HENDERSON, MD, MPH
Professor of Pediatrics, Interim Section Chief, Pediatric Hematology, Oncology and Stem Cell Transplantation, The University of Chicago, Chicago, Illinois, USA

LARS HJORTH, MD
Associate Professor, Department of Paediatrics, Skane University Hospital, Clinical Sciences Lund, Lund University, Lund, Sweden

MELISSA M. HUDSON, MD
Departments of Epidemiology and Cancer Control, Member, Division of Cancer Survivorship, Department of Oncology, St. Jude Children's Research Hospital, Memphis, Tennessee, USA

DAVID M. JOHNSTON, BA
Permits Coordinator, Salt Lake City Waste & Recycling Division, Salt Lake City, Utah, USA

J. MARTIN JOHNSTON, MD
Division of Pediatric Hematology/Oncology, University of Nevada, Reno, Renown Children's Hospital, Reno, Nevada, USA

LINE KENBORG, PhD
Senior Researcher, Childhood Cancer Research Group, Danish Cancer Society Research Center, Copenhagen, Denmark

ANITA KIENESBERGER, MA
Österreichische Kinder-Krebs-Hilfe (ÖKKH), Childhood Cancer International Europe, Wien, Austria

LEONTIEN C.M. KREMER, MD, PhD
Professor, Princess Maxima Center for Pediatric Oncology, Utrecht, Netherlands; Emma Children's Hospital, Amsterdam UMC, Amsterdam, Netherlands

KEVIN R. KRULL, PhD
St. Jude Children's Research Hospital, Memphis, Tennessee, USA

CLAUDIA E. KUEHNI, MD
Head, Childhood Cancer Research Platform, Professor, Swiss Childhood Cancer Registry, Institute of Social and Preventive Medicine, Department of Pediatrics, Paediatric Oncology, Inselspital, Bern University Hospital, University of Bern, Bern, Switzerland

WENDY LANDIER, PhD, CRNP
Professor, Pediatric Hematology/Oncology, Deputy Director, Institute for Cancer Outcomes and Survivorship, University of Alabama at Birmingham, Birmingham, Alabama, USA

ANITA MAHAJAN, MD
Department of Radiation Oncology, The Mayo Clinic, Rochester, Minnesota, USA

MARY L. McBRIDE, MSc
Clinical Professor, BC Cancer, Vancouver, British Columbia, Canada

LILLIAN R. MEACHAM, MD, PhD
Pediatric Endocrinologist, Division of Hematology/Oncology/BMT, Department of Pediatrics, Emory University, Atlanta, Georgia, USA

GISELA MICHEL, PhD
Professor, Department of Health Sciences and Medicine, University of Lucerne, Lucerne, Switzerland

LINDSAY M. MORTON, PhD
Deputy Chief and Senior Investigator, Radiation Epidemiology Branch, Division of Cancer Epidemiology and Genetics, Department of Health and Human Services, National Cancer Institute, National Institutes of Health, Bethesda, Maryland, USA

SOGOL MOSTOUFI-MOAB, MD, PhD, MSCE
Pediatric Endocrinologist and Pediatric Oncologist, Divisions of Endocrinology and Oncology, Departments of Endocrinology and Pediatric Oncology, and Pediatrics, The Children's Hospital of Philadelphia, Philadelphia, Pennsylvania, USA

RENÉE L. MULDER, PhD
Princess Máxima Center for Pediatric Oncology, Utrecht, The Netherlands

PAUL C. NATHAN, MD, MSc
Director, AfterCare Program, Professor, Division of Hematology/Oncology, The Hospital for Sick Children, Professor of Pediatrics and Health Policy, Management and Evaluation, The University of Toronto, Toronto, Canada

KIRSTEN K. NESS, PhD
Member, Department of Epidemiology and Cancer Control, St. Jude Children's Research Hospital, Memphis, Tennessee, USA

FILIPPA NYBOE NORSKER, PhD
Postdoctoral Researcher, Childhood Cancer Research Group, Danish Cancer Society Research Center, Copenhagen, Denmark

KEVIN C. OEFFINGER, MD
Professor, Duke Center for Onco-Primary Care, Duke Cancer Institute, Durham, North Carolina, USA

MARIA OTTH, MD
PhD Student, Childhood Cancer Research Platform, Institute of Social and Preventive Medicine, University of Bern, Bern, Switzerland; Staff Physician, Division of Hematology-Oncology, Department of Pediatrics, Kantonsspital Aarau, Aarau, Switzerland

JOSHUA D. PALMER, MD
Department of Radiation Oncology, The James Cancer Hospital at the Ohio State University Wexner Medical Center, Nationwide Children's Hospital, Columbus, Ohio, USA

MICHAELA PATTON, BA
University of Calgary, Calgary, Alberta, Canada

ARNOLD C. PAULINO, MD
Department of Radiation Oncology, The University of Texas MD Anderson Cancer Center, Houston, Texas, USA

CAMILLA PEDERSEN, PhD
Postdoctoral Researcher, Childhood Cancer Research Group, Danish Cancer Society Research Center, Copenhagen, Denmark

SASKIA PLUIJM, PhD
Princess Maxima Center for Pediatric Oncology, Utrecht, Netherlands

LESLIE L. ROBISON, PhD
Member, St. Jude Children's Research Hospital, Memphis, Tennessee, USA

K. BROOKE RUSSELL, MSc
University of Calgary, Calgary, Alberta, Canada

CARINA SCHNEIDER, MSc
Österreichische Kinder-Krebs-Hilfe (ÖKKH), Childhood Cancer International Europe, Wien, Austria

FIONA SCHULTE, PhD
Assistant Professor, Department of Oncology, Division of Psychosocial Oncology, Cumming School of Medicine, University of Calgary, Psychologist, Hematology, Oncology and Transplant Program, Alberta Children's Hospital, Calgary, Alberta, Canada

RODERICK SKINNER, MB ChB, PhD, FRCPCH
Department of Paediatric and Adolescent Haematology/Oncology, Great North Children's Hospital, Clinical and Translational Research Institute, Newcastle University Centre for Cancer, Newcastle University, Newcastle upon Tyne, United Kingdom

JOP C. TEEPEN, PhD
Postdoctoral Researcher, Princess Máxima Center for Pediatric Oncology, Utrecht, The Netherlands

ZUZANA TOMÁŠIKOVÁ, MSc
Kinderkrebs Schweiz, Childhood Cancer International Europe, Basel, Switzerland

EMILY S. TONOREZOS, MD, MPH
General Internist, Department of Medicine, Memorial Sloan Kettering and Weill Cornell Medical College, Memorial Sloan Kettering Cancer Center, New York, New York, USA

MARIANNE D. VAN DE WETERING, MD, PhD
Pediatric Oncologist, Princess Máxima Center for Pediatric Oncology, Utrecht, The Netherlands

MARRY M. VAN DEN HEUVEL-EIBRINK, MD, PhD
Professor, University of Utrecht, Pediatric Oncologist, Princess Maxima Center for Pediatric Oncology, Prinses Maxima Centrum voor kinderoncologie, Utrecht, The Netherlands

HELENA J. VAN DER PAL, MD, PhD
Specialist for Internal Diseases, Late Effects Specialist, Princess Máxima Center for Pediatric Oncology, Utrecht, The Netherlands

REBECCA J. VAN KALSBEEK, MD
Princess Máxima Center for Pediatric Oncology, Utrecht, The Netherlands

HANNEKE M. VAN SANTEN, MD, PhD
Associate Professor, Pediatric Endocrinologist, Department of Pediatric Endocrinology, Wilhelmina Children's Hospital, UMCU, Princess Máxima Center for Pediatric Oncology, Utrecht, The Netherlands

MARRY M. VD HEUVEL-EIBRINK, MD, PhD
Professor, Pediatric Oncologist, Princess Máxima Center for Pediatric Oncology, Utrecht, The Netherlands

HENK VISSCHER, MD, PhD
Clinical Fellow, Division of Haematology/Oncology, Hospital for Sick Children, Toronto, Ontario, Canada; Pediatric Oncologist, Princess Máxima Center for Pediatric Oncology, Utrecht, The Netherlands

CLAIRE E. WAKEFIELD, PhD
Professor, School of Women's and Children's Health, UNSW Medicine, UNSW Sydney, Sydney, Australia; Behavioural Sciences Unit, Kids Cancer Centre, Sydney Children's Hospital, Randwick, New South Wales, Australia

WILLIAM HAMISH WALLACE, MD, PHD
Professor, Pediatric Oncologist, Department of Pediatric Haematology and Oncology, Royal Hospital for Sick Children, Edinburgh, Scotland

JEANETTE FALCK WINTHER, MD, DMSc
Professor, Childhood Cancer Research Group, Danish Cancer Society Research Center, Copenhagen, Denmark; Department of Clinical Medicine, Faculty of Health, Aarhus University and University Hospital, Aarhus, Denmark

SUZANNE WOLDEN, MD
Department of Radiation Oncology, Memorial Sloan Kettering Cancer Center, New York, New York, USA

AMANDA WURZ, PhD
University of Calgary, Calgary, Alberta, Canada

ADAM YAN, MD
Paediatric Hematology/Oncology Fellow, Division of Haematology/Oncology, The Hospital for Sick Children, Toronto, Canada

Contents

Surviving childhood cancer can be a lifelong challenge: up to 75% of childhood cancer survivors must deal with late effects of their cancer and treatments. Next to keeping the balance between dealing with late-effects and adapting to a life "after cancer" many childhood cancer survivors also face the reality of inadequate or nonexisting follow-up care. Because cure is not enough, patient advocates depict why it is important to #RaiseYourHands4Survivors!

In this article, a father and son describe the experience of childhood leukemia treatment and its aftermath with the unique perspective of a parent who is also a pediatric oncologist. An illness that began with an apparently favorable prognosis was transformed by an early relapse, followed by unexpected complications and difficult treatment decisions. Despite unfavorable statistics, the son is a long-term survivor with an overall excellent quality of life, despite several late events and effects. His father, in the meantime, gained insights that now inform his own practice.

With improvement in cure of childhood cancer came the responsibility to investigate the long-term morbidity and mortality associated with the treatments accountable for this increase in survival. Several large cohorts of childhood cancer survivors have been established throughout Europe and North America to facilitate research on long-term complications of cancer treatment. The cohorts have made significant contributions to the understanding of early mortality, somatic late complications, and psychosocial outcomes among childhood cancer survivors, which has been translated into the design of new treatment protocols for pediatric cancers, with the goal to reduce the potential risk and severity of late effects.

> Childhood cancer disrupts the lives of patients and their families and affects acute and long-term psychological health. This article summarizes (1) psychological challenges, including depression, anxiety, worries, and posttraumatic stress, as well as positive outcomes such as benefit finding and posttraumatic growth in young survivors and parents; (2) health-related quality of life; (3) interventions to support survivors and parents with psychological difficulties; and (4) neurocognitive problems and interventions to help alleviate them. Although many survivors and parents fare well in the long term, many survivors may benefit from interventions. Interventions should be further evaluated and integrated into routine clinical care.

> The authors' objective is to provide a brief update on recent advances in knowledge relating to subsequent primary neoplasms developing in survivors of childhood cancer. This includes a summary of established large-scale cohorts, risks reported, and contrasts with results from recently established large-scale cohorts of survivors of adolescent and young adult cancer. Recent evidence is summarized concerning the role of radiotherapy and chemotherapy for childhood cancer and survivor genomics in determining the risk of subsequent primary neoplasms. Progress with surveillance, screening, and clinical follow-up guidelines is addressed. Finally, priorities for future research are outlined.

> Childhood cancer survivors are at risk for developing cardiovascular disease and pulmonary disease related to cancer treatment. This might not become apparent until many years after treatment and varies from subclinical to life-threatening disease. Important causes are anthracyclines and radiotherapy involving heart, head, or neck for cardiovascular disease, and bleomycin, busulfan, nitrosoureas, radiation to the chest, and lung or chest surgery for pulmonary disease. Most effects are dose dependent, but genetic risk factors have been discovered. Treatment options are limited. Prevention and regular screening are crucial. Survivors should be encouraged to adopt a healthy lifestyle, and modifiable risk factors should be addressed.

> Endocrine late effects, including reproductive disorders and secondary thyroid cancer, have been reported in up to 50% childhood cancer

survivors (CCS) more than 5 years after treatment. Most endocrine disorders are amenable to treatment; awareness of symptoms is therefore of great importance. Recognition of these symptoms may be delayed however because many are nonspecific. Timely treatment of endocrine disorders improves quality of life in CCS and prevents possible consequences, such as short stature, bone and cardiovascular disorders, and depression. At-risk CCS must therefore be regularly and systematically monitored. This article provides a summary of the most commonly reported endocrine late effects in CCS.

Gonadal dysfunction and infertility after cancer treatment are major concerns for childhood cancer survivors and their parents. Uncertainty about fertility or being diagnosed with infertility has a negative impact on quality of survival. In this article, determinants of gonadal damage are reviewed and consequences for fertility and pregnancies are discussed. Recommendations for screening and treatment of gonadal function are provided. These should enable timely treatment of gonadal insufficiency aiming to improve linear growth, pubertal development, and sexual functioning. Options for fertility preservation are discussed.

Childhood cancer survivors (CCSs) are at risk for renal and hepatic complications related to curative cancer treatments. Although acute renal and hepatic toxicities of cancer treatments are well described, data regarding long-term and late-occurring sequelae or their associations with acute sequelae are less robust. This article highlights the literature on the prevalence of and risk factors for late renal and hepatic toxicity in CCSs. Studies investigating these outcomes are needed to inform surveillance practices and the development of future frontline cancer treatment protocols.

Ototoxicity and other neurologic toxicities are potential consequences of exposure to common therapeutic agents used during treatment of childhood cancer, including platinum and vinca alkaloid chemotherapy, cranial radiation, surgery involving structures critical to cochlear and neurologic function, and supportive care medications such as aminoglycoside antibiotics and loop diuretics. This article provides an overview of ototoxicity and other neurologic toxicities related to childhood cancer treatment, discusses the challenges that these toxicities may pose for survivors, and presents an overview of current recommendations for surveillance and clinical management of these potentially life-altering toxicities in survivors of childhood cancers.

Stephanie B. Dixon, Eric J. Chow, Lars Hjorth, Melissa M. Hudson, Leontien C.M. Kremer, Lindsay M. Morton, Paul C. Nathan, Kirsten K. Ness, Kevin C. Oeffinger, and Gregory T. Armstrong

As treatment evolves and the population who survive childhood cancer ages and increases in number, researchers must use novel approaches to prevent, identify and mitigate adverse effects of treatment. Future priorities include collaborative efforts to pool large cohort data to improve detection of late effects, identify late effects of novel therapies, and determine the contribution of genetic factors along with physiologic and accelerated aging among survivors. This knowledge should translate to individual risk prediction and prevention strategies. Finally, we must utilize health services research and implementation science to improve adoption of survivorship care recommendations outside of specialized pediatric oncology centers.

PEDIATRIC CLINICS OF
NORTH AMERICA

THE CLINICS ARE AVAILABLE ONLINE!
Access your subscription at:
www.theclinics.com

Foreword

Childhood Cancer Survival: So Much More Needs to be Done

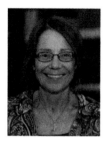

Bonita F. Stanton, MD
Consulting Editor

I completed my pediatric residency during the 1970s. Pediatric residents in that era had the privilege of getting to know children with cancer (and their parents) very well as the children spent so much time in the hospital receiving treatment. For so many of the childhood cancers, despite all our efforts, the ultimate prognoses were not good. The children and their parents endured great pain and illnesses of all kinds. While they may or may not have benefited from many of the treatments available at the time, these children and parents, hopefully benefiting for a least brief intervals themselves, paved the way for the increasing numbers and percentages of successful treatment outcomes that began to emerge over time. As residents, we did all we could to minimize the pain and despair of their time in the hospital. I remember the "on-call tradition" at our children's hospital that emerged over the years. When a child was admitted to the hospital, the nursing staff asked the children or their parents for the name of the resident who was most successful in drawing their blood and/or inserting an intravenous (IV) needle for infusions. That resident would then be paged, and wherever we were on service, it was understood that we would briefly leave our work to draw this child's blood and/or insert his or her IV. Sadly, other than our love and caring for these children with whom we spent so much time, toward the ends of their lives, we often had little else to offer them. Years later, we still have many, many memories of these children and their parents and the sadness that enveloped them (and therefore us), punctuated with the occasional wonderous moment of humor or joy.

But with the passage of time and the remarkable advances in therapy and technology, we have had the joy of watching the average lifespan of children diagnosed as a cancer victim enjoying steadily increasing life expectancy and decreased pain and suffering. We have gaped in awe witnessing the transformation of so many forms of cancer from rapidly fatal system-shut-down to curable diseases. We have had the

https://doi.org/10.1016/j.pcl.2020.10.001
0031-3955/20/© 2020 Published by Elsevier Inc.
pediatric.theclinics.com

privilege of offering our patients individually tailored therapeutic options maximizing life and cures and minimizing pain and suffering.

These successes have not been without their costs, including subsequent development of different forms of cancer and long-term sequalae from the original cancer and/or the treatment thereof that interfere with full recovery or result in shortened lifespans and/or other unwelcome long-term sequalae. Still, the gains and remarkable progress which I have had the joy of witnessing have been substantial.

Unfortunately, this great progress in potential medical outcomes is not equally enjoyed by all children. Children living throughout the globe, and even those from within the United States, are not benefiting equally from these great discoveries and advances in medical care. For example, international differences in the 5-year survival rates for childhood lymphoid leukemia in 2005 to 2009 ranged from 52% in Colombia to 92% in Germany, and for acute myeloid leukemia, from 33% in Bulgaria to 78% in Germany.[1] Outcomes of children (and adults) with cancer in the United States demonstrate significant differences in cancer survival depending on race, socioeconomic status, and age. Particularly discouraging is the observation that these outcome differences appear to be increasing rather than decreasing over time.[2,3]

In summary, this issue of *Pediatric Clinics of North America* is exciting and encouraging as we appreciate the dramatic improvements in cancer survival and quality of life among children over the past several decades. But, at the same time, this issue reminds child health care providers nationally and globally that the advances in health and life are not equally enjoyed. Child health care providers and researchers must take heed of the repeated observations that these gains are not as substantial among children from lower-socioeconomic families and within certain racial groups—and that the differences in lifespan are increasing. These differential outcomes too can be addressed and greatly reduced—but only if we seek to develop therapeutic approaches that consider all the factors resulting in these poorer outcomes.

Bonita F. Stanton, MD
Hackensack Meridian School of Medicine
at Seton Hall University
340 Kingsland Street, Building 123
Nutley, NJ 07110, USA

E-mail address:
bonita.stanton@shu.edu

REFERENCES

1. Bonaventure A, Harewood R, Stiller CA, et al. Worldwide comparison of survival from childhood leukemia for 1995–2009, by subtype, age, and sex (CONCORD-2): a population-based study of individual data for 89 828 children from 198 registries in 53 countries. Lancet Haematol 2017;4(5):e202–17.
2. Tai EW, Ward KC, Bonaventure A, et al. Survival among children diagnosed with acute lymphoblastic leukemia in the United States, by race and age, 2001 to 2009: findings from the CONCORD-2 study. Cancer 2017;123(S24):5178–89.
3. Singh GK, Jemal A. Socioeconomic and racial/ethnic disparities in cancer mortality, incidence, and survival in the United States, 1950–2014: over six decades of changing patterns and widening inequalities. J Environ Public Health 2017;2017: 2819372.

Preface

Surviving Survival—Challenge Accepted: Perspectives on Survivorship in Pediatric Oncology

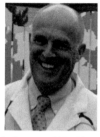
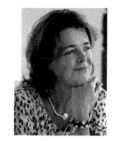

Max J. Coppes, MD, PhD, MBA   Leontine C. M. Kremer, MD, PhD
Editors

Until about a century ago, surviving childhood cancer was unconceivable. Over 7 decades ago, Ladd and Gross[1] noted that in children with renal cancer, while mortality was still high, "a review indicates that about 25% of patients can be cured." Over the next 25 years, standard approaches to specific childhood cancers were developed, initially locally, but soon afterwards involving multiple institutions. This led, initially in North America and Europe, to the creation of very large multidisciplinary study groups that set out to cure childhood cancers through high-quality research. As an example, in the mid-1970s, survival for children with Wilms tumor reached 85% as a result of a combination of cancer surgery, radiation therapy, and chemotherapy.[2] In subsequent decades, this success has spread to other childhood cancers. Today, almost 80% of children and teenagers diagnosed with cancer who have access to appropriate care can expect to become long-term survivors.[3,4]

That of course is great news. There are, however, 2 caveats to the good news. First, over 80% of children do not have access to standard treatments, mostly related to where (the country) they live. As a result, worldwide survival to childhood cancer is only 20%.[5,6] The second qualification to the good news is that for those who have access to appropriate therapies, there is a cost to survival, often considerable. As we learn in the first article, for some survivors, life is disturbingly about "surviving survival." In this issue of the *Pediatric Clinics of North America*, we review the "cost to cure." Radiation therapy and chemotherapy for children with cancer are associated with many health problems later in life. As the number of childhood cancer survivors

https://doi.org/10.1016/j.pcl.2020.09.020
0031-3955/20/© 2020 Published by Elsevier Inc.

(CCS) increased and those who survived started to live longer lives,[7] the cost to cure became evident and increasingly measurable. Studies in the United States and The Netherlands showed that nearly 75% of survivors have one or more health problems years after treatment.[8,9]

To set the stage for reviewing the impact of late effects of childhood cancer treatment, we invited those that live "childhood cancer survival" to share their experience. In many ways, therefore, the first and second articles are the most important ones, setting the stage for all subsequent contributions. Survivors, and parents of survivors, can tell us firsthand what it actually means to have been "lucky to survive." Their experience, as shared in the first 2 articles, is somewhat unnerving and above all educational. While our societies remain focused on winning and scoring additional wins as illustrated by many of the cancer-related slogans ("cancer, we're coming for you"; "cancer: just beat it"; "fight the fight, find a cure"; "it came, we fought, we won"; and "strike out cancer"), survivors invite us to contemplate what lies beyond the "win"; survivors draw attention to the challenges experienced in "surviving survival."

Subsequent contributions cover some of the things we learned early on and how these early lessons influenced a new and still evolving field of medicine, that of long-term childhood cancer survivorship. The content of the field is fueled by insights in the breadth and extent of health problems, such as secondary malignancies and organ-specific damages: renal, hepatic, cardiac, pulmonary, auditory, neurocognitive, and fertility, and other endocrine disorders. We also describe the increased knowledge of treatment-related risk factors, like the different treatment modalities used (eg, surgery, radiotherapy, and chemotherapy), and a beginning insight into susceptibility to late effects, as determined by a patient's genetic background.

This new field of medicine has some unique challenges for the individual health care that needs to be provided to CCS. These are also addressed. First, new models of care and guidelines for surveillance and treatment of late effects have to be developed for delivering optimal survivorship care. How is optimal long-term follow-up care defined for each patient? Where do those caring for CCS get trustworthy information on the most appropriate screening, prevention, and care? This challenging topic is specifically addressed in an article that describes the critical role of Clinical Practice Guidelines for long-term follow-up and how these have been and continue being developed. Second, this field includes many kinds of providers with diverse training, experience, and content knowledge. Most of these providers, including pediatric oncologists, pediatricians, family practitioners, (pediatric) endocrinologists, and obstetricians, have had limited training in childhood cancer late effects. Of all those involved, who serves as the CCS's quarterback? Furthermore, how can a CCS take her or his own responsibility? Third, how do we ensure that best practices are actually applied and used? How do we ensure that sufficient resources are available to address the emerging needs of CCS? Fourth, how do countries ensure the adoption of formal policies that support the ability of the ever-growing population of CCS to live richly filled lives with ample opportunities for personal and professional growth?

We hope that the insightful contributions provided by all authors not only help to optimize the care of CCS but also bring awareness to an ever-growing population that urgently has requested to be acknowledged so that "childhood cancer survivors can be actively engaged in society and live their lives to the fullest."[10]

Max J. Coppes, MD, PhD, MBA
University of Nevada Reno School of Medicine
Renown Children's Hospital
1155 Mill Street
Reno, NV 89502, USA

Leontine C.M. Kremer, MD, PhD
Princess Máxima Center for
Pediatric Oncology, Utrecht
Heidelberglaan 25
Utrecht 3584 CS, The Netherlands

Department of Pediatrics
University of Amsterdam
Amsterdam, The Netherlands

E-mail addresses:
mcoppes@renown.org (M.J. Coppes)
l.c.m.kremer@prinsesmaximacentrum.nl (L.C.M. Kremer)

REFERENCES

1. Ladd WE, Gross RE. Abdominal surgery in infancy and childhood. Philadelphia: WB Saunders; 1941.
2. D'Angio GJ, et al. The treatment of Wilms' tumor: results of the national Wilms' tumor study. Cancer 1976;38:633–46.
3. Howlader N, et al. SEER cancer statistics review, 1975–2012. Bethesda (MD): National Cancer Institute; 2015.
4. Gatta G, et al. Childhood cancer survival in Europe 1999-2007: results of EURO-CARE-5—a population-based study. Lancet Oncol 2014;15:35–47.
5. Howard SC, et al. The My Child Matters programme: effect of public-private partnerships on paediatric cancer care in low-income and middle-income countries. Lancet Oncol 2018;19:e252–66.
6. Gupta S, et al. Treating childhood cancer in low- and middle-income countries. In: Gelband H, Jha P, Sankaranarayanan R, et al, editors. Cancer: disease control priorities, 3rd edition. vol. 3. Washington, DC: The World Bank; 2015.
7. Mariotto AB, et al. Long-term survivors of childhood cancers in the United States. Cancer Epidemiol Biomarkers Prev 2009;18:1033–40.
8. Oeffinger KC, et al. Chronic health conditions in adult survivors of childhood cancer. N Engl J Med 2006;355:1572–82.
9. Geenen MM, et al. Medical assessment of adverse health outcomes in long-term survivors of childhood cancer. JAMA 2007;297:2705–15.
10. Jankovic M, et al. Long-term survivors of childhood cancer: cure and care-the Erice Statement (2006) revised after 10 years (2016). J Cancer Surv 2018;12:647–50.

Surviving Survival— Challenge Accepted!

Perspectives on Survivorship in Pediatric Oncology

Carina Schneider, MSc[a],*, Jaap den Hartogh, MA[b],
Zuzana Tomášiková, MSc[c], Anita Kienesberger, MA[a]

KEYWORDS

- Survivors • Late effects • Long-term follow-up • Patient advocacy
- (Childhood cancer) survivor • Patient-centered care

KEY POINTS

- Cured does not always mean "being well." Up to 75% of survivors deal with late effects. Keeping the balance between coping and living life to the fullest can be a life-long challenge.
- There is a worldwide lack of structure for psychosocial and medical follow-up care. They need to be developed.
- Survivors need comprehensive and age-appropriate information about the risks they can expect due to their cancer and treatments, what to do about their late effects, and where to turn to.
- More research must be carried out to reduce late-effects and optimize long-term care.

INTRODUCTION: BETWEEN THE KINGDOM OF THE SICK AND THE KINGDOM OF THE WELL—CURED FROM CANCER BUT NOT WELL ENOUGH

In a very impressive New York Times blog article, Suleika Jaouad, an American journalist and leukemia survivor commented on Susan Sontag's view that "Everyone who is born holds dual citizenship, in the kingdom of the well and in the kingdom of the sick." She went on commenting that Susan Sontag did not mention that there was also a third kingdom, "no-man's land," that exists between the 2 kingdoms, inhabited by people such as Suleika, who are neither sick nor well.[1]

---

a Österreichische Kinder-Krebs-Hilfe (ÖKKH), Childhood Cancer International Europe, Borschkegasse 1/7, Wien 1090, Austria; b Vereniging Ouders, Kinderen en Kanker, Childhood Cancer International Europe, Schouwstede 2b, Nieuwegein 3431 JB, The Netherlands; c Kinderkrebs Schweiz, Childhood Cancer International Europe, Dornacherstrasse 154, Basel 4053, Switzerland
* Corresponding author.
E-mail address: c.schneider@ccieurope.eu

Pediatr Clin N Am 67 (2020) 1011–1020
https://doi.org/10.1016/j.pcl.2020.07.010
0031-3955/20/© 2020 Elsevier Inc. All rights reserved.

From our work as patient advocates within Childhood Cancer International, we know that there are many survivors who live exactly like this, in this "no-man's land." Some live in the "no-man's land" for a short time after treatment, whereas others live like this for the rest of their lives. Most of us have had some years of follow-up care and are headed into an uncertain future with the realization of possible late effects and hardly any transition programs into the adult health care system to address our forthcoming health and psychosocial issues.

Being diagnosed with and treated for cancer is often hard and it is a long and difficult journey, but many of us are not at all prepared for the even harder road ahead in surviving survival.

Even though being "cured" and called "long-term survivor" may sound great, many of us struggle with several late effects that also affect our psychosocial well-being on a daily basis.

Imagine yourself being a long-term survivor of childhood cancer for one moment.

"Your Hair Will Grow Back in No Time, Don't Worry!"

As treatment starts, the caregivers alert me about the fact that my hair is going to fall out. But they also tell me not to worry because it will come back in no time and it might be even stronger than before and maybe even curly. So, why would I even consider that it will not grow back? Well for some of us, it does NOT grow back and all of a sudden I have alopecia. When I ask why my hair hasn't been coming back normally, the doctor, in an attempt to comfort me, tells me that they don't know for sure, but suspect the reason is one specific chemotherapeutic agent. There is nothing that they can do about it, so they advise me to not comb my remaining hair too often, so that I wouldn't lose even more.

Luckily, after a significant amount of time, I find a way to deal with the fact that I have a cancer history that left me scars, on the outside as well as on the inside. Still, sometimes it can be hard to see how other people react to that fact. Even though others might not see my inside scars, they always see the outside scars, thus confronting me with my own insecurities: "What do they know?", "What do they think?", and "How will they react?"

I will be happy when a person is just genuinely interested in the story behind my scars.

"Do You Want Children?"

When friends tell me that they have decided to have a baby and ask whether I want to have children in the future, I find myself answering that I don't know. Not necessarily because I don't know whether I want children, but because I don't know whether or not I can, because the only thing I do know is that it will be difficult because the treatments may have damaged my reproductive system. At the clinic they told me that, regarding my difficult situation, I should hurry if I really wanted to have children on my own. Pressure is on! But even then, I may worry about the chance that my hypothetical future child might suffer from some sort of impairment due to my cancer history and the prior damage to my reproductive system. Or that a pregnancy could pose a great challenge to my heart, which has been affected by chemotherapy.

So how should I answer my friends' question whether I want to have children?

Maybe it would be easier to think and talk about having children if I had received better education about my fertility throughout treatment and follow-up. But for many of us survivors, it feels that fertility is not a top priority during treatment or follow-up, at least not for our caregivers.

As a result, we have a lack of information and we are left with too many "*maybes*" and "*maybe nots*" to allow ourselves to think about our hypothetical future children.

Before I got sick, I knew exactly if I wanted kids or not, just like I knew that I wanted to become a lawyer, or like I knew that I would run a marathon before I would turn 30 years. I tried to hold on to these ideas and dreams for as long as I could, after having been diagnosed and treated, hoping that I would soon be able to step back into my old life. But then 1 day I may realize that I am too fatigued to keep up with university or that surgery or some serious side effects from chemotherapy will actually prevent me from running a marathon in my life. Similarly, 1 day I may discover that I will have no choice in having a child of my own…… whether I ever wanted one or not.

It can be hard to keep up with my peers who seem to have unlimited energy, whereas I feel drained. At times, I don't really understand why I am not like them, even though I do my best and give everything I have. Accepting that my "new normal" can be a lifelong challenge.

The New Normal

When asked why I changed my plan to become a lawyer, my answer might be as follows. *"With regard to the person I am now, there is a 'before-cancer-me' and an 'after-cancer-me'. In order to cope with what has happened and with the things I could do before and might not be able to do now, the 'after-cancer me had to let go of a big part of the 'before cancer me"*. During the in-between phase, I had to look for an identity that takes into account the positive as well as the negative aspects of having survived childhood cancer. Arriving at a new steady state with this after-cancer-me is challenging. I am trying to make people aware of the daily struggles I undergo. Unfortunately, people do not always understand. In fact, when I tell people that I have survived cancer it sometimes seems that their notion of "after-cancer-me" is one of daily gratitude for the life that I have been given and the motto of my "after-cancer-me" must be: Carpe Diem!

The good thing is that on many days it *is* my motto. But to be honest, on some days I really must make an effort to breathe through fears of relapse and late effects, most of all second malignancies.

The reason why people might think that I do nothing but enjoy life to its fullest, may be more than other people might do, is because I focus on telling them only about all the good things that my cancer experience brought me. That cancer made me grow as a person, made me stronger, made me enjoy what I have, and made me change my priorities and my outlook on life.

What I share with only a very few people in my life, however, is that with the growth and strength sometimes also comes fear, anger, helplessness, at times loneliness, and the loss of light-heartedness.

Keeping a Balance

Many of us carry our inside and outside scars with us. Sometimes, there is not a day without having it on our minds. On good days, it's easy to deal with it. On bad days, this is what being cured means: being neither sick nor well.

When saying that aloud, we don't want anyone to get us wrong: the health care professionals, our families, friends and also myself, we all did everything possible to fight my cancer and have me survive. And yes, I am grateful. I, and many others like myself, live a good life, and we are glad we survived and we enjoy every moment we can. But sometimes it needs to be possible to express that the happy parts of survival are also intertwined with the difficult parts of survival.

It needs to be possible to express that, unfortunately, the harsh reality is that everyone needs to be aware that after treatments and follow-up care, not all survivors will live in the "kingdom of the well."

Unmet Needs

Treatment might have cured our bodies of cancer, but it also left many of us with major challenges: fertility concerns, cardiac problems, neuropsychological issues, orthopedic problems, anxiety, body image issues, endocrine disorders, or even with the risk of developing a new cancer. Worst of all, many of us still do not know what real challenges lay ahead, many of us still do not have adequate care to tackle these issues with us.

And this is why—in the "no man's land between the kingdom of the well and the kingdom of the sick"—we need to be educated and informed about what we might have to deal with. We need to know what we might expect, in order to know what to be aware of, in order to understand why we need to go to our follow-up appointments. We need to be transitioned from pediatric experts to adult experts, providers who know how to deal with our late effects. We need to know where to turn to with our health and psychosocial issues, we need to know where our needs are met with the adequate expertise, know-how, and understanding. Only this way can we take responsibility for our own health and the life we have fought for so hard to keep.

SURVIVORS VOICES—FROM ERICE, ITALY, TO DUBLIN, IRELAND, (...) PanCare, AND CCI

Certainly, the experiences described here do not apply to 100% of childhood cancer survivors (CCS). Not all encounter problems, not all encounter the same problems or experience the same challenges. Still, the majority of survivors are or will be confronted with some kind of physical and psychosocial issues, and the above section depicts experiences that many CCS face in their daily lives. Some survivors certainly show enormous resilience and live their lives no matter what. But as patient advocates it is our responsibility to support those who still need to find ways to cope and regain control over their lives.

This is the reason for the establishment of peer support groups and patient advocates at the local, national, and international level. By exchanging our different experiences, we realized that the problems we face as survivors are very similar around the globe and that was reason enough for national survivor-representatives to get together, team up, and start patient advocacy work on an international level. Within Childhood Cancer International (CCI), a global umbrella organization representing childhood cancer organizations around the world, we ensure that together our voices are heard even louder.

Today, there are many survivor-representatives, parent-representatives, childhood cancer organizations, and medical and psychosocial health care professionals around the globe who are working together to develop structures for long-term care, with the aim to improve the quality of survivorship.

In 1975, Dr Giulio D'Angio was one of the first medical specialists to acknowledge that "cure is not enough."[2] His paper has had a huge impact on pediatric oncology. His assertion that "cure was not enough" was the reason that medical professionals, parents, and survivors came together in Erice (Italy) in 2007, to have a workshop on long-term follow-up care. This workshop led to the so-called Erice Statement: 10 key points summarizing the essential components of cure and care for CCS.[3] The Erice Statement can be seen as the start of what we now know as the PanCare Network,[4] a multidisciplinary pan-European network of professionals, survivors, and their families to improve the care and quality of life of CCS by means of research and guideline development.

Ten years later, in November 2016, 65 pediatric cancer experts, including parents and CCS, from 17 European countries and North America, met again in Erice to review the original statement. An updated version was subsequently published.[5] The original and revised statement most importantly point out that

"There is an additional need for continuing systematic follow-up after cure for surveillance of potential long-term effects of the cancer or its treatment. To this end, every Pediatric Care Unit should have a well-structured "long-term follow-up clinic" with care plans based on risk stratification and evidence-based guidelines and a multidisciplinary team."[3,5]

It is clear that there is still significant work to be done with regard to providing adequate care after the cure of childhood cancer.

Survivor representatives attending a meeting organized by the Childhood Cancer International Survivors Network (CCISN) in Dublin (2016) wrote a declaration in which the views of survivors on survivorship are being pointed out. This so-called Declaration of Dublin (DoD) comprises issues that are encountered by CCS worldwide, including inadequate transition, lack of psychosocial care, discrimination, lack of information—reconfirming that there is still much to be done in to improve quality of survivorship.[6]

Because of this declaration, advances at the advocacy level have been made. The need for a survivor's voice was necessary at the continental level, which led to the establishment of a Europe-wide survivors network under the umbrella of CCI Europe. At the 2017 CCI Europe conference in Rome, 9 survivor representatives from 7 European countries started a network that now has grown to more than 20 representatives and fosters a close collaboration in the field of survivorship care and research in Europe.

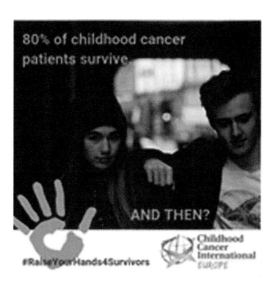

Fig. 1. #RaiseYourHands4Survivors: up to 75% of survivors will suffer from late effects. *Message 1: eighty percent of patients with childhood cancer survive and then?* In Europe, each year 15,000 children and adolescents are diagnosed with cancer. About 80% survive due to multimodal treatment methods. This high cure rate comes with a price: It comes with the price of possible chronic health conditions. According to current research, about 2/3 as many as up to 75% of childhood and adolescent cancer survivors will suffer from at least one adverse late effect of their prior cancer and its treatment. Approximately 1/3 of these survivors will suffer from severe late effects with major impacts on their daily lives.[13,14]

CCI Europe's Survivors Network is involved in various projects. Furthermore, several EU-funded projects on survivorship have been established recently by a collaboration between survivors and health care professionals within PanCare and the European branch of the International Society for Pediatric Oncology (SIOP). These collaborations have resulted in the creation of guidelines, a Survivorship Passport (SurPass), and the EU-funded PanCareFollowUp (PCFU), a project looking at how to best deliver survivorship care. SurPass, which is still in development, will encompass a treatment summary and personalized follow-up recommendations based on cumulative treatment doses.[7]

The aim of PanCareFollowUp is to deliver care according to recently developed guidelines using an innovative model for person-centered care that empowers survivors and supports self-management.[8,9]

The European network of survivor representatives is in constant exchange with other national survivors' groups around the globe, that is, Japan, Hong Kong, Indonesia, India, and Canada, mostly during the annual SIOP/CCI conferences. Here separate survivorship sessions are organized in order to foster exchange of best practice projects. To this point, apart from Europe there are no other continental survivor networks. However, the existing national survivor groups are active and will hopefully soon establish new continental survivor networks.

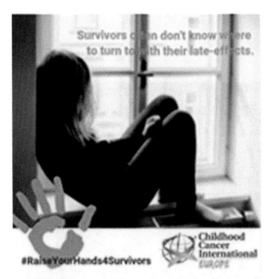

Fig. 2. #RaiseYourHands4Survivors: survivors need to know about their late-effects risk. *Message 2: Know your risk!* Another issue that survivors all around the world report to be facing is not knowing about their personal risk (DoD). For that there might be different reasons, such as for instance the lack of follow-up care solutions in numerous countries, not having detailed information about the personal cancer history by means of treatment summaries handed to the patients, scarcity of financial and personnel resources in hospitals—including high-income countries as well as low- and middle-income countries. The call for comprehensive information and education about personal late-effects risk by patient advocates is becoming louder and louder. Because long-term follow-up care is prevention and early detection and in order to prevent and detect early, we must know how to do so. In order to know how to do that, we must know what to be aware of/expect. Because only if we know what to be aware of/expect can we take the respective measures and do our follow-up.

#RaiseYourHands4Survivors

Another important milestone for survivors was marked by CCI Europe's awareness campaign #RaiseYourHands4Survivors, which was developed in cooperation with the Austrian Childhood Cancer Organization ÖKKH.[10]

Since the formulation of the DoD, patient advocates from CCI Europe and its survivors network have put the survivorship topics in the spotlight. In early 2019, this resulted in the development of a Europe-wide social media campaign, which so far has reached 60,000 people, including survivors, parents, and childhood cancer organizations all around the world.

Fully aware of the inequalities in access to and differences in quality of care—which often depends on the economic situation of the respective country—survival rates vary drastically around the globe. Luckily, there are initiatives that envision tackling this problem.[11]

In some countries, however, survival rates are greater than 80%,[12] leading to the growing necessity for infrastructure to improve quality of survivorship.

Drawing on European numbers and realities, the #RaiseYourHands4Survivors campaign addresses survivors, health care providers, and politicians and points at 4 main messages: the reality of late effects; the need for relevant and credible information; the need for adequate follow-up care; and the need for research.

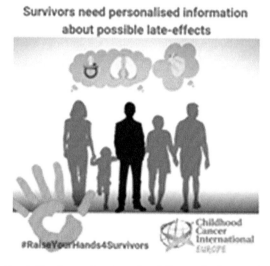

Fig. 3. #RaiseYourHands4Survivors: structures for delivery of adequate long-term follow-up care need to be implemented. *Message 3: Where to turn to?* Knowing the risk is only the first step towards follow-up care. To take the next steps, survivors need to know where to turn to for their follow-up care. Because late-effects research and the rise in survival rates are relatively young, we still lack adequate follow-up care structures globally. Although in some high-income countries, for example,. in the United States and Europe, there are evidence-based follow-up services in place, in many high-income countries and even more so in middle- and low-income countries patient advocates report that there is little to no follow-up care at all. With survival rates going up, the number of survivors with late effects is increasing and with that the necessity for comprehensive follow-up care services is growing rapidly. Survivors need a follow-up care that is easily accessible, individualized, and person-centered. It needs to take into account medical aspects of survivorship as well as psychological, social, and educational/vocational aspects.

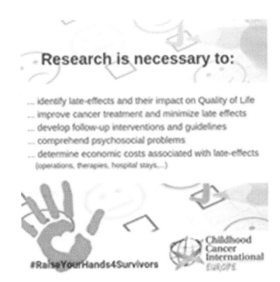

Fig. 4. #RaiseYourHands4Survivors: more research is needed to improve quality of survivorship. *Message 4: More research is needed!* Lastly, more research is needed to find out more about late effects, cancer's implications on mental health and social life. Current therapies need to be improved in order to minimize treatment burden and reduce late effects. Prospective research on long-term effects of new drugs is needed in order to detect relations early and take action. More research on the effectiveness of follow-up services and psychosocial interventions is needed in order to optimize care and improve the quality of life of those 60% to 75% of survivors who deal with late effects.

The campaign comprised more than 20 Facebook posts (**Figs. 1–4**) that were posted during February 15th, the International Childhood Cancer Day (ICCD) and the childhood cancer awareness month September. It also included 2 awareness movies (**Fig. 5**) that have been shot in cooperation with the European Reference Network for Pediatric Cancers (ERN PaedCan) and a petition in support of better follow-up care services that will be brought up before the European Parliament.

SAME BUT DIFFERENT? DIFFERENT, BUT STILL THE SAME!
The Declaration of Dublin

Across the globe, survival rates differ significantly. Although in high-income countries approximately 80% of the diagnosed children and adolescents with cancer can be

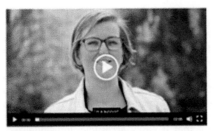
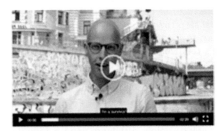

Fig. 5. #RaiseYourHands4Survivors awareness movies [Available at https://ccieurope.eu/survivors/].

cured, in some middle- and low-income countries the cure rate is only as high as 20%.[11]

This, however, does not change the fact that most of those who do survive will have late effects and that they will need full disclosure about their risks and adequate follow-up care. The day before the SIOP/CCI conference in Dublin in 2016, almost 40 survivor representatives—patient advocates—from numerous countries, including Austria, Germany, Hong Kong, India, Ireland, Japan, the Netherlands, and South Africa, voiced their requests:

Surviving childhood cancer can be a lifelong challenge, regardless of geographical, religious, ethnic, financial, and cultural backgrounds. We, the global CCI Survivors Network, ask medical and psychosocial professionals and all other stakeholders to acknowledge the challenges and needs of survivors.

Survivors of childhood cancer may develop medical and psychosocial late effects that severely impact their quality of life. Therefore, comprehensive long-term follow-up care is essential. We ask that adequate long-term follow-up clinics are established, where survivors can have access to personalized follow-up care. We ask for more research on late effects so that survivor care services can be improved.

Inadequate transition from childhood cancer care to adult medical care can result in a lack of knowledge and understanding of the impact and consequences of childhood cancer by the treating health professional(s). It is essential that these health professionals have a thorough understanding of the needs of cancer survivors. We request for full disclosure and sharing of our medical history and potential risks to our current and future health.

We emphasize the importance of trustworthy and empathetic psychosocial support during and after treatment. We ask all involved with our long-term care to be forthcoming and honest with us and to take our issues seriously.

In some countries, survivors are stigmatized and experience discrimination. We ask for equal opportunities in society including, but not limited to, education, employment and insurance.

Although cancer is a major cause of death amongst children around the world, it is important to convey to the general public that childhood cancer is often curable and that the survivors' population is increasing globally each year. We urge you to work with us to educate the general public in order to dispel misconceptions and myths about childhood cancer.

With the support and commitment of all stakeholders, childhood cancer survivors can be actively engaged in society and live their lives to the fullest.'
    —The declaration of Dublin. The CCISN. Dublin, October 18th, 2016[6]

ACKNOWLEDGMENTS

Thank you to all survivor representatives from the CCISN involved in the making of the Declaration of Dublin; to the Austrian Childhood Cancer Organization for developing the campaign together with CCI Europe; to the ERN PaedCan for the possibility to produce the awareness movies; and to SIOPE, PanCare, and the global network of CCI for their continuous partnership. For more information visit us at: CCI Europe www.ccieurope.eu; CCI www.childhoodcancerinternational.org; PanCare www.pancare.eu; SIOPE www.siope.eu; ERN PaedCan http://paedcan.ern-net.eu/; www.pancarefollowup.eu; www.survivorshippassport.org; To watch the awareness movies, go to: https://ccieurope.eu/survivors/

DISCLOSURE

The authors have nothing to disclose.

REFERENCES

1. Jaouad S. Lost in Transition after Cancer. In: Life, interrupted. 2015. Available at: https://well.blogs.nytimes.com/2015/03/16/lost-in-transition-after-cancer/. Accessed November, 13, 2019.
2. D'Angio GJ. Pediatric cancer in perspective: Cure is not enough. Cancer 1975; 35(S3):866–70.
3. Haupt R, Spinetta JJ, Ban I, et al. Long term survivors of childhood cancer: Cure and care. The Erice Statement. Eur J Cancer 2007;43:1778–80.
4. Jankovic M, Haupt R, Spinetta JJ, et al. Long-term survivors of childhood cancer: cure and care-the Erice Statement (2006) revised after 10 years (2016). J Cancer Surviv 2018;12(5):647–50.
5. Hjorth L, Haupt R, Skinner R, et al. Survivorship after childhood cancer: PanCare: A European Network to promote optimal long-term care. Eur J Cancer 2015;51: 1203–11.
6. Childhood Cancer International Survivors Network. The Declaration of Dublin. Available at: https://www.childhoodcancerinternational.org/understanding-childhood-cancer/facts-on-survivorship/. Accessed November 13, 2019.
7. Haupt R, Essiaf S, Dellacasa C, et al. The 'Survivorship Passport' for childhood cancer survivors. Eur J Cancer 2018;102:69e81.
8. PanCareFollowUp. What is PanCareFollowUp?. Available at: http://pancarefollowup.eu/about/. Accessed November 13, 2019.
9. Loonen J, Blijlevens NM, Prins J, et al. Cancer survivorship care: person centered care in a multidisciplinary shared care model. Int J Integr Care 2018;18(1):4.
10. CCI Europe. RaiseYourHands4Survivors. Petition. Available at: www.ccieurope.eu/petition. Accessed: November 13, 2019.
11. World Health Organization WHO. Cancer in Children. Available at: https://www.who.int/news-room/fact-sheets/detail/cancer-in-children. Accessed: November 23, 2019.
12. Gatta G, Botta L, Rossi S, et al. Childhood cancer survival in Europe 1999–2007: results of EUROCARE-5—a population-based study. Lancet Oncol 2014;15: 35–47.
13. Oeffinger KC, Mertens AC, Sklar CA, et al. Chronic health conditions in adult survivors of childhood cancer. N Engl J Med 2006;355:1572–82.
14. Hudson MM, Mertens AC, Yasui Y, et al. Health status of adult long-term survivors of childhood cancer. JAMA 2003;290(12):1583–92.

When Childhood Cancer Becomes a Family Affair, It Really Hits Home

David M. Johnston, BA[a], J. Martin Johnston, MD[b],*

KEYWORDS

- Childhood acute lymphoblastic leukemia • Relapsed acute leukemia
- Childhood cancer survivorship • Late effects

KEY POINTS

- Survival statistics for childhood cancer cannot predict individual outcomes. Optimism tempered by realism is the most effective strategy for patient and family management.
- The story of cancer survivorship has many articles, some with ambiguous endings.
- Cancer survivors must not be identified by that designation alone. They should continue to pursue a life trajectory that transcends "survival."
- A physician/parent experiences his child's illness and medical care with overlapping and at times conflicting perspectives.

WHEN YOUR FATHER IS A PEDIATRIC ONCOLOGIST: A PATIENT'S VIEW
Memories of Memories

While on a recent trip to Reno, I spent the better part of a day digging through boxes of my childhood belongings, things that had been moved from our former home in Georgia out to my parents' new house in Nevada. Most of the memorabilia I hadn't seen in years, if not decades. I was looking for something specific, something I never found—a photo album filled with faces of former Kindergarten and first-grade classmates. Instead, I uncovered several more interesting items, in particular a few manila envelopes at the bottom of a box labeled "David," stuffed full of 20-year-old letters and cards from family and friends of my parents, all on the matter of my leukemia treatment. Apologies. Prayers. Get well soon's. Some of them were addressed to me, but most were not. Many of these senders I didn't know or remember, having to ask my dad to connect these tattered lines and help me make some sense of the who and when and where and why. Beyond the obvious sympathy for my parents

[a] 2150 South McClelland Street, Salt Lake City, UT 84106, USA; [b] Division of Pediatric Hematology/Oncology, University of Nevada, Reno, Renown Children's Hospital, 1155 Mill Street, Reno, NV 89502, USA
* Corresponding author.
E-mail address: Martin.Johnston@Renown.org

Pediatr Clin N Am 67 (2020) 1021–1031
https://doi.org/10.1016/j.pcl.2020.07.001
0031-3955/20/© 2020 Elsevier Inc. All rights reserved.

welling up within me as I perused these pieces, parsing personal sentiment from these senders' notes proved nearly impossible, my distance from that child version of me, the impasse.

Today, reflecting on my time in and out of the hospital over those years of treatment is equally disorienting. Memories of my time in treatment are piecemeal at best, some animated only by familial stories told time and again. There are some vague visions of rooms where I'd get my blood drawn (by the sharpest needles in the hospital, my 6-year-old self would have promised you). A visit from University of Wisconsin football players. Days hooked up to my wheelabout IV pump. A Halloween night spent in the hospital. Occasional visits from extended family. Even as I catalog these episodes, I can't decide if these are true memories or simply images I've crafted in my mind, painted with the help of a few date-stamped photos and stories from the people who saw the whole ordeal much more vividly, traumatically than I could have as a child. Namely, my parents.

I'm fortunate for this, to struggle to remember these times of seeming-imminent tragedy. Times that I know kept my parents up many nights for years and forced them to face the terrifying possibility of losing a child. Times that warranted letters from so many people, all thinking and praying and wishing for my getting well soon. To this day, the only reason I know these times were so difficult is because I've been told just as much and because I saw it in the reactions of my family around me.

Having been diagnosed on my third birthday and not quite 6 years old by the time I finished treatment, my direct relationship with my survivorship has always been minimal. What have stayed with me much more are the various medical issues I have had to handle in the years following treatment. Hand-me-downs from years of chemo and radiation and the various other treatments I received that helped to save my life at the time. These memories—*true* memories—are of needing to explain my scars to kids in my elementary classes, balance and stamina struggles as a child and into adulthood, self-administered growth hormone shots in my early teens, anxieties tied to my needing extra time for papers and exams in college, and, through it all, an on-again-off-again sense of self-doubt. Those are the memories that are much more vivid, memories most definitely real. Every survivor's story is different. I won't pretend to speak for all of us at once. I know I was particularly fortunate, even if I didn't understand it at the time, to have a father in the field of pediatric oncology. I know that what I struggled through during my treatment, and what I've had to deal with since are minuscule in the face of many other survivors' more harrowing stories. Still, I hope what I share here can help the medical personnel who work with patients with cancer undergoing treatment and with survivors in the years that follow. Perhaps these words can even help family and friends in understanding a little more of what survival really means to the survivor.

What Are Those Scars on Your Neck?

It's funny to be so marked up with scars from surgeries so many years ago. As a kid I took pride in such questions as, "What are those scars on your neck?" I wore it a bit like a badge. Sure, I didn't run as fast or have the energy of others, but I had some sweet scars. This was a common question, particularly with moving schools and cities, an expected question as I grew older and made new friends in new places. With older classmates, it always took a little longer to broach the subject. (In contrast to fifth graders, high schoolers actually have a bit of a social filter.) Still, at the pool or the beach, with scars more prominently visible, it would eventually come up.

As proud as I was of my scars, such physical markers make it impossible to forget the physical trauma that affected me so many years ago. Though I know now that there are all kinds of skin treatments or surgeries that could cover these up, I don't see myself ever doing it. For better or worse, these are my badges. These are and forever will be a significant part of my identity, and I welcome questions about scars and treatments and the like. Plus, when I do meet other cancer patients or survivors, or their friends or families, it creates an easier entry to conversations about those very difficult years.

Won't Come Easy

There's a lot of talk in school of "natural talent" or "natural athleticism." I always felt the opposite of this, and it drove me mad at times. Physicality never came easy for me. Peewee soccer and little league were exhausting for me, much more than it ever seemed for other kids. I struggled to learn to ride a bike until after my 10th birthday (and I'm still not comfortable on a bike at age 28). With skiing, I never even tried to keep up with school friends who were jumping off cliffs by age 12.

From early childhood, even up into high school, I wanted to play football. In sixth grade a buddy who was playing football himself devised a game where we would take turns passing a football to each other before trying to run back the opposite way without being tackled by our former quarterback. It was thrilling. We'd talk for hours about different teams and players, various football positions, and where I might fit in if I were on a team. Linebacker? I might have to get a little faster to the ball. Tight end? Maybe if I was a little taller.

Ultimately, it never happened. The most immediate and daunting blockade to my football debut was certainly my mother, who as a speech pathologist had many patients with traumatic brain injury. And of course there was my dad, the doctor, who was quick to support the 'never playing football' argument. I did participate on the YMCA swim team for a few years and then on my high school's swim team freshman year. After a meager attempt at running track, I wound up throwing discus and putting the shot. These sports played to my strengths, even if I never performed as I had hoped.

Sports are, of course, a big deal in school, but as much as I wanted to be as good as those I saw excelling at sports, I never put in the time or energy to make it a reality. Part of me expected that, at some point, athleticism would just… happen. That's the way, superficially, it seemed to work with my sporty peers. Another part of me, though, was plagued with self-doubt.

I count a lack of self-confidence among personal deficits to this day. In my school years, this self-doubt manifested as a single, driving thought: even if I dedicated the hours necessary, could I even achieve the heights of my more athletic peers? Surely much of this notion was built up in my own psyche, but how much of it might be the product of doctors and family tempering my expectations so frequently over the years? "You're going to have to work much harder than other kids to do what they do," was repeated to the point of exhaustion. The intent of such a pointer was not meant to discourage, but the encouragement—"You can do anything you want, just be prepared to work harder for it"—was, I think, lost on me. Instead, I heard it more like, "Don't expect to ever do as well as others. How could you, with *your* medical history?" After all I went through as a kid, after the medications and the surgeries and the neuropathies and everything, how could I?

Growing Pains

Some time around sixth grade I learned from my doctor that I wasn't growing quite right. The way it was described to me at the time—and the way I still feel most comfortable describing it to others without mucking up the science—was that my bone age was older than I was. Not by a small margin, but by a matter of years. What this meant was that my bones were getting ready to "fuse," and upon fusing, the most I could hope to grow might be another inch. Needless to say, five-foot-two me was not thrilled by this.

The solution was laid out—take one pill to stop this fusion and give myself a shot every night until my growth was back on track. This lasted almost 2 years.

I never quite adjusted to this shot part. I got good at giving myself the shot. Really good. Still, the necessity of this—at sleepovers, summer camps, you name it—was enough to drive me a bit crazy at times. It was embarrassing and bothersome and generally not normal.

Whether my growth problems were tied to my leukemia treatment may not be certain, though this is the leading theory. A whacky pituitary was likely to blame, thrown out of normalcy by radiation treatments. Regardless of how these growth issues came about, though, this was yet another in a long series of medical issues that were beyond beginning to wear on me. Why couldn't I just grow normally? *Be* normal? None of my other friends had to give themselves shots every night just to grow.

The idea that I was somehow broken or busted or otherwise not normal was perpetuated by this complication and others over the years. In this case, during socially formative years, where all I wanted, like other young teens, was to "fit in" and be popular. This felt like just another hurdle to getting there.

Extra Time

Through high school, I finally felt, mostly, medically normal. I was still unathletic and was reveling in my nerdiness—with a group of friends opting for Friday night video game sessions versus football games and after parties—so I was hardly cool or popular. Still, things felt solid for me. Cue the curveball.

My senior year, I was invited to be part of an Atlanta-based research program on the long-term effects of radiation and chemo treatment for cancer. This entailed a series of exams over the course of a day to determine what, if any, cognitive and intellectual "impairments" I was having at 18 and how these might relate to past treatments. By the end of the day, my shortcomings were clear: my struggles were those of executive function; time management and multitasking being my most lagging areas. This news wasn't earth-shattering; I had felt difficulties with timed assignments in school before. What surprised me was just *how* bad I was in these areas. I know these results didn't completely portray my ability. I had been excited to participate in the study, but when test time came I felt distracted and overwhelmed by all these tests that kept coming, one after another. I was exhausted by the end of the day. I knew I had more trouble focusing on these exams than I did in classrooms. Still, the results were there, low percentiles and all. So what do I do with all this?

I struggled with that question, of whether to use this to my advantage, to seek extra time and other exemptions in my college classes. I wished badly that this question could just be erased, the decision ignored. Did I really deserve to receive extra time? Isn't this something that students with *real* learning disabilities receive? I hadn't received such privileges previously; enacting it now felt somehow like abusing system. I was ready to leave my past treatments behind me. I was 18, an adult, and didn't want to be held back by my childhood health issues anymore.

I decided to put the decision on hold and went off to college prepared to do as well as I could and reassess after the first semester. As expected of a college curriculum, everything was much harder. The homework load was heavier, the papers were longer, the exams expecting more. However, the thoughts brought up during my

Atlanta exams persisted: do these struggles in college reflect intellectual ability, or just processing speeds and managing exam times?

Ultimately, I opted to request extra time. This did prove helpful, for tests in particular. Through college, though, and to this day, I ask myself: wouldn't *anybody* benefit from more time on exams? An extra week to get a paper in? Maybe I had a medical "right" to this, but maybe I just needed to learn to adapt.

Lost Summer Days and New Normals

My first seizure occurred during work hours. It was Earth Day 2018 and I was working at 2 different Earth Day events with my Salt Lake County Recycling Office teammates. After a morning at the zoo, I split from the group to make a presentation at a business's own environmental showcase conference. With that session winding down a few hours later, and only a few employees circling the conference room, I suddenly found myself on the floor, paramedics standing over me, taking my pulse, telling me I'd blacked out and seized. They were preparing to put me in an ambulance to the ER.

I didn't know what to say. I started arguing with them, questioning which behaviors or symptoms they'd seen that would indicate a seizure. No, not what the eventgoer saw from across the room—what did *you* see? Did *you* see me shaking? No? Oh really....

I had never considered seizures as something I could ever have. There was no explanation for it then (and there's still no clear explanation for it now). As I was processing what I'd been told, hooked up in an ambulance en route to the hospital, the pitiful thought squeaked up again, for the first time in a long while: Why me?

My MRI revealed 2 things: a number of cavernous malformations, visible as little white spots, and a larger, unexplainable marking, first referred to as a "mass," later simply as a lesion or an abnormal signal in the gray matter, since it's apparently not a tumor. It likely indicates, I am told, some degree of demyelination. In the scan, it's a *big* spot, many times larger than even the largest malformation. More than big enough to keep me up at night every now and then, especially since what it is, isn't known.

Shortly after my seizure, an older neurologist told me that, neurologically speaking, I was *normal* and that I should just live my life. And I did, mostly, for a while. Once I started driving again 3 months later and work and life resumed mostly as if this whole seizure thing was some sort of fever dream, I started to feel all right. In August, 2019, while out late with friends at a casino in Wendover, Nevada, I had my second seizure. Fifteen months after the first. Now, 8 months later, I don't think I've fully recovered, emotionally, from that one. As I don't yet know specific triggers, I must take all precautions. Some are medically recommended: I hardly drink anymore, I certainly don't go out for drinks with friends, I don't stay up late, and I prioritize sleep. Some are more anxieties: I've struggled to get back into a weightlifting routine, fearing such stress might trigger another episode; even hiking and backpacking, things I love, now cause anxiety that I'm working to overcome. There may be no logic to these fears, medically, but they're still obstacles, mental checkpoints I need to clear. And I will clear them. I'll keep on tuning meds and adjusting habits and pushing boundaries and doing my damnedest to heed the advice of that old neurologist, to live my life as if I'm normal, even if I'm not. I know I'm not. And maybe that's OK.

Fair Share (Medical Exhaustion)

Perhaps because I was so young when I was diagnosed and went through treatment, I rarely found myself asking, "Will I relapse?" I consider myself incredibly fortunate in this regard. The whole notion of relapsing feels distant to me, the same way the treatment at the time does and did. Even as a kid, only a few years after remission, this fear rarely crossed my mind. Except, of course, at doctors' appointments, where everyone—except me—saw the seriousness of the situation and the need to ponder such questions.

Though this fear may not persist, there are plenty of others that do. Mostly I fear the unknown. And that's probably why I'm sick of hospitals.

I understand doctors and treatments and medicines have done so much to keep me healthy, to make my life as good as it is. Beyond affording me survival of my leukemia, I've received incredible care that's helped me through all sorts of challenges, from neuropathies and growth problems to Lyme disease (don't even ask) and epilepsy. Still, I'm sick of clinics and nurses and doctors and shots and scans and everything else that comes with these seemingly constant appointments.

That's where the anxiety comes in, that slight peak in my heart rate that sneaks in just between turning over the clipboard to the receptionist and getting my "vitals" checked. It often lingers until, at last, I meet with the doctor. It subsides for a few hours, reassurances and doctor's office vernacular keeping it at bay, only to invade my thoughts at home once more as I'm cooking dinner or getting ready for bed or trying to distract myself from the daily grind with an episode of *New Girl*. This isn't a specific anxiety. It's often impossible for me to say definitively, "That's what I'm afraid of." Right now, seizures are what's most on my mind, but more often it's just this fear of the unknown. Of what lurks around the corner, in the shadows. The fear that yet another curveball is coming my way.

Tempered Expectations (Not Anymore)—[Conclusions]

In January, in honor of a new decade, I completed a month-long, self-help–inspired project of logging goals for the 2020s. One goal I did not record on my list, but should have: malleability. I've never taken the punches all that well, but it's time for that to change. Something I did not take into account in creating these goals? My seizures. Nor my possibly lacking executive functions. Nor my lack of athleticism.

These are obstacles, they're not barriers. It may take time and energy, but I will cross them.

WHEN A PEDIATRIC ONCOLOGIST'S OWN SON IS A PATIENT: A PARENT'S VIEW

I call it, "The best credential that I never wanted."

As a pediatric oncologist, it's clear that being the father of a childhood cancer survivor gives me a certain advantage over my colleagues. When I meet a new patient with cancer and his or her family, I don't *immediately* tell them that my now adult son, David, was treated for leukemia as a child; this is clearly not the first thing they want to know. But at some point in our initial conversations about their own child's diagnosis, treatment plan, and prognosis, it becomes relevant. When I do tell them, the obvious point is that I have walked in their shoes; I can truly empathize with what they are experiencing. Making that connection with the family is great, but, more important, I want them to know that surviving childhood cancer is not an abstraction. It's a living, breathing fact.

I also use David's story as a means of discussing probabilities, statistics, and prognostication.

When David was diagnosed with "high risk" T-cell acute lymphoblastic leukemia in March 1995, the projected event-free survival for such patients was on the order of 80%. To a parent, this sounds like money in the bank. But after 17 months of "augmented Berlin-Frankfurt-Münster" chemotherapy, David—still on maintenance treatment—suffered an "early extramedullary relapse" of T-cell acute lymphoblastic leukemia, a disease notorious for bad relapses. David's likelihood for survival had suddenly plummeted. Even worse, when his reinduction chemotherapy (in anticipation of an eventual allogeneic marrow transplant) was complicated by systemic aspergillosis and bilateral fungal pneumonia, all seemed lost.

Today, David is alive and his leukemia remains in second remission, more than 22 years off treatment. He defied the odds twice: first by relapsing and later by not dying. Kaplan-Meier survival curves are statistical constructs, not oracles.

So now David is a "survivor." What is that like for him? I will let David share his own thoughts. But this is the story of another survivor, his father, the oncologist.

Relapse Fears

When David was going through second-line treatment, his brother Greg, along with his second-grade classmates, was asked to draw a self-portrait. His picture's perspective was from behind and he portrayed himself in the act of drawing a stick-figure boy. The drawing within the drawing was unfinished but "Greg" had put his pencil down. His teacher, curious, asked why the stick-figure was incomplete and Greg responded, "Because I don't know if he's going to live."

It's a cliché to say that having a child diagnosed with cancer is every parent's worst nightmare. Once your child *has* cancer, there is a new worst nightmare and it's called "relapse." After living that second nightmare once, David seemed, unfortunately, a likely candidate to do it again. Even his 7-year-old brother could sense that. Nonetheless, when, against all odds, he had been off all treatment for just over a year, I began to consider a career move. At that point, my wife Annette and I were, without saying as much, still almost *expecting* a second relapse—unconsciously we were probably *waiting*—but we still had life decisions to make. After much discussion, we agreed and I accepted a new position in Boise, Idaho.

We had been in Boise for only a few weeks when I got a phone call from David's school nurse: he was in her office with a severe headache and he looked "really sick." I *felt* sick. I told her I was on my way, then asked my partner, David's new oncologist, to arrange for bloodwork, a lumbar puncture, and a brain MRI study—STAT! When the dust had settled, David had a sinus infection and we had a surge in confidence about his prognosis.

Parents ask me: When did you *stop* worrying about a relapse? My stock answer is that the worry-meter never goes to zero. Most parents have an unconscious list of worries, in some sort of rank order. "My child will get run over." "My child will drown." "My child will get cancer." For us unlucky few, "My child's cancer will *relapse*" becomes #1 on the list and there it stays until at some point, if all goes well, its ranking begins to fall and eventually it drops out of the top 25.

From the oncologist's perspective, "cure" is a problematic concept, but the term is certainly more succinct (and optimistic) than "extended remission in the absence of ongoing therapy."

Unpredictable Vaccine Response

Not long after we moved to Boise, David developed a persistent cough. After 2 or 3 visits to his pediatrician (and after I had raised the possibility more than once), he was finally diagnosed with pertussis. This, despite having received appropriate catch-up immunizations.

This episode left us with one funny anecdote: David indignantly reported to Annette one afternoon that one of the teachers had "squeezed" him ("Hard!") in the school lunchroom, in what was no doubt an attempted Heimlich maneuver.

Endocrine Effects

Surveys of childhood cancer survivors demonstrate that the great majority have one or more chronic medical conditions and roughly one-half of these are "grade 3 or 4."[1] Among these, endocrine disorders are quite common.

Prior to his leukemia diagnosis, David had grown along the 75th percentile for height but, with all of his medical issues, this had declined to the 10th percentile at age 7. He stayed there until he was 10 years old, when his growth began to accelerate. This seemed a good sign at first but, as he approached the 50th percentile around age 12, I was concerned: could David be growing *too* fast? (David's pubertal development, I would later learn, was also accelerating, but even if your Dad is a pediatrician, some things are kept private. Like, privates.)

We consulted an endocrinologist. X-rays confirmed that David's bone age was 21 months ahead of his chronologic age, which meant that he had 21 fewer months to keep growing than we might otherwise have expected. Doing the math, it looked like he was destined to top out at about 5 feet 2 inches. Given his parents' and older brother's heights, this seemed undesirable. The endocrinologist offered a somewhat novel treatment: oral letrozole would theoretically slow down bone maturation, allowing David's growth plates to remain open and functioning, while injections of supplemental growth hormone would accelerate growth while it could still happen.

A year and a half of daily injections (and $1000 a month out-of-pocket) were not ideal, but the combination therapy worked as advertised. Today, ironically, David is the tallest member of our family, about an inch taller than his Dad.

I often tell my patients with *constitutional* short stature that, "It doesn't matter how tall you are, as long as your feet reach the ground." From a father's perspective, however, I must acknowledge that our society is not so sanguine on this issue. Being a cancer survivor is, on one hand, a source of pride but it is also, in some people's eyes, a sign that one is "damaged." Why stand out by being noticeably shorter than one's family members?

Intellectual and Developmental Concerns

Survivors of childhood leukemia—even those who receive only front-line therapy—are at increased risk for learning disabilities and (usually subtle) intellectual impairment.[2] In David's case, after suffering a central nervous system relapse, there was a broad consensus that craniospinal radiation therapy must be included in second-line treatment. It was less clear, however, *how much* radiation should be used. Given the guarded prognosis, we erred on the side of higher doses and David received 2340 cGy of whole-brain radiation. At the time, he was just barely 5 years old and it was clear that we were placing him at risk for "late effects." *If* he lived long enough.

Over the years, David underwent 2 separate neuropsychological evaluations. The first time, he was 7 years old. The psychologist told Annette that David's overall intelligence put him "in the group of people who are most successful in life." While there was no obvious "fingerprint" of damage from radiation, he cautioned us that this could change over time. David's results did indicate difficulty with respect to time management and multitasking. When Annette asked how this might someday express itself, the psychologist put it this way: "Someday, his wife will tell David that dinner is ready in 15 minutes and he'll reply, 'Great. I'm just going to clean the garage first.'"

We decided to pursue a subsequent assessment when David was a high school senior and 18 years old. At the time, he was enrolled in a college-preparatory high school and was doing very well, later to graduate *cum laude* as a member of the National

Honor Society.[a] We were thus stunned by portions of the report that showed considerable neurocognitive deficits and seemed not to reflect the young man we knew. In particular, scores indicative of "initiation" were strikingly low. The assessment, which we had sought to gain helpful guidance, instead became a source of distress and frank disbelief.

As a physician, I try to respect "objective" neuropsychological testing, but as a father I want it known that a good attitude, hard work, and a supportive family are equally vital.

Following the second evaluation, we were told that David's scores qualified him for accommodations at school, such as extra time for finishing standardized tests. Contrary to his parents' advice, David opted not to pursue this. As he put it, "In real life, they don't give you accommodations." So, David took college entrance exams right beside his peers, did just fine, and gained acceptance at a well-regarded (and quite competitive) regional liberal arts college. Once he enrolled, however, it became clear that college-level work did present more challenges than anticipated by him or us. Annette and I worried about the psychological toll this was taking on David. With our prodding, he approached the college's counseling office, they reviewed the situation, and David was finally given "a break" in the form of extra time to complete exams and some assignments. During graduation events, we heard from more than one of David's professors how impressed they were by his academic work. As were his parents.

At age 28, David lives independently, holds down a well-paying job, and has thoughts of attending graduate school.

Neurologic Issues

August 2018. David called me at work to report that he was being loaded into an ambulance after (he was told) suffering a *grand mal* seizure. All he knew was that he had fallen out of his chair and awoke surrounded by a huddle of concerned work mates, who told him he had been "twitching." He was headed for the hospital. I caught the next plane to Salt Lake City.

An initial head computed tomography scan suggested a small intracranial bleed, but David's brain MRI revealed this to be an old (calcified) hemorrhage arising from one of numerous tiny vascular lesions—presumably an after-effect of cranial radiation and, arguably, not so concerning. Much more ominously, however, there was a large, irregular but reasonably well-circumscribed, white matter lesion in the left cortex. The suggested diagnosis was low-grade glioma.

The other shoe, it seemed, had finally dropped.

We were now consulting a neurologist, a neurosurgeon, *and* a neuro-oncologist. Given the various MRI abnormalities, there was little question but that David should start anticonvulsant treatment and plan to stay on it for life. That was the (relatively) easy part. As for the cortical lesion, it was unclear whether this was the source of David's seizure but for now it "needed to be watched." *Maybe* it wasn't a tumor at all (the neuro-oncologist was quite suspicious but also conceded that he was, after all, an *oncologist*; the neurosurgeon was less convinced but in no rush to biopsy). We would see....

David's next MRI scan took place on my 60th birthday. By far the best present I received that year was his unchanged scan. We are now approaching 2 years since

---

[a] A nationwide organization for high school students in the United States. Selection is based on 4 criteria: academic achievement, leadership, service, and character.

his seizure and all subsequent scans have shown no progression of the lesion, which may represent demyelination or cortical dysplasia.

The Future

Early in my career as a pediatric oncologist, I mused occasionally on "what it would be like" if the child of a friend or a relative were diagnosed with cancer. "That would be really strange and upsetting," I thought. But it never occurred to me that one of my own sons would be diagnosed with childhood leukemia. Let alone be treated twice.

David is now well into adulthood. He is a remarkable young man, who is doing well medically and otherwise, but there is no denying his past medical history. What are the concerns, moving forward? Moreover, his parents aren't getting any younger. What will be *our* role in managing these concerns?

We have already had our glioma scare (apparently, a false alarm) but David remains at some slight increased risk for second malignancies. Thankfully, the window for treatment-related malignancies is, statistically speaking, largely behind us.[3]

David received 3 different anthracycline chemotherapeutics, with a cumulative dose of more than 400 mg/m^2 (doxorubicin equivalents), as well as 600 cGy of spinal radiation therapy. All together, this places him at significant risk for delayed cardiotoxicity. Thankfully, serial echocardiograms have shown no evidence of decreased myocardial function, but unlike second cancers this particular "late effect" does not appear within a specific period. The heart failure risk curve for anyone continues uphill with the only question being its slope. My advice to David remains: take good care of your heart. You can't undo the past, but there is plenty of evidence that you can mitigate your future cardiac risk by avoiding tobacco, maintaining a healthy weight, exercising regularly, and monitoring (and treating, if necessary) blood pressure and cholesterol levels.[4]

Will David exhibit more significant postradiation neurocognitive effects when he is older? As with myocardium, our brains don't improve with age and exposure to therapeutic radiation doesn't help.[5] Our obvious hope is that David will continue to exceed expectations, as has been his habit. Annette and I also know that, in our eventual absence, his brother Greg still has David's back. (Greg occasionally refers to how "we" took care of David when he was sick.)

Finally, I have the same 400-pound-gorilla question as any parent: what will my son *do* with his life?

David is fortunate to be a survivor and to be so healthy and "normal." He is, however, aware that he cannot define himself solely as a survivor. David has heard for many years that he has to "do something as an encore" to surviving cancer and, if I am any judge, he will continue to develop his career, pursue his other interests, and lead a productive life in whatever arena(s) he chooses.

Will David be a father someday? (This from his parents: "Get married first.") He had normal pubertal/sexual development, but whether his fertility has been affected remains unknown. Given his complex treatment history, any predictions would be speculative, but I do believe he would make a wonderful father.

My patients' parents invariably ask whether I chose a career in oncology *because* of David's illness. No, I must concede, I had in fact just finished my training and started my oncology career when, as I like to put it, God decided that I wasn't educated enough. I fully expect that David will continue to educate me about cancer survivorship until the day I die.

DISCLOSURE

The authors have nothing to disclose.

REFERENCES

1. Phillips SM, Padgett LS, Leisenring WM, et al. Survivors of childhood cancer in the United States: prevalence and burden of morbidity. Cancer Epidemiol Biomarkers Prev 2015;24(4):653–63.
2. Zhou C, Zhuang Y, Lin X, et al. Changes in neurocognitive function and central nervous system structure in childhood acute lymphoblastic leukaemia survivors after treatment: a meta-analysis. Br J Haematol 2020;188(6):945–61.
3. Yavvari S, Makena Y, Sukhavasi S, et al. Large population analysis of secondary cancers in pediatric leukemia survivors. Children (Basel) 2019;6(12):130.
4. Armenian S, Bhatia S. Predicting and preventing anthracycline-related cardiotoxicity. Am Soc Clin Oncol Educ Book 2018;38:3–12.
5. Schuitema I, Deprez S, Van Hecke W, et al. Accelerated aging, decreased white matter integrity, and associated neuropsychological dysfunction 25 years after pediatric lymphoid malignancies. J Clin Oncol 2013;31(27):3378–88.

Late Effects in Childhood Cancer Survivors: Early Studies, Survivor Cohorts, and Significant Contributions to the Field of Late Effects

Filippa Nyboe Norsker, PhD[a], Camilla Pedersen, PhD[a],
Gregory T. Armstrong, MD, MSCE[b], Leslie L. Robison, PhD[b],
Mary L. McBride, MSc[c], Michael Hawkins, DPhil[d],
Claudia E. Kuehni, MD[e,f], Florent de Vathaire, PhD[g],
Julie Berbis, PhD[h], Leontien C. Kremer, MD, PhD[i],
Riccardo Haupt, MD[j], Line Kenborg, PhD[a,*],
Jeanette Falck Winther, MD, DMSc[a,k,1]

KEYWORDS

- Childhood cancer survivors • Survivor cohorts • Cancer research • Late effects
- Long-term complications

Continued

[a] Childhood Cancer Research Group, Danish Cancer Society Research Center, Strandboulevarden 49, 2100 Copenhagen, Denmark; [b] Department of Epidemiology & Cancer Control, St. Jude Children's Research Hospital, 262 Danny Thomas Place, Mail Stop 735, Memphis, TN 38105, USA; [c] Cancer Control Research, BC Cancer, 675 West 10th Avenue, Room 2.107, Vancouver, BC, V5Z 1L3, Canada; [d] Centre for Childhood Cancer Survivor Studies, Institute of Applied Health Research, Robert Aitken Building, University of Birmingham, Birmingham B15 2TT, UK; [e] Swiss Childhood Cancer Registry, Institute of Social and Preventive Medicine, University of Bern, Mittelstrasse 43, CH-3012 Bern, Switzerland; [f] Paediatric Oncology, Inselspital, Bern University Hospital, University of Bern, Freiburgstrasse 18, CH-3010 Bern, Switzerland; [g] Centre for Research in Epidemiology and Population Health, INSERM Unit 1018, Institut Gustave Roussy, University of Paris-Saclay, 114 Rue Edouard Vaillant, 94800 Villejuif, France; [h] Assistance Publique Hopitaux de Marseille, Aix-Marseille University, EA 3279 CEReSS, Health Service Research and Quality of Life Center, Faculté de Médecine 27, Bd Jean Moulin 13005 Marseille, France; [i] Princess Maxima Center for Pediatric Oncology, University Medical Center Utrecht, Utrecht University, Heidelberglaan 25, 3584 CS Utrecht, The Netherlands; [j] IRCCS Istituto Giannina Gaslini, Via Gerolamo Gaslini, 5, 16147 Genova, Italy; [k] Department of Clinical Medicine, Faculty of Health, Incuba Skejby, building 2, Palle Juul-Jensens Boulevard 82, 8200 Aarhus N, Denmark
[1] Shared last authorship.
* Corresponding author.
E-mail address: kenborg@cancer.dk

Pediatr Clin N Am 67 (2020) 1033–1049
https://doi.org/10.1016/j.pcl.2020.07.002
0031-3955/20/© 2020 Elsevier Inc. All rights reserved.

pediatric.theclinics.com

Continued

KEY POINTS

- Overview of childhood cancer survivor cohorts across Europe and North America including their historical background.
- Selected publications with significant clinical impact for the treatment and follow-up of patients with childhood cancer within each childhood cancer survivor cohort.
- An up-to-date summary of the contributions to the research from childhood cancer survivor cohorts in Europe and North America.

INTRODUCTION

With improvement in cure has come the responsibility to investigate the long-term morbidity and mortality associated with the treatment modalities leading to this increase in survival.[1,2] Treatment-related effects on normal growth and development, neuropsychological functioning, and reproductive capacity are some of the main concerns raised by parents and by patients themselves.[3] These concerns were already expressed more than 40 years ago by Dr Giulio J. D'Angio:*"It is clear that the child cured of cancer must be followed for life, not so much because late recurrence of disease is feared as to permit detection of the delayed consequences of radio- and chemotherapy. Careful studies of these late effects must be conducted."*[4]

To facilitate research on health later in life, several large cohorts of childhood cancer survivors have been established throughout Europe and North America in recent decades.[5,6] These cohorts have facilitated a vast amount of research on late effects and continue to provide the basis for investigating many different health-related aspects of cancer and cancer treatment at a young age. Some of the pioneering research of late effects after childhood cancer were the studies from the Late Effects Study Group, which was initiated in the early 1970s.[7] These studies, investigating the risk of second malignant neoplasms (SMNs), and the role of first primary tumor type, genetic predisposition, and radiotherapy treatment, demonstrated the value and need of establishing large and well-designed cohorts of childhood cancer survivors.[7–9]

In 2001, the *Journal of Clinical Oncology* published 2 landmark studies on subsequent mortality and its causes in childhood cancer survivors: a Scandinavian population-based study[10] and an American hospital-based study.[11] Both studies showed that 5-year survivors had a 10.8-fold increased mortality rate, but although modern treatments had reduced mortality from the primary cancer, there was an increased rate of long-term treatment-related deaths. These studies provided an important resource for understanding risk factors associated with increased mortality and morbidity. They also allowed the identification of treatment modifications that could reduce the noted treatment-related consequences for future patients with childhood cancer.[10,11] Years later, in 2016 and 2018, 2 studies from the North American Childhood Cancer Survivor Study (CCSS) confirmed that adjusted treatment regimens designed to reduce the potential risk and severity of late effects have indeed led to fewer late effects as well as better survival rates.[12–14]

When cure is no longer the only goal, multidisciplinary and international collaborative studies must be designed to improve the outcomes for this large and steadily growing cohort of long-term survivors of childhood cancer. It is, however, a challenge to develop strategies for the long-term follow-up of survivors addressing their needs.[15] Early efforts to describe late effects were largely

Table 1
Characteristics of North American childhood cancer survivor cohorts

Characteristics	CCSS	SJLIFE	CAYACS
Country or province	United States and Canada	United States	British Columbia, Canada
Year of establishment	1994	2007	2005
Period of cancer diagnosis	1970–1999	1962–2012	1970–2010
Cohort size	37,593 (25,664 active participants)	8245 (6004 active participants)	8735
Survival at entry	$\geq$5 y	$\geq$5 y	0 y
Age at cancer diagnosis, y	0–20	0–24	0–24
Type of cancer	Leukemia, CNS, Hodgkin lymphoma, non-Hodgkin lymphoma, neuroblastoma, soft tissue sarcoma, Wilms, bone tumors	All types	All types
Study design	Hospital-based retrospective cohort with prospective follow-up	Hospital-based retrospective cohort with prospective follow-up	Retrospective population-based cohort with prospective follow-up
Obtained information	Surveys, medical records	Clinical assessments, surveys, medical records	Registries, administrative databases, medical records
Comparison population	Siblings, general population	Frequency matched community controls, general population	Random sample from the general population of British Columbia
Therapeutic exposures	Yes (>90%)	Yes (100%)	Yes
Collection of germline DNA	For some (<60%)	Yes (>95%)	NA

Abbreviations: CAYACS, Childhood, Adolescent, Young Adult Cancer Survivors; CCSS, Childhood Cancer Survivor Study; CNS, central nervous system; NA, not available; SJLIFE, St Jude Lifetime Cohort Study.

conducted through single-institution and smaller consortia studies. However, by the mid-1980s, it became increasingly clear that these approaches had inherent limitations, including small sample size, incompletely characterized populations, and limited length of follow-up. Consequently, over the past 25 years, several cohorts of childhood cancer survivors have been established across Europe and North America. In this article, we provide an overview of these cohorts and point out some of their most significant contributions to the area of late effects. Characteristics of the childhood cancer survivor cohorts are presented in **Tables 1** and **2**.

Table 2
Characteristics of European childhood cancer survivor cohorts

Characteristics	BCCSS	ALiCCS	SCCSS	FCCSS	LEA	LATER Study	OTR
Country or region	England, Wales, Scotland	Denmark, Finland, Iceland, Norway, Sweden	Switzerland	Selected regions in France	France (the participating pediatric-oncology centers cover nearly 75% of all childhood acute leukemia survivors diagnosed since 1980)	Netherlands	Italy
Year of establishment	1998	2010	2007	2015	2004	2006	1980
Period of cancer diagnosis	1940–1991 in original cohort; 1940–2006 in extended cohort	1943–2012	1976–2018 (ongoing)	1946–1999	1980–2019 (ongoing)	1963–2002	1960–2004
Cohort size	17,981 in original cohort; 34,490 in extended cohort	33,160	5737	7670	14,201	6165	14,201
Survival at entry	≥5 y	≥1 y	≥5 y	≥5 y	≥2 y	≥5 y	End of treatment
Age at cancer diagnosis, y	0–14	0–19	0–20	0–19	0–18	0–18	0–19
Type of cancer	All types	All types	All types	All but leukemia	Leukemia	All types	All types

Study design	Retrospective population-based cohort study	Retrospective population-based cohort study	Retrospective population-based cohort study with prospective follow-up	Hospital-based retrospective cohort with prospective follow-up	Retrospective hospital- and local register-based cohort study with prospective follow-up	Hospital-based retrospective cohort study with prospective follow-up	Retrospective and prospective national hospital-based from AIEOP clinics with prospective follow-up
Obtained information	Registries, surveys, medical records	Nordic registries, medical records	Registries, surveys, medical records	National hospital and medical insurance databases, clinical visits, surveys	Registries, clinical visits, surveys, medical records	Registries, clinical visits, surveys, medical records	Regional registries, hospital data
Comparison population	General population	Matched population comparisons	Siblings and population comparisons	From national statistics	Comparisons from a national database of health care	Siblings and matched population controls	Population data
Therapeutic exposures	Crude in main cohort; detailed in case-control studies	Detailed in case-cohort studies	Crude in main cohort, detailed in nested studies	Yes (<95%), including whole body dose reconstruction for radiotherapy	Crude in main cohort; detailed in case-control studies	Yes	Crude for all; detailed for a selected group (in survivorship passports)
Collection of germline DNA	NA	NA	Yes	Yes (60%)	NA	Yes (50%)	N/A

Childhood cancer cohorts: AIEOP, Associazione Italiana di Ematologia e Oncologia Pediatrica; ALiCCS, Adult Life after Childhood Cancer in Scandinavia; BCCSS, British Childhood Cancer Survivor Study; DCCSS, Dutch Childhood Cancer Survivorship LATER Cohort Study; FCCSS, French Childhood Cancer Survivor Study; LATER Study, Dutch Childhood Cancer Survivorship LATER Cohort Study; LEA, The French Childhood Cancer Survivor Study for Leukaemia; NA, not available; OTR, The Italian Study on off-therapy Childhood Cancer Survivors; SCCSS, Swiss Childhood Cancer Survivor Study.

CHILDHOOD CANCER SURVIVOR COHORTS IN EUROPE AND NORTH AMERICA
The North American Childhood Cancer Survivor Study

The CCSS was the first large childhood cancer survivor cohort to be initiated and was funded by the US National Cancer Institute in 1994.[6] The CCSS is a unique resource because of its large size combined with comprehensive data and banked biologic samples, thus overcoming some of the limitations from earlier studies. CCSS originally included more than 20,000 5-year survivors diagnosed from 1970 to 1986 before age 21 years and treated at 26 clinical centers in the United States and Canada.[16] Subsequently, the cohort was expanded to include 37,593 eligible survivors diagnosed through 1999 with 25,664 participating.[17] More than 370 peer-reviewed publications investigating various aspects of pediatric cancer and its treatment on later health have been carried out within the CCSS cohort.[16]

One of the early significant contributions of the CCSS was published in 2001.[18] CCSS investigators noted a modest increased frequency of SMN in survivors even for the subgroups of survivors carrying the greatest risks. However, given the trajectory of the cumulative incidence curve, with no evidence of plateau, survivors were at increased risk for SMNs across their lifespan. A subsequent CCSS study, published in 2006, showed that almost three-fourths of childhood cancer survivors treated in the 1970s and 1980s had a chronic health condition with more than 40% having serious health problems.[19] The incidence of health conditions increased with time, emphasizing the need for ongoing close monitoring of survivors as an important part of their overall health care.[19] Last, a study published in 2016 confirmed that more recent pediatric cancer treatment regimens designed to reduce the potential risk and severity of late effects, in fact do so. Thus, along with increased promotion of approaches for early detection and improvements in medical care for late effects, this study presented quantitative evidence that the strategy of lowering therapeutic exposures has contributed to extending the lifespan for many survivors of childhood cancer.[12]

St. Jude Lifetime Cohort Study

The St. Jude Children's Research Hospital initiated the St. Jude Lifetime Cohort Study (SJLIFE) in 2007, with the aim of establishing a lifetime cohort of survivors to perform prospective medical assessment of health outcomes. The SJLIFE study is a retrospective cohort design with prospective clinical follow-up and ongoing accrual of 5-year survivors of all childhood cancers diagnosed and treated at St. Jude Children's Research Hospital since its opening in 1962.[20] As of March 2020, more than 6000 survivors have been enrolled into the SJLIFE cohort, as well as 735 age-matched, sex-matched, and race-matched controls. This unique cohort, funded by St. Jude and a grant from the US National Cancer Institute, has published more than 120 peer-reviewed manuscripts, describing various aspects of the long-term consequences experienced by cohort participants.

In 2013, SJLIFE investigators estimated that at age 45 years, the cumulative prevalence of any chronic health condition was 95.5% and 80.5% for a serious/disabling or life-threatening chronic condition.[21] This publication also detailed the yield from conducting risk-based screening. A few years after, in 2017, a subsequent study demonstrated that by age 50 years, a survivor would experience, on average, 17.1 chronic health conditions of any grade, of which 4.7 were severe/disabling, life-threatening, or fatal.[22] Last, using whole genome sequencing of 3006 survivors, SJLIFE investigators assessed the prevalence of pathogenic/likely pathogenic mutations in 60 cancer predisposition genes with autosomal dominant inheritance and moderate to high penetrance and evaluated the association with risk of subsequent neoplasms.[23]

Mutations were identified in 5.8% of survivors and were associated with significantly increased rates of subsequent breast cancer and sarcoma among irradiated survivors and with increased rates of developing any subsequent neoplasm among nonirradiated survivors. These findings support referral of all survivors for genetic counseling with potential clinical genetic testing.

The Childhood, Adolescent, and Young Adult Cancer Survivors Research Program

A multidisciplinary research team in British Columbia (BC), Canada, initiated the first steps toward the establishment of the Childhood, Adolescent, and Young Adult Cancer Survivors Research Program (CAYACS) research program with the overall aim to study late effects and health care outcomes in childhood cancer survivors by linking different data sources in BC.[24] The initial study was funded by the Canadian Institutes for Health Research from 2001 to 2004 and used the benefits of population files with complete follow-up and data linkage to reduce the risk of misclassification of patients with cancer and outcomes. This work formed the basis for the CAYACS research program, funded by the Canadian Cancer Society Research Institute from 2005 to 2015, which so far has resulted in 20 peer-reviewed studies. The cohort includes all residents in BC diagnosed with cancer from 1970 to 2010 before 25 years of age and examines health, education, and income outcomes with appropriate population-based control groups.

Based on CAYACS, the risk for hospitalization-related late morbidity was found to be highest in survivors of leukemia, central nervous system (CNS) tumors, bone and soft tissue sarcomas, and kidney cancer. Importantly, hospitalizations due to other diseases than cancer became more prevalent over time.[25] Significant findings from CAYACS have also brought awareness of the late complications in survivors among stakeholders. The results from a comprehensive study showing lower educational attainment among childhood cancer survivors[26] were disseminated to system funders and policymakers (BC Ministry of Education), program managers, and teachers to act on the educational challenges in the survivors. The CAYACS has also been a leading resource to estimate the health care costs for patients with childhood cancer, useful for evidence-informed policy development and health care delivery of follow-up and management.[27]

The British Childhood Cancer Survivor Study

Studies from the early 1990s reporting an increased risk of secondary cancers[28,29] and causes of increased late mortality in childhood cancer survivors[30] led to the establishment of the British Childhood Cancer Survivor Study (BCCSS). The aim of the BCCSS was to obtain estimates of the risk for *selected* adverse health and social outcomes occurring among survivors and their offspring and to investigate variation of such risks in relation to different risk factors, including type of childhood cancer and its treatment.[31] Hence, the BCCSS was established in 1998[31] including almost 18,000 5-year survivors of all types of childhood cancer diagnosed before age 15 years in England, Wales, and Scotland. To date, more than 70 peer-reviewed studies have been published based on BCCSS data.

Some of the most significant contributions achieved through the BCCSS cohort to date were the results from a study published in 2010, reporting that second cancers and cardiovascular outcomes accounted for 50% and 25% of the excess number of deaths in adult survivors of childhood cancer.[32] This important information allowed for developing strategies to decrease early mortality. The year after, a study reported that most of the excess second cancers observed among long-term survivors were also the common cancers in the general population and that abdominal irradiation was associated with a similar risk of bowel cancer to that experienced by individuals with 2 affected first-degree relatives.[33] Last, a study from 2017 provided a risk stratification tool for specific causes of death, SMNs and nonfatal non-neoplastic outcomes for childhood cancer survivors. These data were used in a new Service Specification by the National Health Service England concerning the clinical follow-up of survivors throughout England.[34]

Adult Life After Childhood Cancer in Scandinavia

In the early 1990s and 2000s, Nordic, population-based studies on SMNs and late mortality in childhood cancer survivors were published.[10,35,36] The risk estimates from these studies were lower than those previously reported in most hospital-based studies, emphasizing the necessity of conducting large, population-based studies. Further, the early studies of late effects were mainly conducted in US populations.[7–9] To determine whether the US findings were applicable elsewhere, other countries initiated their own programs. This led to the population-based Nordic Adult Life after Childhood Cancer in Scandinavia (ALiCCS) research program[37] initiated in 2010 comprising 33,160 1-year survivors of all childhood cancers diagnosed between 1943 and 2008 in Denmark, Finland, Iceland, Norway, and Sweden. Due to the size and age of the survivor cohort as well as the meticulous registration in the Nordic registries, the ALiCCS program enables studies of specific cancer types and rare medical disorders in both adulthood and senescence. To date, more than 20 peer-reviewed studies have been published.

One of the first ALiCCS studies provided an exhaustive endocrine risk profile of childhood cancer survivors treated in northern Europe. At age 60 years, survivors had a cumulative risk of more than 40% for endocrine disorders requiring a hospital contact.[38] Another study, linking long-term neuroblastoma survivors with patient and clinical registries, illustrated the high risk of late effects, particularly among survivors of high-risk neuroblastoma, who are some of the most intensively treated patients within pediatric oncology and for whom very little is known about later adverse health outcomes[39]. Recently, it was shown that 5-year survivors of a CNS tumor had an increased risk of nervous system diseases. Due to a complete hospital history for each survivor, both before and after diagnosis, it was possible to show that the risk of epilepsy was highly increased several years before the cancer diagnosis, emphasizing the importance of following children with epilepsy for CNS tumors.[40]

Swiss Childhood Cancer Survivor Study

The Swiss Childhood Cancer Survivor Study (SCCSS) is a nationwide population-based cohort study established in 2007 including 5737 5-year survivors of childhood cancer diagnosed between 1976 and 2018 with ongoing enrollment of study participants. The aim of this collaborative is to evaluate long-term consequences of childhood cancer, with a special focus on the incidence of late effects, risk factors for late effects, health care use, and medical follow-up, as well as health-related behaviors and their determinants. Before the official establishment of the SCCSS, a first multi-center hospital-based study was conducted in 1992 to 1994 in which detailed information on somatic, psychosocial, and socioeconomic outcomes in survivors was collected. Since 2007, regular national questionnaire surveys, supplemented by nested hospital-based studies, have been conducted on a national level.[41] To date, more than 170 peer-reviewed studies have been published based on SCCSS data.

The population-based approach with detailed clinical information and questionnaire data enables studies elucidating many different aspects of late complications. In the SCCSS, pulmonary diseases, particularly pneumonia and chest wall abnormalities, were reported to be up to 4 to 6 times more common in survivors than in siblings,[42] indicating that long-term monitoring is required to give insight into the progression of lung disease, risk factors, and potential prevention. Another study reported that the prevalence of self-reported hearing loss among survivors was high (10%), especially after a CNS tumor (25%). The burden of hearing loss was stabilized in survivors treated more recently, suggesting a positive impact of new treatment regimens with less ototoxic radiation and more carefully dosed platinum compounds.[43] Most survivors reported low levels of psychological distress; although one-fourth of survivors still reported distress to a degree that makes closer observation and potentially counseling worthwhile.[44]

The French Childhood Cancer Survivor Study

The basis for the French Childhood Cancer Survivor Study (FCCSS) started with 2 single-center studies of 634 5-year survivors treated for solid tumors in childhood at Gustave Roussy in Paris between 1942 and 1969. One study reported the long-term risk for SMNs[45] and the other assessed the role of chemotherapy and radiation dose and site on this risk.[46] The results revealed that the relative risk of SMN was highly increased in survivors treated with both radiation and chemotherapy. These early findings led to an expansion of the cohort including several treatment centers in France as well as 3 centers from Great Britain to study the risk of different late complications in 4122 5-year survivors in the Euro2K cohort, including cardiac disease[47] and diabetes.[48] In 2015, the FCCSS combined the 3172 French survivors from the Euro2K treated between 1942 to 1985 and 4498 survivors treated between 1985 to 2000 at the Gustave Roussy and at the Curie Center.[49] To date, 68 peer-reviewed studies have been published based on FCCSS data.

The FCCSS has contributed important knowledge on different late complications due to the very detailed level of treatment information. One study reported on the association between radiation dose to the tail of the pancreas as part of the cancer treatment and diabetes as a late complication[48] whereas another study demonstrated that both anthracyclines and heart radiation doses were highly associated with cardiac disease: 2 important results with clinical implications for follow-up of childhood cancer survivors.[50]

The French Childhood Cancer Survivor Study for Leukemia

The French Childhood Cancer Survivor Study for Leukemia (LEA) cohort is a French multicenter follow-up program exclusively including children treated for acute leukemia since 1980. LEA was initiated in 2004 with the aim to study the medical, socioeconomic, behavioral, and environmental determinants of health outcomes in patients treated for childhood acute leukemia. The 5160 patients included were treated at 17 pediatric hematology and oncology centers throughout France, covering approximately 80% of all French children diagnosed with acute leukemia.[51] Until now, 31 studies have been published based on data from the LEA cohort.

The combination of clinical and therapeutic information retrieved from medical records, physical and laboratory examinations, and questionnaire data makes LEA an important source for studying a wide range of late complications in childhood acute leukemia survivors. One study reported an increased risk for reduced femoral bone mineral density among adult survivors with gonadal deficiency who received hematopoietic stem cell transplantation, which might increase their risk for fractures later in life.[52] Another study disclosed a higher risk for metabolic syndrome among survivors, independent of the treatment received suggesting that early detection, followed by changes in lifestyle, might prevent cardiovascular events among survivors.[53] Finally, a study of late cardiomyopathy in 185 survivors of acute myeloid leukemia revealed that the development of late cardiomyopathy is associated with previous history of relapse and cumulative dose of anthracyclines.[54]

Dutch Childhood Cancer Survivorship LATER Cohort Study

Since 2006, the LATER study group, a collaboration among health care providers, researchers, survivors, and the Dutch Childhood Oncology Group has been establishing the Dutch Childhood Cancer Survivorship LATER Cohort Study. The aims of the LATER Study are to determine the risk and severity of therapy-related health problems in childhood cancer survivors and to gain insight into genetic and personal risk factors for health problems. Furthermore, the LATER Study aims to identify diagnostic tests to detect and treat late effects at an early stage and to understand which possible interventions can improve the quality of life in survivors. For the first part of the LATER Study, data were collected from questionnaires and linkage studies for more than 6000 survivors alive 5 years after diagnosis and diagnosed between 1965 and 2001 and their siblings. For the LATER part 2 study data from a visit to the outpatient clinic between 2016 and 2020 of nearly 2500 survivors and 750 siblings were collected. The unique combination of information from medical records, questionnaires, clinical examinations, and clinical material enables the LATER Study to generate new knowledge for improving the care of childhood cancer patients and survivors. To date more than 30 papers have been published based on the LATER Study cohort.

A study on subsequent breast cancer, sarcoma, and solid cancers, following treatment with different chemotherapeutical agents, suggested that doxorubicin exposure increased the risk of all solid cancers and breast cancer, whereas exposure to cyclophosphamide increased the risk of sarcomas. These results may be used to adjust future treatment protocols for patients with childhood cancer and for setting up surveillance guidelines for survivors.[55] Another important LATER study underscored the crucial role of primary care physicians in the care of childhood cancer survivors. The study pointed to the need for collaboration across care professions and the importance of having a care plan for every survivor that can be used by different health care providers.[56] Last, in a collaborative study combining data from 3 survivorship cohorts (the LATER Study, SJLIFE, and CCSS), the risk of late-onset cardiomyopathy in childhood cancer survivors was examined. The study revealed that daunorubicin was associated with decreased risk for cardiomyopathy compared with doxorubicin, whereas epirubicin was approximately isoequivalent. The current hematologic-based doxorubicin dose equivalency of mitoxantrone (4:1), however, appeared to underestimate the association of mitoxantrone with long-term risk of cardiomyopathy.[57]

The Italian Study on Off-Therapy Childhood Cancer Survivors

The Italian Study on Off-Therapy Childhood Cancer Survivors (OTR) was established in 1980 as a multi-institutional register of off therapy pediatric patients treated at one of the institutions of the Italian Association of Pediatric Hematology and Oncology (AIEOP). The main purpose of the OTR was to improve the understanding of the clinical need for long-term follow-up of childhood cancer survivors. In 1989, AIEOP started a cancer register, where all children with cancer were included since diagnosis. Through linkage with the cancer register, the OTR has identified off therapy patients since 1996.[58]

The OTR is an important resource for studying childhood cancer survivors from Southern Europe. So far, 7 studies of late complications based on the OTR have been published. The late mortality among 5-year survivors compared with the general Italian population has been described, providing insight into the specific causes of death among Italian childhood cancer survivors.[59] The OTR group initiated an international consensus paper together with the International Berlin-Frankfurt-Munster Early and Late Toxicity Educational Committee to generate a statement of cure and care for survivors of childhood cancer.[60] This important document became the basis for the European PanCare Foundation established in 2008.

European Consortia

The aim of the PanCare network (www.pancare.eu) established in 2008 as a multidisciplinary European network of professionals, survivors, and their families is to reduce the frequency, severity, and impact of late effects of cancer treatment in children and adolescents with cancer as well as to ensure optimal long-term care.[61] PanCare is presently the backbone of late effect studies in Europe. Within Europe, complementing the large-scale cohort studies using population-based registries, are the well-established hospital-based cohort studies, which benefit from detailed information on individual patients rarely available to population-based cohort studies such as treatment information and outcomes of clinical tests.

In recent years, great strides have been taken to coordinate efforts to exploit these advantages in the European context through the establishment of 3 EU-funded collaborative research projects by investigators from several European countries, that is, PanCareSurFup focusing on cardiac disease, subsequent primary neoplasms, and late mortality in survivors as well as development of guidelines to improve lives for survivors (www.pancaresurfup.eu)[62]; PanCareLIFE focusing on female infertility, cisplatin-induced ototoxicity, and quality of life (www.pancarelife.eu); and PanCareFollowUp aiming at setting up state-of-the-art late effect clinics based on international guidelines for surveillance of late effects and a new innovative model for integrated care for survivors (www.pancarefollowup.eu). These large consortia have several advantages including very large cohort studies combining both register-based and hospital-based data with data from surveys, clinical case-control studies with detailed treatment information and dosimetry evaluation, as well as genetic evaluations.

A recent study from the PanCareSurFup consortium reported a fourfold increased risk of developing subsequent primary leukemia in childhood cancer survivors, which remained significantly elevated beyond 20 years from first primary malignancy.[62] Further, 2 sister studies provided new insight into the risk of SMNs, demonstrating a 22-fold increased risk of subsequent soft-tissue sarcomas[63] and a 30-fold increased risk for bone cancers when compared to population norms.[64] A study from PanCareLIFE[65] investigating genetic variation of cisplatin-induced ototoxicity in pediatric patients confirmed the previously observed association between cumulative dose of cisplatin and risk of ototoxicity and found an association between the single nucleotide polymorphisms ACYP2 rs1872328 and SLC22A2 rs316019 and ototoxicity in a meta-analysis. Further, an intervention study successfully raised the level of fertility preservation knowledge in parents of older patients as well as parents with higher educational levels and further improved patient and parent empowerment.[66]

DISCUSSION

The responsibility to investigate the long-term morbidity and mortality that came along with the treatment modalities leading to the improvements in cure has led to the establishment of an impressive number of childhood cancer survivor cohorts throughout Europe and North America. These cohorts complement each other with their different designs and methodology and have facilitated a vast amount of research on a wide spectrum of long-term adverse health consequences of the life-saving cancer treatments.[2] Published findings on late effects have led to a more thorough understanding of the lifelong, often very complex and serious disease pattern that childhood cancer survivors encounter after finishing treatment. These findings all stress that survivors need tailored follow-up care to identify health problems after treatment at an early stage.

In this article, we provided an overview of childhood cancer survivor cohorts across Europe and North America that have emerged since the mid-1990s, including the historic background for the establishment of these cohorts as well as some of the most significant contributions to the research area of late effects. A summary of these contributions is presented in **Box 1**.

Implementing follow-up care for childhood cancer survivors has proven challenging across the globe. Findings from a recent survey, providing the current state of survivorship care in 18 countries across 5 continents, indicated that a large proportion of pediatric-age survivors were seen by a physician being familiar with late effects, whereas far fewer survivors had access to an expert after transition to adulthood, stressing that long-term follow-up is still only available for a small proportion of children diagnosed with cancer.[15,67]

Box 1
Summarization of findings with significant clinical implications for the treatment and/or follow-up of patients with childhood cancer

- At approximately the turn of the century, the increased risk of early mortality and second malignant neoplasms following childhood cancer was established across various cohorts of childhood cancer survivors in Europe and the United States

- Main risk factors for early mortality were second malignant neoplasms and cardiovascular complications, thus providing insight into preventive strategies for reducing mortality

- The incidence of chronic health conditions in survivors treated in the 1970s and 1980s was high with almost all survivors experiencing some degree of health problems in middle age

- Numerous recent studies showed no indication of a plateau for the increased risk of adverse health conditions, calling for lifelong follow-up

- Findings of hospital-based studies on the risk of late complications were confirmed in population-based studies with complete follow-up and prospectively collected outcome information

- Identification of high-risk populations according to cancer treatment, cancer type, demographics, socioeconomics, and genetic predisposition has formed the basis for risk stratification of childhood cancer survivors to be used in the clinical follow-up

- Recent studies confirm that lowered therapeutic exposures has contributed to lifespan extension and fewer late effects in more recently treated survivors

- Evidence-based recommendations for the organization of long-term follow-up care for childhood and adolescent cancer survivors have been developed through the work of the International Harmonization Guideline Group

Lack of harmonized evidence-based guidelines might partly explain why survivors do not receive optimum care. Thus, in 2010, a worldwide collaboration to harmonize guidelines for long-term follow-up of childhood and young adult cancer survivors was initiated, the International Harmonization Guideline Group, providing uniform surveillance guidelines in collaboration with PanCare based on a large expert panel (www.ighg.org).[68,69] Another reason is the challenge of providing comprehensive, risk-based survivorship care.

These issues will be addressed by PanCareFollowUp, a third EU-funded consortium initiated in 2019. With the aim of improving follow-up care for adult survivors of childhood cancer, a new intervention will be developed, the PanCareFollowUp Care, a person-centered approach to survivorship care based on international clinical guidelines for surveillance of late effects empowering survivors to play an active role in their own health management. Setting up state-of-the-art late effect clinics in 4 European countries, Belgium, Czech Republic, Italy, and Sweden, the impact of this Care intervention will be assessed in terms of effectiveness measured as quality of life, physical and psychosocial outcomes, value, cost-effectiveness, acceptability, and feasibility (www.pancarefollowup.eu).

Despite the wealth of information published about adverse outcomes in childhood cancer survivors, our current understanding of several important areas of long-term health is still limited. To address knowledge deficits in childhood cancer survivors, longitudinal systematic medical assessment is needed to elucidate the pathophysiology of cancer treatment-related morbidity, identification of biomarkers of subclinical organ dysfunction, and characterization of high-risk groups who may benefit from interventions to preserve health. Further, because late effects are by definition effects of treatments given in the past, future studies set up to detect treatment-induced adverse effects of contemporary drugs used to treat pediatric cancers are essential, as for example, the potential adverse effects of immunotherapy used as part of some treatments today.

The overall goal of ongoing and future collaborations based on these large and rich survivor cohorts is to provide every childhood cancer survivor with better care and long-term health for survivors to reach their full potential, and to the degree possible, enjoy the same quality of life and opportunities as their peers.

DISCLOSURE

The authors have nothing to disclose.

REFERENCES

1. Gatta G, Botta L, Rossi S, et al. Childhood cancer survival in Europe 1999-2007: results of EUROCARE-5–a population-based study. Lancet Oncol 2014;15(1):35–47.

2. Robison LL, Hudson MM. Survivors of childhood and adolescent cancer: life-long risks and responsibilities. Nat Rev Cancer 2014;14(1):61–70.

3. Wallace HGD. Introduction. In: Wallace HGD, editor. Late effects of childhood cancer. 1st edition. New York: Oxford University Press; 2004. p. 1–2.

4. D'Angio GJ. Pediatric cancer in perspective: cure is not enough. Cancer 1975; 35(3 suppl):866–70.

5. Winther JF, Kenborg L, Byrne J, et al. Childhood cancer survivor cohorts in Europe. Acta Oncol 2015;54(5):655–68.

6. Robison LL, Mertens AC, Boice JD, et al. Study design and cohort characteristics of the Childhood Cancer Survivor Study: a multi-institutional collaborative project. Med Pediatr Oncol 2002;38(4):229–39.

7. Meadows AT, Baum E, Fossati-Bellani F, et al. Second malignant neoplasms in children: an update from the Late Effects Study Group. J Clin Oncol 1985;3(4): 532–8.

8. Meadows AT, D'Angio GJ, Mike V, et al. Patterns of second malignant neoplasms in children. Cancer 1977;40(4 Suppl):1903–11.

9. Mike V, Meadows AT, D'Angio GJ. Incidence of second malignant neoplasms in children: results of an international study. Lancet 1982;2(8311):1326–31.

10. Moller TR, Garwicz S, Barlow L, et al. Decreasing late mortality among five-year survivors of cancer in childhood and adolescence: a population-based study in the Nordic countries. J Clin Oncol 2001;19(13):3173–81.

11. Mertens AC, Yasui Y, Neglia JP, et al. Late mortality experience in five-year survivors of childhood and adolescent cancer: the Childhood Cancer Survivor Study. J Clin Oncol 2001;19(13):3163–72.

12. Armstrong GT, Chen Y, Yasui Y, et al. Reduction in late mortality among 5-year survivors of childhood cancer. N Engl J Med 2016;374(9):833–42.

13. Gibson TM, Mostoufi-Moab S, Stratton KL, et al. Temporal patterns in the risk of chronic health conditions in survivors of childhood cancer diagnosed 1970-99: a report from the Childhood Cancer Survivor Study cohort. Lancet Oncol 2018; 19(12):1590–601.

14. Turcotte LM, Liu Q, Yasui Y, et al. Temporal trends in treatment and subsequent neoplasm risk among 5-year survivors of childhood cancer, 1970-2015. JAMA 2017;317(8):814–24.

15. Winther JF, Kremer L. Long-term follow-up care needed for children surviving cancer: still a long way to go. Lancet Oncol 2018;19(12):1546–8.

16. Robison LL, Armstrong GT, Boice JD, et al. The Childhood Cancer Survivor Study: a National Cancer Institute-supported resource for outcome and intervention research. J Clin Oncol 2009;27(14):2308–18.

17. webpage CCSS. Demographic and cancer treatment of participants in the expansion, original and overall cohorts. Available at: https://ccss.stjude.org/content/dam/en_US/shared/ccss/documents/data/treatment-exposure-tables.pdf. Accessed October 29, 2019.

18. Neglia JP, Friedman DL, Yasui Y, et al. Second malignant neoplasms in five-year survivors of childhood cancer: childhood cancer survivor study. J Natl Cancer Inst 2001;93(8):618–29.

19. Oeffinger KC, Mertens AC, Sklar CA, et al. Chronic health conditions in adult survivors of childhood cancer. N Engl J Med 2006;355(15):1572–82.

20. Hudson MM, Ehrhardt MJ, Bhakta N, et al. Approach for classification and severity grading of long-term and late-onset health events among childhood cancer survivors in the st. jude lifetime cohort. Cancer Epidemiol Biomarkers Prev 2017;26(5):666–74.

21. Hudson MM, Ness KK, Gurney JG, et al. Clinical ascertainment of health outcomes among adults treated for childhood cancer. JAMA 2013;309(22):2371–81.

22. Bhakta N, Liu Q, Ness KK, et al. The cumulative burden of surviving childhood cancer: an initial report from the St Jude Lifetime Cohort Study (SJLIFE). Lancet 2017;390(10112):2569–82.

23. Wang Z, Wilson CL, Easton J, et al. Genetic risk for subsequent neoplasms among long-term survivors of childhood cancer. J Clin Oncol 2018;36(20): 2078–87.

24. McBride ML, Rogers PC, Sheps SB, et al. Childhood, adolescent, and young adult cancer survivors research program of British Columbia: objectives, study design, and cohort characteristics. Pediatr Blood Cancer 2010;55(2):324–30.

25. Lorenzi MF, Xie L, Rogers PC, et al. Hospital-related morbidity among childhood cancer survivors in British Columbia, Canada: report of the childhood, adolescent, young adult cancer survivors (CAYACS) program. Int J Cancer 2011; 128(7):1624–31.

26. Lorenzi M, McMillan AJ, Siegel LS, et al. Educational outcomes among survivors of childhood cancer in British Columbia, Canada: report of the Childhood/Adolescent/Young Adult Cancer Survivors (CAYACS) Program. Cancer 2009;115(10): 2234–45.

27. McBride ML, de Oliveira C, Duncan R, et al. Comparing childhood cancer care costs in two Canadian Provinces. Healthc Policy 2020;15(3):76–88.

28. Hawkins MM, Wilson LM, Stovall MA, et al. Epipodophyllotoxins, alkylating agents, and radiation and risk of secondary leukaemia after childhood cancer. BMJ 1992;304(6832):951–8.

29. Hawkins MM, Wilson LM, Burton HS, et al. Radiotherapy, alkylating agents, and risk of bone cancer after childhood cancer. J Natl Cancer Inst 1996;88(5):270–8.

30. Robertson CM, Hawkins MM, Kingston JE. Late deaths and survival after childhood cancer: implications for cure. BMJ 1994;309(6948):162–6.

31. Hawkins MM, Lancashire ER, Winter DL, et al. The British Childhood Cancer Survivor Study: Objectives, methods, population structure, response rates and initial descriptive information. Pediatr Blood Cancer 2008;50(5):1018–25.

32. Reulen RC, Winter DL, Frobisher C, et al. Long-term cause-specific mortality among survivors of childhood cancer. JAMA 2010;304(2):172–9.

33. Reulen RC, Frobisher C, Winter DL, et al. Long-term risks of subsequent primary neoplasms among survivors of childhood cancer. JAMA 2011;305(22):2311–9.

34. Frobisher C, Glaser A, Levitt GA, et al. Risk stratification of childhood cancer survivors necessary for evidence-based clinical long-term follow-up. Br J Cancer 2017;117(11):1723–31.

35. Garwicz S, Anderson H, Olsen JH, et al. Second malignant neoplasms after cancer in childhood and adolescence: a population-based case-control study in the 5 Nordic countries. The Nordic Society for Pediatric Hematology and Oncology. The Association of the Nordic Cancer Registries. Int J Cancer 2000;88(4):672–8.

36. Olsen JH, Garwicz S, Hertz H, et al. Second malignant neoplasms after cancer in childhood or adolescence. Nordic Society of Paediatric Haematology and Oncology Association of the Nordic Cancer Registries. BMJ 1993;307(6911): 1030–6.

37. Asdahl PH, Winther JF, Bonnesen TG, et al. The Adult Life After Childhood Cancer in Scandinavia (ALiCCS) Study: design and characteristics. Pediatr Blood Cancer 2015;62(12):2204–10.

38. de Fine Licht S, Winther JF, Gudmundsdottir T, et al. Hospital contacts for endocrine disorders in Adult Life after Childhood Cancer in Scandinavia (ALiCCS): a population-based cohort study. Lancet 2014;383(9933):1981–9.

39. Norsker FN, Rechnitzer C, Cederkvist L, et al. Somatic late effects in 5-year survivors of neuroblastoma: a population-based cohort study within the Adult Life after Childhood Cancer in Scandinavia study. Int J Cancer 2018;143(12):3083–96.

40. Kenborg L, Winther JF, Linnet KM, et al. Neurologic disorders in 4858 survivors of central nervous system tumors in childhood—an Adult Life after Childhood Cancer in Scandinavia (ALiCCS) study. Neuro Oncol 2019;21(1):125–36.

41. Kuehni CE, Rueegg CS, Michel G, et al. Cohort profile: the Swiss childhood cancer survivor study. Int J Epidemiol 2012;41(6):1553–64.

42. Kasteler R, Weiss A, Schindler M, et al. Long-term pulmonary disease among Swiss childhood cancer survivors. Pediatr Blood Cancer 2018;65(1). https://doi.org/10.1002/pbc.26749.

43. Weiss A, Sommer G, Kasteler R, et al. Long-term auditory complications after childhood cancer: A report from the Swiss Childhood Cancer Survivor Study. Pediatr Blood Cancer 2017;64(2):364–73.

44. Michel G, Rebholz CE, von der Weid NX, et al. Psychological distress in adult survivors of childhood cancer: the Swiss Childhood Cancer Survivor study. J Clin Oncol 2010;28(10):1740–8.

45. de Vathaire F, Schweisguth O, Rodary C, et al. Long-term risk of second malignant neoplasm after a cancer in childhood. Br J Cancer 1989;59(3):448–52.

46. de Vathaire F, Francois P, Hill C, et al. Role of radiotherapy and chemotherapy in the risk of second malignant neoplasms after cancer in childhood. Br J Cancer 1989;59(5):792–6.

47. Tukenova M, Guibout C, Oberlin O, et al. Role of cancer treatment in long-term overall and cardiovascular mortality after childhood cancer. J Clin Oncol 2010; 28(8):1308–15.

48. de Vathaire F, El-Fayech C, Ben Ayed FF, et al. Radiation dose to the pancreas and risk of diabetes mellitus in childhood cancer survivors: a retrospective cohort study. Lancet Oncol 2012;13(10):1002–10.

49. Demoor-Goldschmidt C, Allodji RS, Journy N, et al. Risk factors for small adult height in childhood cancer survivors. J Clin Oncol 2020;38(16):1785–96.

50. Haddy N, Diallo S, El-Fayech C, et al. Cardiac diseases following childhood cancer treatment: cohort study. Circulation 2016;133(1):31–8.

51. Berbis J, Michel G, Baruchel A, et al. Cohort Profile: the French childhood cancer survivor study for leukaemia (LEA Cohort). Int J Epidemiol 2015;44(1):49–57.

52. Le Meignen M, Auquier P, Barlogis V, et al. Bone mineral density in adult survivors of childhood acute leukemia: impact of hematopoietic stem cell transplantation and other treatment modalities. Blood 2011;118(6):1481–9.

53. Oudin C, Berbis J, Bertrand Y, et al. Prevalence and characteristics of metabolic syndrome in adults from the French childhood leukemia survivors' cohort: a comparison with controls from the French population. Haematologica 2018;103(4): 645–54.

54. Barlogis V, Auquier P, Bertrand Y, et al. Late cardiomyopathy in childhood acute myeloid leukemia survivors: a study from the L.E.A. program. Haematologica 2015;100(5):e186–9.

55. Teepen JC, van Leeuwen FE, Tissing WJ, et al. Long-term risk of subsequent malignant neoplasms after treatment of childhood cancer in the DCOG LATER study cohort: role of chemotherapy. J Clin Oncol 2017;35(20):2288–98.

56. Streefkerk N, Heins MJ, Teepen JC, et al. The involvement of primary care physicians in care for childhood cancer survivors. Pediatr Blood Cancer 2019;66(8): e27774.

57. Feijen EAM, Leisenring WM, Stratton KL, et al. Derivation of anthracycline and anthraquinone equivalence ratios to doxorubicin for late-onset cardiotoxicity. JAMA Oncol 2019;5(6):864–71.

58. Zurlo MG, Pastore G, Masera G, et al. Italian registry of patients off therapy after childhood acute lymphoblastic leukemia. Results after first phase of data collection. Cancer 1986;57(5):1052–5.

59. Bagnasco F, Caruso S, Andreano A, et al. Late mortality and causes of death among 5-year survivors of childhood cancer diagnosed in the period 1960-1999 and registered in the Italian Off-Therapy Registry. Eur J Cancer 2019;110: 86–97.

60. Haupt R, Spinetta JJ, Ban I, et al. Long term survivors of childhood cancer: cure and care. The Erice statement. Eur J Cancer 2007;43(12):1778–80.

61. Byrne J, Alessi D, Allodji RS, et al. The PanCareSurFup consortium: research and guidelines to improve lives for survivors of childhood cancer. Eur J Cancer 2018; 103:238–48.

62. Allodji RS, Hawkins MM, Bright CJ, et al. Risk of subsequent primary leukaemias among 69,460 five-year survivors of childhood cancer diagnosed from 1940 to 2008 in Europe: A cohort study within PanCareSurFup. Eur J Cancer 2019;117: 71–83.

63. Bright CJ, Hawkins MM, Winter DL, et al. Risk of soft-tissue sarcoma among 69 460 five-year survivors of childhood cancer in Europe. J Natl Cancer Inst 2018; 110(6):649–60.

64. Fidler MM, Reulen RC, Winter DL, et al. Risk of subsequent bone cancers among 69 460 five-year survivors of childhood and adolescent cancer in Europe. J Natl Cancer Inst 2018;110(2). https://doi.org/10.1093/jnci/djx165.

65. Clemens E, Broer L, Langer T, et al. Genetic variation of cisplatin-induced ototoxicity in non-cranial-irradiated pediatric patients using a candidate gene approach: The International PanCareLIFE Study. Pharmacogenomics J 2019; 20(2):294–305.

66. Borgmann-Staudt A, Kunstreich M, Schilling R, et al. Fertility knowledge and associated empowerment following an educational intervention for adolescent cancer patients. Psychooncology 2019;28(11):2218–25.

67. Tonorezos ES, Barnea D, Cohn RJ, et al. Models of care for survivors of childhood cancer from across the globe: advancing survivorship care in the next decade. J Clin Oncol 2018;36(21):2223–30.

68. Kremer LC, Mulder RL, Oeffinger KC, et al. A worldwide collaboration to harmonize guidelines for the long-term follow-up of childhood and young adult cancer survivors: a report from the International Late Effects of Childhood Cancer Guideline Harmonization Group. Pediatr Blood Cancer 2013;60(4):543–9.

69. Michel G, Mulder RL, van der Pal HJH, et al. Evidence-based recommendations for the organization of long-term follow-up care for childhood and adolescent cancer survivors: a report from the PanCareSurFup Guidelines Working Group. J Cancer Surviv 2019;13(5):759–72.

Radiotherapy and Late Effects

Joshua D. Palmer, MD[a], Matthew D. Hall, MD, MBA[b], Anita Mahajan, MD[c],
Arnold C. Paulino, MD[d], Suzanne Wolden, MD[e], Louis S. Constine, MD[f,g,h],*

KEYWORDS

- Pediatric cancer • Radiotherapy • Late effects • Radiobiology

KEY POINTS

- The incidence of childhood cancer survivors is increasing.
- Radiation therapy has important late effects.
- Radiation late effects are organ system dependent.
- Health screening and survivorship are important to identify late effects of radiation therapy.

INTRODUCTION

The cure rate for childhood cancer now exceeds 80%[1,2] in developed countries, but the multimodality therapy associated with this improved survival can lead to adverse long-term health-related outcomes that manifest months to years after completion of cancer treatment. Normal tissue damage following radiotherapy varies across the age spectrum. Specific to children, sensitivity to radiation injury directly relates to the developmental dynamics and maturational status of the organ, its regenerative potential, and ultimately the extent to which it has begun to senesce. Although radiation-induced impairment of growth and maturation is specific to younger children, organ

[a] Department of Radiation Oncology, The James Cancer Hospital at the Ohio State University Wexner Medical Center, Nationwide Children's Hospital, Columbus, OH, USA; [b] Department of Radiation Oncology, Miami Cancer Institute and Nicklaus Children's Hospital, Miami, FL, USA; [c] Department of Radiation Oncology, The Mayo Clinic, Rochester, MN, USA; [d] Department of Radiation Oncology, The University of Texas MD Anderson Cancer Center, Houston, TX, USA; [e] Department of Radiation Oncology, Memorial Sloan Kettering Cancer Center, New York, NY, USA; [f] Department of Radiation Oncology, University of Rochester, Rochester, NY, USA; [g] Department of Pediatrics, University of Rochester, Rochester, NY, USA; [h] Department of Radiation Oncology, The Judy DiMarzo Cancer Survivorship Program, James P. Wilmot Cancer Institute, University of Rochester Medical Center, PO Box 647, Rochester, NY 14642, USA
* Corresponding author. Department of Radiation Oncology, The Judy DiMarzo Cancer Survivorship Program, James P. Wilmot Cancer Institute, University of Rochester Medical Center, PO Box 647, Rochester, NY 14642.
E-mail address: Louis_Constine@urmc.rochester.edu

Pediatr Clin N Am 67 (2020) 1051–1067
https://doi.org/10.1016/j.pcl.2020.08.001
0031-3955/20/© 2020 Elsevier Inc. All rights reserved.

damage with tissue-specific dysfunction in repair processes is common to both children and adolescents. The Childhood Cancer Survivor Study demonstrated that childhood cancer survivors have a 1 in 10 chance of treatment-related mortality after 30 years.[3] Moreover, 50% of survivors experience at least one severe or fatal health condition by age 50 years, a 5 times greater risk than their siblings.[4] It is critical for caretakers and the radiation oncologists who treat children with cancer to appreciate the risk to these specific organs at risk. In this review, the authors discuss the biology of late radiotherapy effects, the impact of age on late effects, commonly affected organ systems, and the importance of screening to detect late effects.

RADIOTHERAPY USE IN PEDIATRIC ONCOLOGY
Radiotherapy Modalities Used in Pediatric Cancer

Preventing or ameliorating late adverse effects of radiotherapy requires an understanding of normal tissue tolerance. Radiotherapy tolerance is influenced by total dose and fractionation, dose rate, overall treatment time, machine energy, and the volume of tissue irradiated, which is a function of treatment technique. The earliest usage of radiation therapy was with 2-dimensional (2D) approaches that consisted of a limited number of beams with boundaries drawn on orthogonal radiographs. Beam shaping was limited and based largely on bony anatomy, and commonly used treatment plans were simple shapes such as squares, rectangles, and diamonds. In this era, treatment was delivered with low conformality and exposed adjacent organs with the same high doses intended for the tumor. Acute and late side effects rates limited the dose that could be safely delivered to tumor and resulting cure rates.

Computed tomography (CT) enabled more modern planning using 3D conformal radiation therapy (3D-CRT). 3D-CRT allows tumor volumes and all organs at risk to be delineated, so that normal tissues can potentially be shielded from high doses of radiation. Thus, acute and late side effects can be reduced while delivering a tailored dose of radiation to the target. Treatment planning systems have also improved, allowing for more complex beam arrangements and the ability to calculate the volume of an organ exposed to different radiation doses and correlate that information with toxicities.

Beyond CT, improvements in volumetric imaging have also led to superior definition of tumor, using metabolic and MRI. Advances in tumor identification and target volume delineation have led to the use of more highly conformal therapies and the application of high-fidelity patient positioning using improved immobilization devices and frequent on-treatment imaging (radiography, CT imaging, or more recently MRI).

Contemporary radiotherapy techniques modulate the intensity profile of radiation within a beam of radiation with the use of multileaf collimators, known as intensity-modulated radiation therapy (IMRT). The use of IMRT allows significantly improved conformality and the ability to deliver higher doses to tumor while maintaining acceptable normal tissue toxicity. However, a potential disadvantage is the exposure of significantly larger volumes of normal tissues to low and intermediate doses.

Particle therapy, including proton therapy, uses the charged nucleus of an atom to deliver therapeutic radiation while taking advantage of reduced total integral radiation exposure to normal tissues. Although photons deliver radiation dose along the entire beam path, proton therapy (and other heavy ions) has an advantage of stopping at a certain depth and not delivering dose past the tumor volume (no exit dose). Proton therapy can be delivered with 3D or intensity modulation (intensity-modulated proton therapy [IMPT]) to allow highly conformal treatment to tumor and low doses to adjacent normal tissues.

Stereotactic radiosurgery represents another modality where target tumors are treated with small margins and a hypofractionated radiation dose schedule given in 1 to 5 treatments. This involves narrow "rifle shot–like" beams delivering ablative doses to the tumor and requires rigorous patient immobilization and highly accurate targeting and treatment delivery. Although significant experience exists using photon-based techniques, proton therapy is increasingly applied using these techniques. Although this technique can deliver potentially curative radiotherapy to well-circumscribed targets, microscopic tumor infiltration in adjacent normal tissues is not treated. Thus, this approach has limited applicability in standard pediatric situations.

Finally, brachytherapy refers to radioactive sources being inserted directly into tumor or tumor bed. This is an alternative method of delivering highly conformal radiation to tumor with a rapid dose falloff. Coverage of infiltrative margins of the tumor can be underdosed using this technique, and its application remains limited to centers with sufficient patient volume and physician experience using this modality.

Trends in Radiation Modality Usage over Time

The use of radiation therapy to treat patients with pediatric cancer has declined over time between the 1970s and 2000s.[5] The tumors with the greatest decline in radiation use are acute lymphoblastic leukemia, non-Hodgkin lymphoma from 57% to 10% to 15%, and retinoblastoma from 30% to 2%, in 1976 and 2008, respectively.[5] Additional large decreases have been seen with central nervous system (CNS) tumors, from 70% to 39%, and neuroblastoma, from 60% to 25%. In a report from the Surveillance, Epidemiology, and End Results of children treated from 1973 to 2008, the overall utilization rate of radiation is 27.3% across all diagnosis, with the lowest being retinoblastoma at 2%, and highest in Wilms tumors at 53%.[5] As previously implied, overall, there is a trend toward an increasing use of highly conformal techniques (**Figs. 1** and **2**). As of 2020, an estimated 100 proton centers will be open or in development around the world with more than one-third located in the United States.[6] The most frequent tumor types treated with proton therapy are CNS tumors and sarcomas.[6]

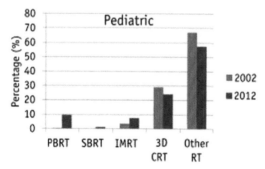

Fig. 1. Pediatric patients receiving either 3D-CRT, 2D radiation therapy/brachytherapy (other radiation therapy [RT]), IMRT, stereotactic body radiation therapy (SBRT), or proton beam radiation therapy (PBRT) in 2002 versus 2012. "Other RT" includes conventional radiation therapy, brachytherapy, and palliative treatment courses. (*From* Waddle MR, Sio TT, Van Houten HK, et al. Photon and Proton Radiation Therapy Utilization in a Population of More Than 100 Million Commercially Insured Patients. International Journal of Radiation Oncology*Biology*Physics. 2017;99(5):1078-1082. https://doi.org/10.1016/j.ijrobp.2017.07.042; with permission.)

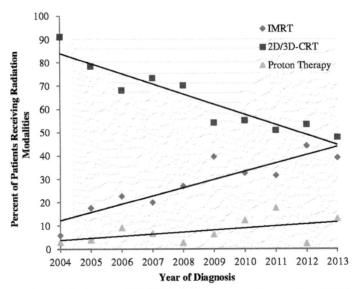

Fig. 2. National trends in the use of 3D-CRT, IMRT, and proton therapy from 2004 to 2013, by year of diagnosis. During this study time period from 2004 to 2013, there was a significant decrease in use of 2D/3D-CRT from 91.2% to 47.8%, with a subsequent increase in IMRT utilization from 5.9% to 39.1% and increase in PT utilization from 2.9% to 13.0%. (*From* Khan AJ, Kann BH, Pan W, Drachtman R, Roberts K, Parikh RR. Underutilization of proton therapy in the treatment of pediatric central nervous system tumors: an analysis of the National Cancer Database. Acta Oncol. 2017;56(8):1122-1125. https://doi.org/10.1080/0284186X.2017. 1287948; with permission.)

BIOLOGICAL EFFECTS OF RADIOTHERAPY

The mechanism of action of radiotherapy on target cells is damage to DNA strands mediated by oxygen-derived free radicals. When photons are absorbed, they impart energy in the medium by recoiling electrons. Direct effects of radiation are caused by the interaction of electrons hitting a DNA strand producing a break. Indirect effects are more common with the recoil electron interacting with a molecule of water producing a hydroxyl radical that will impact the DNA strand and cause a strand break.[7] A single stand break is readily repaired; however, if a double strand break occurs, then mitotic death will ensue[7] (**Fig. 3**).

PATHOGENESIS OF TUMORIGENESIS AND LATE RADIOTHERAPY INJURY

During the postnatal period, cell proliferation and differentiation into different organ systems provides a fertile environment for tumorigenesis. It is during spurts in the rapidly growing tissues and organs that mutations might be readily amplified, particularly during the adolescent phase. During these phases, additional factors driving oncogenesis include the accumulation of toxic and environmental insults that are more frequently expressed in tissues that maintain the largest proliferative potential. This may, in part, explain why blood and lymphoid tissue cancers are the most common in childhood[8,9] (see **Fig. 3**).

The biological impact of ionizing radiation that leads to late radiation toxicity stems from a complex cascade of events within the treated organ parenchyma, vasculature, connective tissue, and the resulting local immune system response.[10–14] The response

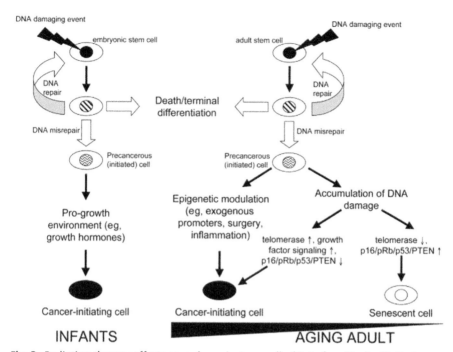

Fig. 3. Radiation therapy effects on embryonic stems cells. (*Data from* Trosko JE. Review paper: cancer stem cells and cancer nonstem cells: from adult stem cells or from reprogramming of differentiated somatic cells. Vet Pathol. 2009;46(2):176-193. https://doi.org/10. 1354/vp.46-2-176 and Mimeault M, Batra SK. Recent insights into the molecular mechanisms involved in aging and the malignant transformation of adult stem/progenitor cells and their therapeutic implications. Ageing Res Rev. 2009;8(2):94-112. https://doi.org/10.1016/j.arr. 2008.12.001.)

of parenchymal cells to radiation is organ specific and can result in cell loss and hypoplasia via direct cytotoxic effects or recruitment of nonproliferative cells into the cell cycle, leading to cell death. This loss of normal physiologic units within the organ can lead to a decrease in organ system function.[10] Radiation exposure can also provoke early differentiation of fibroblasts that lead to collagen deposition.[11] Macrophages are often recruited, leading to delayed radiation fibrosis through the production of transforming growth factor β and/or reactive oxygen species and further downstream effects.[12] Many radiation late effects are observed in the setting of chronic inflammatory changes. In addition, radiation-induced endothelial cell damage in vasculature can lead to leaky vessels, loss of capillaries, and vascular occlusion.[10,15] These effects are usually irreversible and may worsen over time.[13] Fibrogenic pathways are heavily involved in the development of late radiation response, but organ cell depletion and cell loss are also very important. In many cases, though, organ damage and late toxicity are multifactorial and result from numerous damage and repair pathways.[14] The latency, or time to onset of late toxicity, is thought to be inversely related to radiation dose, whereas their progression directly depends on radiation dose.[10]

RADIATION TECHNIQUES TO MITIGATE TOXICITY

Recent advances in radiation delivery may further reduce the risk of acute and late organ dysfunction and toxicity. For tumors within the thoracic cavity (mediastinum, lung, chest wall), organ motion due to breathing is a complicating factor, which historically required larger planning target volumes to be used due to respiratory motion. Techniques such as deep inspiration breath-hold in which radiation delivery only occurs during one phase of breathing allow for less exposure to normal tissues such as the heart and lungs that can be better shielded at end-inspiration. In addition, respiratory motion and positional uncertainty are nullified. Additional options for thoracic and abdominal tumors include abdominal compression, which limits breathing/organ motion. The use of 4D CT imaging, or acquiring treatment planning imaging while monitoring the phases of breathing, provides for more detailed delineation of the tumor and adjacent tissues.

Patient positioning can also help to mitigate treatment toxicity. Examples include prone patient positioning on a belly board to treat abdominal/pelvic targets in order to have the bowel "fall away" from the target. Another technique involves instructing patients to have a full bladder (or using a foley catheter) to maintain consistent bladder filling to push healthy bowel away from the radiation target. As discussed earlier, advanced radiation modalities have also demonstrated improved toxicity profiles for various pediatric tumors. The use of IMRT compared with 2D and 3D techniques has advantages in brain tissue exposure for germinoma and many other brain tumor subtypes.[16] Proton therapy can reduce organ doses and provide an improved toxicity profile for craniospinal irradiation compared with photon therapy due to lack of radiation in the thoracic and abdominal cavities.[17] The use of radiosurgery allows for lower high-dose exposure to normal tissues for pediatric brain tumors compared with IMPT.[18]

IMPACT OF AGE ON RADIATION INJURY

Pediatric cancers are thought to be inherently different from adult malignancies due to the plasticity found during development that normally drives organogenesis and organ development but can also promote cancer formation. Organogenesis and tissue maturation reflect cellular proliferation from a pluripotent stem cell to terminally differentiated cells. There are 3 main developmental periods: infancy/early childhood, late childhood, and puberty. Infancy/early childhood (1–6 years of age) is a time when most tissues are rapidly dividing. Late childhood (6 years old through puberty) is a time when some tissues are dominated by proliferation, others by hypertrophy, and still others by quiescence until hormonal changes begin during puberty. Puberty includes the years after late childhood and before adulthood when there is an acceleration in tissues due to hormonal surges.[8,19]

During these time periods the organ systems can be segregated into 5 categories typified by different patterns/rates of growth (hematologic, lymphoid tissue, CNS, musculoskeletal, and gonadal germ cells) (see **Fig. 3**).[19,20]

1. Early in development the hematologic system (blood cell formation and bone marrow) continues to expand, beginning in utero through birth and peaking around 5 to 10 years of age.
2. Lymphoid tissues expand in multiple organs/compartments (spleen, lymph nodes, thymus, appendix, bone marrow, and Peyer patches) with growth peaking between the ages of 6 and 12 years.
3. The CNS begins its growth prenatally, but most active myelination and synaptogenesis occurs between the ages of 1 and 5 years, and continues for the next 20 or 30 years.
4. Musculoskeletal growth is bimodal with the first 5 years demonstrating rapid growth and the second sequenced growth spurt occurring during puberty. Skeletal

muscle has some capacity for regenerative growth; for example, smooth muscle is highly regenerative, whereas cardiac cells undergo hypertrophic rather than regenerative growth. Similar tissues with bimodal growth are the integumentary and gastrointestinal systems.

5. Gonadal germ cells are quiescent at birth and through the first 10 years of age but become active due to hormonal stimulation that occurs during puberty, typically at 12 to 18 years of age.[8,19,20]

Importantly, the phases of growth in normal tissues and organ systems coincide with the peak years of malignancies derived from these tissues. Rapidly dividing cells are preferentially damaged from ionizing radiation, which is important for radiation therapy efficacy, but during different developmental phases, this may also lead to increased risk of damage to these organ systems[8,9,21] (**Fig. 4**).

COMMON ORGAN SYSTEMS EFFECTED
Central Nervous System

Radiotherapy can cause significant late effects in the brain and other cranial substructures. The prevalence of late effects measured in the St Jude Lifetime Cohort Study was measured in patients who survived 10 years or more from diagnosis.[4,22] The effects of surgery and chemotherapy can be additive or synergistic with radiotherapy.[22] In several investigations, the prevalence of neurocognitive impairment was seen in 46.1% of patients receiving antimetabolite chemotherapy, 56.1% of patients treated with cranial radiation, and 63% of patients who underwent neurosurgical intervention.[22–24] Radiotherapy factors most associated with neurocognitive decline are volume of brain irradiated, dose delivered, and age of the patient. Radiation doses to

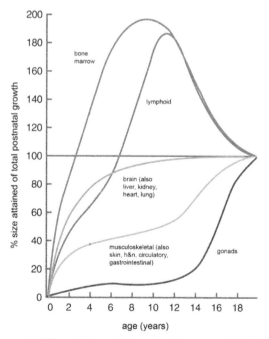

Fig. 4. Growth curves of different tissues during development. (*Modified from* Tanner JM. The Assessment of Growth and Development in Children. Arch Dis Child. 1952;27(131):10-33; with permission.)

the whole brain associated with cognitive decline are as low as 18 Gy[23,24] (**Table 1**), although patients treated to this dose also receive chemotherapy. In its absence, cognitive decline is observed after higher dose, usually greater than 25 to 35 Gy. Necrosis of brain tissue is rare less than doses of 50 Gy.[24]

Eye and Ear

In previous reports, the prevalence of developing cataracts was 37.5% for patients receiving busulfan, 17% after corticosteroids, and 27.3% after radiation exposing the lens.[22] Threshold radiation doses for cataractogenesis are generally considered to be greater than 2 Gy, and smaller individual fraction sizes are less damaging. The risk of clinically significant cataracts is associated with higher doses but may take years to manifest.[25,26] Glaucoma developed in 1.2% of patients at 10 years after ocular radiation therapy.[22,27] The prevalence of reduced visual acuity was 7.2%.[22,27] Radiation doses greater than 40 to 45 Gy to the retina and optic nerve are associated with an increased risk for loss of visual acuity.[28] The prevalence of hearing loss was 67.1% with cisplatin/carboplatin chemotherapy and 64.3% with radiation doses greater than 30 Gy with chemotherapy and greater than 45 Gy with radiation therapy alone[22,29] (**Fig. 5**).

Endocrine System

Radiotherapy to the endocrine system may lead to numerous downstream effects compromising general and reproductive health. Various hormonal deficiencies can develop following radiotherapy to the hypothalamic/pituitary axis (HPA), including deficiencies of growth hormone (GH), adrenocorticotropic hormone (ACTH), luteinizing hormone (LH), follicle-stimulating hormone (FSH), and thyroid-stimulating hormone (TSH).[30] Radiation doses greater than 60 Gy are associated with high rates of panhypopituitarism.[30,31] GH levels are most sensitive to the effects of radiotherapy; the prevalence of GH deficiency following radiotherapy at doses greater than 18 Gy to the HPA is 51%.[22,32] For radiation doses greater than 40 Gy, the prevalence of ACTH deficiency is 19.5%, FSH deficiency 30.8%, LH deficiency 26.2%, and TSH deficiency 25%[22,30,32] (see **Table 1**). In a recent analysis, Jalali and colleagues[33,34] found that patients receiving greater than or equal to 27 Gy to any portion of the HPA had a 4-fold increase in endocrinopathy risk. In addition, 5 years postradiation, 78.8%, 42.8%, 18.2%, and 14% had GH, thyroid hormone, ACTH, and gonadotropin deficiency after greater than or equal to 40 Gy mean dose to the pituitary and hypothalamus.[35]

The prevalence of being overweight or obese are quite high after receiving radiation to the HPA, 29.4% and 48.3%, respectively.[22] The prevalence of diabetes mellitus is 7.8%[22] as a component or result of a metabolic syndrome. The prevalence of primary ovarian failure with alkylating agents is 10.5% and is several fold higher with radiation to the female reproductive system with a prevalence of 33.2%.[22,30] The ovaries are actually more sensitive in older children due to the declining number of oocytes, with doses of 5 to 10 Gy impairing fertility in adolescents but younger children retaining fertility with even higher doses.[33,36] The rate of male germ cell failure is 31.7% with alkylating agents and 45.3% with radiation to the male reproductive system,[22] even with doses as low as 5 Gy.[37] The prevalence of low testosterone is 11.7% with alkylating agents and 27% with radiation to the male reproductive system[22] although with higher doses of 20 to 40 Gy are high risk for developing compromised hormone synthesis (see **Fig. 5**).

Table 1
Summary of late-effect evidence for each disease site

Organ System	Dose Greater Than Which Risks Increase	Toxicities	Other Risk Factors
Cardiovascular	>10 Gy (low doses to large volumes of the heart increase the risk) >30 Gy	Cardiac dysfunction Cardiomyopathy (>20 Gy with chemotherapy) Myocardial infarction/conduction abnormality/valve damage	Anthracycline exposure Diabetes Hypertension Obesity Smoking
Central nervous system	>18 Gy >60 Gy >50 Gy	Cognitive deficits Large-vessel stroke Myelitis	Young age at time of diagnosis High doses of methotrexate
Neuroendocrine and special senses	>60 Gy >18 Gy >20 Gy >40 Gy >50 Gy >10–18 Gy >45 Gy	Panhypopituitarism GH deficiency Precocious puberty LH or FSH deficiency TSH deficiency ACTH deficiency Hyperprolactinemia Optic nerve Retina conjunctivae Cataracts Ototoxicity	Diabetes insipidus Hearing loss Late orbital complications
Musculoskeletal Growth and development	>20 Gy >18–20 Gy >40–50 Gy	Muscular hypoplasia Spinal growth abnormality Osteonecrosis or fracture	Larger volumes irradiated
Pulmonary	>12–14 Gy	Pulmonary fibrosis Decrease in pulmonary function tests	Chemotherapy (bleomycin, CCNU, methotrexate)
Digestive system	>40–50 Gy >30 Gy	Enteritis Fibrosis of bowel Liver failure	Doxorubicin or actinomycin-D

(continued on next page)

Table 1
(continued)

Organ System	Dose Greater Than Which Risks Increase	Toxicities	Other Risk Factors
Genitourinary	>20 Gy or >15 Gy with chemotherapy	Kidney dysfunction (decrease in GFR)	Platinum-based chemotherapy, ifosfamide, methotrexate

Abbreviation: ACTH, adrenocorticotropic hormone; CCNU, lomustine; FSH, follicle-stimulating hormone; GFR, glomerular filtration rate; GH, growth hormone; LH, luteinizing hormone; TSH, thyroid-stimulating hormone

Modified from Palmer et al Pediatric Blood and Cancer 2020.

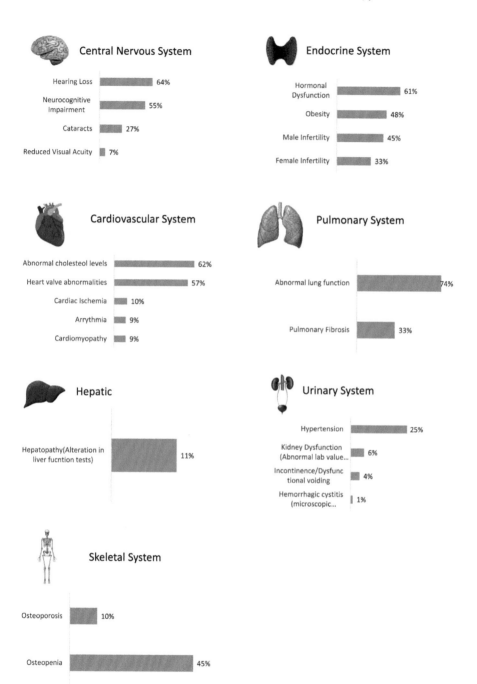

Fig. 5. Frequency of late radiation-related side effects based on organ system. (*Data from* Hudson MM, Ness KK, Gurney JG, et al. Clinical Ascertainment of Health Outcomes among Adults Treated for Childhood Cancer: A Report from the St. Jude Lifetime Cohort Study. JAMA. 2013;309(22):2371-2381. https://doi.org/10.1001/jama.2013.6296.)

Cardiovascular System

Radiotherapy exposure can lead to the injury of various substructures of the heart. An important contributing factor to these cardiovascular late effects is anthracycline/anthraquinone exposure.[22,38–40] Radiation doses greater than 30 Gy are clearly associated with cardiomyopathy risk, but when radiation is combined with chemotherapy (anthracycline/anthraquinone) this toxicity already occurs with doses of 20 Gy.[39–41] A decrease in left ventricular systolic function is noted in 6.6% of patients exposed to anthracycline/anthraquinone, whereas radiation alone is associated with a 6% prevalence.[22,42] Radiation doses as low as 5 to 10 Gy to large volumes of the heart may lead to cardiac dysfunction.[39,43] Valvular heart disease on echocardiogram is noted in 29% of childhood cancer survivors and 56.7% of patients with a history of radiation to the heart. Arrhythmias noted on electrocardiogram are observed in 7.4% of childhood cancer survivors with a 6.2% risk after exposure to anthracycline/anthraquinones and a slightly higher prevalence of 9.2% with radiation.[22,40] The prevalence of any conduction disorder was 14.2% in childhood cancer survivors; anthracycline/anthraquinones are specifically associated with a prevalence of 14.3%, and radiation exposure to the heart had a slightly lower prevalence of 13%.[22] The risk of ischemic events was 5.7% of childhood cancer survivors with an increased prevalence of 9.4% for those with radiation to the heart.[22,44] Dyslipidemia is seen in approximately 50% of childhood cancer survivors overall, but cisplatin/carboplatin exposure connotes a slightly higher prevalence of 53.9%, and radiation to the HPA has a prevalence of 61.8%[22,38,45] (see **Fig. 5**).

Pulmonary System

Radiation therapy to the lung can lead to late effects that can manifest clinically and be quantified with pulmonary function testing (PFT) and chest imaging (chest radiograph, CT). Radiation doses greater than 12 to 14 Gy to the whole lung are associated with lung dysfunction and fibrosis[46] (see **Table 1**). Contributing factors to the development of late pulmonary dysfunction are chemotherapy and surgery.[11,22] The prevalence of abnormal PFTs is 75% for patients after exposure to busulfan, 68.8% after exposure to carmustine/lomustine, and 73.3% to bleomycin.[22,47] The prevalence of abnormal PFTs after lung radiotherapy is 74.4% and after thoracotomy 53.2%.[22,48] The prevalence of pulmonary fibrosis on chest imaging is 25% for busulfan, camustine/lomustine, and thoracotomy and 22.6% for bleomycin.[22] The prevalence of pulmonary fibrosis is slightly higher after radiation to the lung at 33.4%[22,46] (see **Fig. 5**).

Hepatic/Gastrointestinal

The liver is a resilient organ that can continue to function well when large components undergo surgical resection or damage. The prevalence of hepatopathy as measured by serum liver function tests is 13.1% with mercaptopurine/thioguanine and slightly less at 11.4% with radiation (>30 Gy) to the liver[22,49] (see **Fig. 5**). Radiation damage to the bowel leading to enteritis or bowel fibrosis/narrowing has been demonstrated with radiation doses greater than 40 to 50 Gy[48,50] (see **Table 1**).

Urinary System

Radiation exposure to the urinary system (kidneys, ureters, and bladder) can lead to late effects that affect urinary function and blood pressure. Contributing factors include chemotherapy and surgery.[22,49] The prevalence of hypertension for patients receiving chemotherapy was 8.4% with ifosfamide, 15.7% for cisplatin/carboplatin, and 22.5% for methotrexate.[22] Radiotherapy alone portends a prevalence of 24.7%, and surgery (nephrectomy) has the highest prevalence of hypertension with 28%.[22] Kidney dysfunction can occur with radiation doses greater than 20 Gy or greater than 15 Gy with chemotherapy[48,51,52] (see **Table 1**). The prevalence of kidney dysfunction assessed by serum blood testing (complete metabolic panel) or urinalysis was 11.2% for ifosfamide, 15.7% for cisplatin/carboplatin, and 3.6% for methotrexate.[22,53] Radiation exposure to the kidney alone has a prevalence of kidney dysfunction that is relatively low at 6.4% when compared with chemotherapy and nephrectomy without radiation exposure at 17%.[22] The use of IMRT carries a slightly lower risk of renal dysfunction,[54] with mean kidney doses of 15 Gy to the affected side and 11 Gy to the unaffected side.[54] The prevalence of hemorrhagic cystitis was rare with 0.6% for cyclophosphamide/ifosfamide and 1.0% after radiation alone to the bladder. The prevalence of urinary incontinence was 4.3% with radiation to the bladder and 4.0% with pelvic/spinal surgery[22,49] (see **Fig. 5**).

Skeletal System

Radiation therapy to the skeletal system can lead to impairment of bone growth/development and a diminution of bone integrity. The latter is thought to occur based on altered bone remodeling.[55] Other factors that may affect bone strength and growth are methotrexate exposure and corticosteroids.[20,56] Radiation doses greater than 20 Gy are clearly associated with skeletal hypoplasia. Radiation doses greater than 40 to 50 Gy are associated with osteonecrosis and/or fracture[56] (see **Table 1**). The prevalence of osteopenia in patients who received methotrexate chemotherapy is 37.5%, corticosteroids is 36.6%, and radiation therapy alone to the HPA is 41.5%.[22] Prevalence of osteoporosis was lower, with methotrexate connoting a risk of 8.1%, corticosteroids 8.4%, and radiation to the HPA 12.8%[22,56] (see **Fig. 5**).

SUMMARY

Radiotherapy and chemotherapy can result in clinically significant long-term physical, intellectual, emotional, social, and occupational sequelae for survivors of childhood cancer. Although these treatment modalities have dramatically increased survival rates for most pediatric malignancies, it is essential to balance therapeutic benefits against potential harms in therapy selection.

The physiologic mechanisms of damage caused by radiotherapy and chemotherapy to normal tissues are increasingly understood. However, the variation in response to therapy among individuals to the same therapeutic exposures remains an evolving science. Although many children and adolescents are treated with the same radiotherapy doses, fields, and volumes, significant variability is observed in the proportions that develop toxicities. Cytotoxic chemotherapy can enhance radiotherapy effects. In contrast, our understanding of host-related factors, such as genetic susceptibility including inherited differences in radiation sensitivity to normal tissue or genes of xenobiotic metabolism, nucleotide provision, or DNA repair, remain limited. In addition, morbidity and premature mortality have been examined with respect to treatment exposures but not yet in association with other factors such as diet, sun exposure, alcohol, and tobacco use that are significant confounders related to major health problems in an aging population. Importantly, new patterns of late morbidity and mortality may emerge as survivors continue to age. It is only through continued diligent study that such patterns will emerge that may lead to improvements in treatment delivery and prevention of late morbidity.

DISCLOSURE

J.D. Palmer declares grant funding from Varian Medical Systems and speaking fees from Depuy Synthes (outside the submitted work).

REFERENCES

1. Jemal A, Siegel R, Xu J, et al. Cancer statistics, 2010. CA Cancer J Clin 2010; 60(5):277–300.
2. Howlader N, Noone AM, Krapcho M, et al, editors. SEER Cancer Statistics Review, 1975-2016, National Cancer Institute. Bethesda (MD). Available at: https://seer.cancer.gov/csr/1975_2016/. Based on November 2018 SEER data submission, posted to the SEER web site, April 2019. Accessed November 24, 2019.
3. Armstrong GT, Liu Q, Yasui Y, et al. Late mortality among 5-year survivors of childhood cancer: a summary from the childhood cancer survivor study. J Clin Oncol 2009;27(14):2328–38.
4. Armstrong GT, Kawashima T, Leisenring W, et al. Aging and risk of severe, disabling, life-threatening, and fatal events in the childhood cancer survivor study. J Clin Oncol 2014;32(12):1218–27.
5. Jairam V, Roberts KB, Yu JB. Historical Trends in the use of radiation for pediatric cancers: 1973–2008. Int J Radiat Oncol Biol Phys 2013;85(3):e151–5.
6. Journy N, Indelicato DJ, Withrow DR, et al. Patterns of proton therapy use in pediatric cancer management in 2016: An international survey. Radiother Oncol 2019;132:155–61.
7. Hall EJ. Radiation biology for pediatric radiologists. Pediatr Radiol 2009;39(Suppl 1):S57–64.
8. Rubin P, Williams JP, Devesa SS, et al. Cancer genesis across the age spectrum: associations with tissue development, maintenance, and senescence. Semin Radiat Oncol 2010;20(1):3–11.
9. Paulino AC, Constine LS, Rubin P, et al. Normal tissue development, homeostasis, senescence, and the sensitivity to radiation injury across the age spectrum. Semin Radiat Oncol 2010;20(1):12–20.
10. Dörr W. Radiobiology of tissue reactions. Ann ICRP 2015;44(1_suppl):58–68.
11. Rodemann HP, Bamberg M. Cellular basis of radiation-induced fibrosis. Radiother Oncol 1995;35(2):83–90.
12. Hakenjos L, Bamberg M, Rodemann HP. TGF-beta1-mediated alterations of rat lung fibroblast differentiation resulting in the radiation-induced fibrotic phenotype. Int J Radiat Biol 2000;76(4):503–9.
13. Zhao W, Robbins MEC. Inflammation and chronic oxidative stress in radiation-induced late normal tissue injury: therapeutic implications. Curr Med Chem 2009;16(2):130–43.
14. Bentzen SM. Preventing or reducing late side effects of radiation therapy: radiobiology meets molecular pathology. Nat Rev Cancer 2006;6(9):702–13.
15. Constine L, Tarbell N, Halperin E. Pediatric radiation Oncology. 6th edition. Wolters Kluwer; 2016.
16. Dosimetric advantage of intensity-modulated radiotherapy for whole ventricles in the treatment of localized intracranial germinoma. - PubMed - NCBI. Available at: https://www.ncbi.nlm.nih.gov/pubmed/21640515. Accessed November 23, 2019.
17. A review of dosimetric and toxicity modeling of proton versus photon craniospinal irradiation for pediatrics medulloblastoma: Acta Oncologica: Vol 56, No 8.

Available at: https://www.tandfonline.com/doi/full/10.1080/0284186X.2017. 1324207. Accessed November 23, 2019.

18. Radiation Therapy for Pediatric Brain Tumors using Robotic Radiation Delivery System and Intensity Modulated Proton Therapy. - PubMed - NCBI. Available at: https://www.ncbi.nlm.nih.gov/pubmed/31542454. Accessed November 23, 2019.
19. Tanner JM. The Assessment of Growth and Development in Children. Arch Dis Child 1952;27(131):10–33.
20. Tanner JM. Growth and Maturation during Adolescence. Nutr Rev 1981;39(2): 43–55.
21. Krasin MJ, Constine LS, Friedman DL, et al. Radiation-related treatment effects across the age spectrum: differences and similarities or what the old and young can learn from each other. Semin Radiat Oncol 2010;20(1):21–9.
22. Hudson MM, Ness KK, Gurney JG, et al. Clinical ascertainment of health outcomes among adults treated for childhood cancer: a report from the St. Jude Lifetime Cohort Study. JAMA 2013;309(22):2371–81.
23. Kadan-Lottick NS, Zeltzer LK, Liu Q, et al. Neurocognitive functioning in adult survivors of childhood non-central nervous system cancers. J Natl Cancer Inst 2010; 102(12):881–93.
24. Ellenberg L, Liu Q, Gioia G, et al. Neurocognitive status in long-term survivors of childhood CNS malignancies: a report from the Childhood Cancer Survivor Study. Neuropsychology 2009;23(6):705–17.
25. Chodick G, Sigurdson AJ, Kleinerman RA, et al. The risk of cataract among survivors of childhood and adolescent cancer: a report from the childhood cancer survivor study. Radiat Res 2016;185(4):366–74.
26. de Blank PMK, Fisher MJ, Lu L, et al. Impact of vision loss among survivors of childhood central nervous system astroglial tumors. Cancer 2016;122(5):730–9.
27. Whelan KF, Stratton K, Kawashima T, et al. Ocular late effects in childhood and adolescent cancer survivors: A report from the childhood cancer survivor study. Pediatr Blood Cancer 2010;54(1):103–9.
28. Bhandare N, Jackson A, Eisbruch A, et al. Radiation therapy and hearing loss. Int J Radiat Oncol Biol Phys 2010;76(3 Suppl):S50–7.
29. Constine LS, Woolf PD, Cann D, et al. Hypothalamic-pituitary dysfunction after radiation for brain tumors. N Engl J Med 1993;328(2):87–94.
30. Darzy KH, Shalet SM. Hypopituitarism following radiotherapy. Pituitary 2009; 12(1):40–50.
31. Krull KR, Li C, Phillips NS, et al. Growth hormone deficiency and neurocognitive function in adult survivors of childhood acute lymphoblastic leukemia. Cancer 2019. https://doi.org/10.1002/cncr.31975.
32. Fahrner B, Prosch H, Minkov M, et al. Long-term outcome of hypothalamic pituitary tumors in Langerhans cell histiocytosis. Pediatr Blood Cancer 2012;58(4): 606–10.
33. Nandagopal R, Laverdière C, Mulrooney D, et al. Endocrine late effects of childhood cancer therapy: a report from the Children's Oncology Group. Horm Res 2008;69(2):65–74.
34. Jalali R, Maitre M, Gupta T, et al. Dose-Constraint Model to Predict Neuroendocrine Dysfunction in Young Patients With Brain Tumors: Data From a Prospective Study. Practical Radiation Oncology 2019;9(4):e362–71.
35. Vatner RE, Niemierko A, Misra M, et al. Endocrine deficiency as a function of radiation dose to the hypothalamus and pituitary in pediatric and young adult patients with brain tumors. J Clin Oncol 2018;36(28):2854–62.

36. Sklar CA. Growth and neuroendocrine dysfunction following therapy for childhood cancer. Pediatr Clin North Am 1997;44(2):489–503.

37. Kazlauskaite R, Evans AT, Villabona CV, et al. Corticotropin tests for hypothalamic-pituitary- adrenal insufficiency: a metaanalysis. J Clin Endocrinol Metab 2008;93(11):4245–53.

38. Armstrong GT, Oeffinger KC, Chen Y, et al. Modifiable risk factors and major cardiac events among adult survivors of childhood cancer. J Clin Oncol 2013;31(29):3673–80.

39. Bates JE, Howell RM, Liu Q, et al. Therapy-related cardiac risk in childhood cancer survivors: an analysis of the childhood cancer survivor study. J Clin Oncol 2019;JCO1801764. https://doi.org/10.1200/JCO.18.01764.

40. Hahn E, Jiang H, Ng A, et al. Late cardiac toxicity after mediastinal radiation therapy for hodgkin lymphoma: contributions of coronary artery and whole heart dose-volume variables to risk prediction. Int J Radiat Oncol Biol Phys 2017;98(5):1116–23.

41. van der Pal HJ, van Dalen EC, van Delden E, et al. High risk of symptomatic cardiac events in childhood cancer survivors. J Clin Oncol 2012;30(13):1429–37.

42. Mansouri I, Allodji RS, Hill C, et al. The role of irradiated heart and left ventricular volumes in heart failure occurrence after childhood cancer. Eur J Heart Fail 2018. https://doi.org/10.1002/ejhf.1376.

43. Haddy N, Diallo S, El-Fayech C, et al. Cardiac diseases following childhood cancer treatment: cohort study. Circulation 2016;133(1):31–8.

44. Chow EJ, Chen Y, Hudson MM, et al. Prediction of ischemic heart disease and stroke in survivors of childhood cancer. J Clin Oncol 2018;36(1):44–52.

45. Armenian SH, Hudson MM, Mulder RL, et al. Recommendations for cardiomyopathy surveillance for survivors of childhood cancer: a report from the International Late Effects of Childhood Cancer Guideline Harmonization Group. Lancet Oncol 2015;16(3):e123–36.

46. McDonald S, Rubin P, Maasilta P. Response of normal lung to irradiation. Tolerance doses/tolerance volumes in pulmonary radiation syndromes. Front Radiat Ther Oncol 1989;23:255–76 [discussion: 299–301].

47. Josephson MB, Goldfarb SB. Pulmonary complications of childhood cancers. Expert Rev Respir Med 2014;8(5):561–71.

48. Skou A-S, Glosli H, Jahnukainen K, et al. Renal, gastrointestinal, and hepatic late effects in survivors of childhood acute myeloid leukemia treated with chemotherapy only–a NOPHO-AML study. Pediatr Blood Cancer 2014;61(9):1638–43.

49. Bhakta N, Liu Q, Ness KK, et al. The cumulative burden of surviving childhood cancer: an initial report from the st. jude lifetime cohort study. Lancet 2017;390(10112):2569–82.

50. Goldsby R, Chen Y, Raber S, et al. Survivors of childhood cancer have increased risk of gastrointestinal complications later in life. Gastroenterology 2011;140(5):1464–71.e1.

51. Mitus A, Tefft M, Fellers FX. Long-term follow-up of renal functions of 108 children who underwent nephrectomy for malignant disease. Pediatrics 1969;44(6):912–21.

52. Ritchey ML, Green DM, Thomas PR, et al. Renal failure in Wilms' tumor patients: a report from the National Wilms' Tumor Study Group. Med Pediatr Oncol 1996;26(2):75–80.

53. Dawson LA, Kavanagh BD, Paulino AC, et al. Radiation-associated kidney injury. Int J Radiat Oncol Biol Phys 2010;76(3 Suppl):S108–15.

54. Beckham TH, Casey DL, LaQuaglia MP, et al. Renal function outcomes of high-risk neuroblastoma patients undergoing radiation therapy. Int J Radiat Oncol Biol Phys 2017;99(2):486–93.

55. Dhakal S, Chen J, McCance S, et al. Bone density changes after radiation for extremity sarcomas: exploring the etiology of pathologic fractures. Int J Radiat Oncol Biol Phys 2011;80(4):1158–63. Available at: https://www.ncbi.nlm.nih.gov/pubmed/?term=Dhakal+S%3B+Chen+J%3B+McCance+S%3B+Rosier+R%3B+O%27Keefe+R%3B+Constine+LS.+%22Bone+density+changes+after+radiation+for+extremity+sarcomas%3A+exploring+the+etiology+of+pathologic+fractures.%22+International+journal+of+r. Accessed November 24, 2019.

56. Fletcher BD. Effects of pediatric cancer therapy on the musculoskeletal system. Pediatr Radiol 1997;27(8):623–36.

The Critical Role of Clinical Practice Guidelines and Indicators in High-Quality Survivorship After Childhood Cancer

Renée L. Mulder, PhD[a],*, Rebecca J. van Kalsbeek, MD[a],
Melissa M. Hudson, MD[b,c], Roderick Skinner, MB ChB, PhD[d],
Leontien C.M. Kremer, MD, PhD[a]

KEYWORDS

- Childhood cancer survivors • Quality of care • Clinical practice guidelines
- Quality indicators

KEY POINTS

- Evidence-based medicine integrates research evidence with clinical expertise, patient values, and costs within clinical decision making.
- Guidelines for the follow-up care of survivors of childhood cancer are harmonized worldwide by the International Late Effects of Childhood Cancer Guideline Harmonization Group (www.ighg.org).
- Clinical practice guidelines facilitate translation of research evidence into clinical practice.
- Quality of care is evaluated and promoted with valid quality indicators that assess processes, structures, and/or outcomes of care.

INTRODUCTION

Continuing advances in the treatment of childhood cancer during the last 50 years have contributed to greatly increased survival rates.[1,2] However, improvement in prognosis has been accompanied by the occurrence of late, treatment-related complications.[3,4] Consequently, the number of childhood cancer survivors at high risk for premature morbidity and mortality is growing.

[a] Princess Máxima Center for Pediatric Oncology, Utrecht, The Netherlands; [b] Department of Epidemiology and Cancer Control, St. Jude Children's Research Hospital, Memphis, TN, USA; [c] Department of Oncology, St. Jude Children's Research Hospital, Memphis, TN, USA; [d] Department of Paediatric and Adolescent Haematology/Oncology, Great North Children's Hospital, Newcastle University Centre for Cancer, Newcastle upon Tyne, UK
* Corresponding author. Princess Máxima Center for Pediatric Oncology, Heidelberglaan 25, Utrecht 3584 CS, The Netherlands.
E-mail address: R.L.Mulder@prinsesmaximacentrum.nl

Pediatr Clin N Am 67 (2020) 1069–1081
https://doi.org/10.1016/j.pcl.2020.07.003
0031-3955/20/© 2020 Elsevier Inc. All rights reserved.

Late adverse effects of cancer treatment contribute to an increased incidence of chronic diseases in adult survivors of childhood cancer and may ultimately reduce life expectancy.[5]

Long-term follow-up care is important to facilitate early detection of late effects and timely initiation of interventions to preserve and improve health. Childhood cancer survivors and health care providers need guidance to increase awareness and proactive surveillance of cancer-related and treatment-related health risks to initiate timely intervention. Moreover, those caring for childhood cancer survivors need resources to address the emerging needs of their patients at risk for therapy-related late complications. To provide high-quality care for childhood cancer survivors and optimize their quality of life and life expectancy, clinicians must stay informed about this field and its developments, including data generated by a rapidly expanding area of research. Keeping up, however, is challenging because the number of survivorship studies has increased substantially in recent decades, and quadrupled since 1996.[6] These data underscore the need for more reliable and relevant information to translate this information into evidence-based clinical practice guidelines (CPGs). The steps required to achieve this include synthesizing evidence into evidence summaries and systematic reviews, developing clinical policy from evidence into evidence-based CPGs, disseminating and implementing CPGs, and evaluating their impact on quality of care and survivor health outcomes. These elements form the cornerstones of evidence-based medicine (EBM), as shown in the quality of care cycle (**Fig. 1**).

EVIDENCE-BASED MEDICINE

The term "evidence-based medicine" was introduced by the EBM Working Group in 1992. They defined EBM as "the process of integrating clinical expertise with the best research evidence to make high-quality decisions about the care of individual patients."[7] A clinical decision based on the EBM principles combines high-quality clinical research with clinical expertise, patient values (eg, preferences and expectations), and social considerations (eg, cost).[8,9] The introduction of EBM has informed clinical decision-making in health care by clarifying the quality of the evidence available and knowledge gaps related to specific clinical topics.

Cochrane Collaboration

In 1993 the Cochrane Collaboration was founded in response to the introduction of EBM. The mission of the Cochrane Collaboration is to improve the availability of the best evidence in health care by facilitating the preparation and maintenance of systematic reviews. Cochrane systematic reviews help clinicians evaluate all of the evidence concerning a particular clinical problem using standardized methodology for searching and appraising the literature and for reporting the results.[10] The Cochrane Collaboration, which represents the largest provider of systematic reviews for health care, has produced approximately 6000 systematic reviews available in the Cochrane Library. Cochrane Childhood Cancer has been registered within the Cochrane Collaboration since 2006 (www.ccg.cochrane.org). The aim of Cochrane Childhood Cancer is to perform and sustain systematic reviews about interventions and diagnosis in childhood and young adult patients with cancer and survivors with respect to prevention, treatment, supportive care, psychosocial care, palliative and terminal care, nursing care, and late adverse effects. Systematic reviews form the basis of evidence-based CPGs.

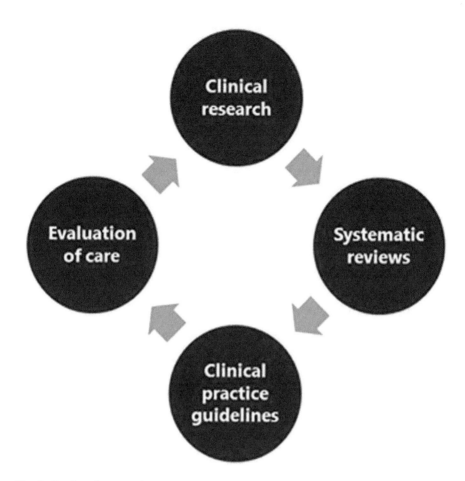

Fig. 1. Quality of care cycle.

EVIDENCE-BASED CLINICAL PRACTICE GUIDELINES

Translation of evidence into clinical practice is essential to deliver high-quality clinical care. Guidelines can facilitate bridging the gap between research and clinical practice. CPGs are increasingly used to assist clinical and health care policy decision-making.[11] As defined by the US Institute of Medicine, CPGs are "statements that include recommendations intended to optimize patient care that are informed by a systematic review of evidence and an assessment of the benefits and harms of alternative care options."[12] CPGs help the practitioner provide clinical care based on the best available evidence.

CPGs are seen as powerful tools to improve quality of care. Their main aim is to improve health care processes and health outcomes. Guidelines recommending proven effective interventions and discouraging ineffective ones may reduce morbidity and mortality. In many fields of medicine, care that is consistent with evidence-based recommendations has led to improved patient outcomes and more efficient care delivery.[11,13–18] Guidelines facilitate uniform care, thereby reducing variability in daily health care practice. They can also contribute to the reduction of inconsistencies in health care decisions between physicians, and promote effective care, communication, and collaboration among health care professionals, and among health care professionals and patients.[11] Finally, CPGs can contribute to reduced health care costs by standardizing care, increasing the efficiency of care provision, and reducing unnecessary or inefficient components of health care. CPGs can decrease expenses for hospitalization, drug prescriptions, surgery, and other procedures.[11]

Before the wider implementation of CPGs, clinical practice was usually guided by nonsystematic observations based on clinical experience. Systematic development of CPGs within a well-defined program started in the late 1970s, with these first efforts featuring consensus-based recommendations. The US National Institutes of Health initiated the development of "consensus statements" by convening consensus conferences.[19] During the 1980s, several organizations outside the United States adopted this program to develop their national and regional consensus statements and standards for good medical care. Since the introduction of the principles of EBM in the 1990s, the method of evidence-based guideline development has become the international standard in which the best available evidence, clinical judgments, and patients' perspectives are integrated.[12,14]

CHILDHOOD CANCER SURVIVORSHIP CARE GUIDELINES

Over recent decades several North American and European groups have developed evidence-based CPGs for long-term follow-up of childhood cancer survivors.[20–23] The main goal of these CPGs is to facilitate opportunities for early detection and timely intervention to treat or prevent late effects. In addition, these survivorship guidelines highlight surveillance tests that may be unnecessary or inadvisable because of the potential for overdiagnosis, psychological distress, or lack of availability of appropriate interventions.[24]

Despite all efforts, the recommendations between existing survivorship guidelines differ, sometimes greatly, in terms of risk groups, and surveillance modalities and intervals. This may have resulted from differences in methodologies used for guideline development, and diversity in clinical expertise and cultural variation. To combine international expertise, reduce duplication of work, and further improve survivorship care, a worldwide collaboration was initiated in 2010 to harmonize the existing CPGs for long-term follow-up of survivors of childhood and young adult cancer: the International Late Effects of Childhood Cancer Guideline Harmonization Group (IGHG; www.ighg.org).[25] Its main goal is to establish a common vision and integrated strategy for the surveillance of late effects in childhood and young adult cancer survivors worldwide. The IGHG focuses on harmonizing surveillance of the more highly prevalent persistent and late-onset adverse effects experienced by childhood cancer survivors and provides recommendations regarding which patients need surveillance, what surveillance modalities should be used, when surveillance should be initiated, at what frequency surveillance should be performed, and what should be done when abnormalities are identified. The IGHG is a multidisciplinary collaboration that includes late effects experts in pediatric and radiation oncology, pediatric and medical subspecialties, primary care, nursing, and patient advocates. In addition, the effort involves individuals with formal training in evidence-based guideline development. The recommendations are developed to permit implementation in a variety of different health care and resource settings.

So far, the IGHG has developed guidelines related to surveillance for subsequent breast cancer,[26] cardiomyopathy,[27] premature ovarian insufficiency,[28] male gonadotoxicity,[29] subsequent thyroid cancer,[30] ototoxicity, and obsteric care.[31,55] In addition, many guidelines are currently under development (**Box 1**).

Evidence-Based Methods International Late Effects of Childhood Cancer Guideline Harmonization Group Guidelines

The IGHG guidelines are developed following consideration of the available evidence, benefits and harms of the particular surveillance intervention, and knowledge and expertise of health care professionals and patients. Guideline development involves three phases: (1) the preparation phase, (2) the development phase, and (3) the finalization phase.

For the preparation phase a guideline panel is convened and the scope of the guideline defined. Diversity is an essential feature of a guideline panel. Its exact composition should be tailored to the guideline topic and reflect the range of stakeholders involved.

The development phase consists of five steps:

1. Evaluation of concordant and discordant guideline areas among recommendations in existing survivorship guidelines.
2. Formulation of clinical questions in the PICO format (participants, interventions, control group, and outcome). The questions should be clear, focused, and closely define the boundaries of the topic. They serve as a starting point for the systematic literature search that aims to identify all the available evidence.
3. Identification of available evidence by systematic literature searches based on predefined inclusion and exclusion criteria.
4. Summarization of the evidence using standardized data-extraction forms including the methodologic quality of the included evidence. For each clinical question a

---

Box 1
Overview of clinical practice guidelines of the International Guideline Harmonization Group that are currently available and in progress

Available IGHG guidelines
  Breast cancer surveillance[26]
  Cardiomyopathy surveillance[27]
  Premature ovarian insufficiency surveillance[28]
  Male gonadotoxicity surveillance[29]
  Thyroid cancer surveillance[30]
  Ototoxicity surveillance[31]

IGHG guidelines currently being developed[55]
  Central nervous system neoplasms surveillance
  Coronary artery disease surveillance
  Hypothalamic-pituitary dysfunction surveillance
  Fatigue surveillance
  Mental health surveillance
  Psychosocial problems surveillance
  Metabolic syndrome surveillance
  Pulmonary dysfunction surveillance
  Bone toxicity surveillance
  Nephrotoxicity surveillance
  Thyroid dysfunction surveillance
  Neurocognitive problems surveillance
  Colorectal cancer surveillance
  Hepatic toxicity surveillance

conclusion of evidence is formulated. The quality of the total body of evidence is graded using the Grades of Recommendation, Assessment, Development and Evaluation Working Group (GRADE) methodology.

5. Formulation and grading of the recommendations using the GRADE Evidence to Decision (EtD) framework. The EtD framework ensures that all important criteria for making a decision are considered and informs the guideline panel about the relative pros and cons of the interventions or options being considered. This approach makes the decision-making process structured and transparent. The panel discusses the benefits, harms, patient values, and other important factors, and formulates recommendations. Recommendations are classified into three categories: (1) strong recommendation to do (green), (2) moderate recommendation to do (yellow), and (3) recommendation not to do (red).

In the finalization phase the guideline is written, including a specific description of the process and the considerations made in formulating recommendations. The manuscript is sent out for external review by experts in the field and patient advocates, and subsequently published in peer-reviewed journals.

The development of CPGs does not guarantee improvement in the quality of care. The success of a guideline not only depends on the clinical context and rigor of methodology, but also on dissemination and implementation strategies.[32]

DISSEMINATION AND IMPLEMENTATION OF CHILDHOOD CANCER SURVIVORSHIP CARE GUIDELINES

After the IGHG recommendations are developed and published, they are integrated into the existing region/country-specific survivorship guidelines. Within the United States, the Children's Oncology Group (COG) Long-Term Follow-Up Guidelines for Survivors of Childhood, Adolescent and Young adult Cancers (COG-LTFU Guidelines) provide risk-based, exposure-related recommendations for screening and management of late effects resulting from therapeutic exposures used during treatment of pediatric malignancies.[33] The COG-LTFU Guidelines include 165 sections that detail potential late effects observed following specific chemotherapeutic agents, radiation treatment fields exposing targeted organs and tissues, blood product transfusions, hematopoietic cell transplantation, and surgical procedures. In addition, the COG-LTFU Guidelines offer surveillance recommendations for survivors who are at excess risk of subsequent neoplasms related to pediatric cancer treatment. They are updated on a 5-year cycle by system-based task forces that assess the quality of the evidence emerging in the literature and present recommendations for guideline revisions for approval by a multidisciplinary late effects expert panel. The COG-LTFU Guidelines are disseminated through a Web site (www.survivorshipguidelines.org) that includes surveillance recommendations, patient educational materials (Health Links), and other resources to facilitate risk-based survivorship care, such as the World Wide Web–based Passport of Care that provides tailored late effects screening recommendations to individual survivors based on their therapeutic exposures.[34] In addition, COG members have disseminated guideline recommendations through local, regional, and national academic and community forums and in numerous scholarly publications. COG investigators are highly committed and engaged in the global harmonization of surveillance recommendations for childhood cancer survivors advocated by the IGHG.

Development and dissemination of long-term follow-up guidelines across Europe has been led by the PanCare society (Pan-European Network for Care of Survivors after Childhood and Adolescent Cancer, www.pancare.eu).[35] Two EU-funded projects have played particularly important roles. PanCareSurFup (PanCare Survivor Follow-Up Studies, www.pancaresurfup.eu) contributed strongly to the development of evidence-based surveillance CPGs in the IGHG consortium, and also worked independently to develop evidence-based CPGs for the delivery of LTFU care. A CPG for models of long-term follow-up care has been published, and CPGs for requirements for transition of care from the pediatric to adult health care setting and health promotion are under development. The PanCareFollowUp project (pancarefollowup. eu) is developing consensus-based surveillance guidelines for those late effects topics not addressed by published or imminent IGHG guidelines.

Dissemination of the evidence- and consensus-based CPGs has been achieved by presentations at the biannual PanCare meetings, the international PanCareSurFup closing conference (held in Brussels in May 2016), and several European and international late effects and other specialist conferences. The guidelines will also be accessible on the PanCare and PanCareFollowUp Web sites. Finally, many PanCare members have publicized and disseminated the CPGs within their own countries. It is important that dissemination include provision of appropriate and readily understandable information for survivors and their families. PanCare has established a PLAIN Information Group to develop lay language summaries of the guideline recommendations. In addition, PanCare helped to develop the Survivorship Passport (SurPass), a World Wide Web–based tool that provides a treatment summary and individual recommendations for surveillance of late effects, to empower survivors to seek the care they need.[35]

EVALUATION OF THE QUALITY OF CARE

The last essential feature of the on-going process of quality improvement is the evaluation of the quality of care delivered. Although developing and distributing CPGs is important in optimizing clinical care, insight into actual care given and received is necessary to achieve successful implementation. Quality of care is defined as "whether individuals can access the health care structures and processes of care which they need and whether the care received is effective."[36] The Institute of Medicine elaborates on this by stating that high-quality care should also be safe, patient-centered, timely, efficient, and equitable.[37] The quality of the actual care delivered is measured with so-called quality indicators. Quality indicators are "measurable elements of practice performance for which there is evidence of consensus that they can be used to assess quality and hence change in quality, of care provided."[38] They are statements that are used to precisely quantify structural, procedural, and outcome-related aspects of care quality.[39,40]

Indicator measurement and monitoring has many purposes. Quality indicators make it possible to document the quality of care; make comparisons (benchmarking) over time between health care institutions; make judgments and set priorities; support accountability, regulation, and credibility; support quality improvement; and support patient choice of care services.[41] They give a reliable reflection of the quality of the care provided. By comparing the delivered care with the recommended care in CPGs, identification of suboptimal care can guide improvement of the quality of care.

Three types of quality indicators are distinguished, referring to the process and structure of medical care and the outcome of delivered care (**Table 1**). Process indicators assess what the provider did for the patient and how well this was done. Process measures are direct measures of the quality of care, provided that an association has been demonstrated between a given process and outcome. For example, the proportion of survivors treated with greater than or equal to 35 Gy radiotherapy to a

Table 1
Examples of a recommendation, indicator, review criterion, and standard

	Process	Structure	Outcome
Recommendation	Survivors treated with chest radiation ≥35 Gy should receive cardiomyopathy surveillance using echocardiography with assessment of left ventricular systolic function, to begin no later than 2 y after completion of therapy, repeated at 5 y after diagnosis and continued every 5 y thereafter[27]	Every pediatric oncology center should have a long-term follow-up clinic[52]	Survivors should receive cardiomyopathy surveillance to minimize the burden of cardiovascular disease[27]
Indicator	Survivors treated with chest radiation ≥35 Gy receiving an echo of the heart within 2 y after completion of therapy *Indicator numerator:* Survivors treated with chest radiation ≥35 Gy having received an echo of the heart within 2 y after completion of therapy *Indicator denominator:* All survivors treated with chest radiation ≥35 Gy	The presence of a long-term follow-up clinic for survivorship care at pediatric oncology centers *Indicator numerator:* Presence of a long-term follow-up clinic for survivorship care at the pediatric oncology centers *Indicator denominator:* All pediatric oncology centers	The cumulative incidence of clinical heart failure among survivors treated with chest radiation ≥35 Gy *Indicator numerator:* Survivors treated with chest radiation ≥35 Gy with clinical heart failure at or before the age of 45 y *Indicator denominator:* All survivors treated with chest radiation ≥35 Gy that attained the age of 45 y or older
Review criterion	Has this survivor treated with chest radiation ≥35 Gy received an echo of the heart at 2 y after completion of therapy?	Does this pediatric oncology center have a long-term follow-up clinic to provide survivorship care?	Has this survivor treated with chest radiation ≥35 Gy had clinical heart failure at or before the age of 45 y?
Standard	*Target standard:* 80% of survivors treated with chest radiation ≥35 Gy should receive an echo of the heart within 2 y after completion of cardiotoxic therapy *Achieved standard (hypothetical):* 50% of survivors treated with chest radiation ≥35 Gy has received an echo of the heart within 2 y after completion of cardiotoxic therapy	*Target standard:* 80% of the pediatric oncology centers should have a long-term follow-up clinic to provide survivorship care *Achieved standard:*[53] 38% of survivors receive long-term follow-up care under the guidance of a cancer survivorship expert service or cancer center	*Target standard:* Cumulative incidence of clinical heart failure in survivors treated with chest radiation ≥35 Gy should be 3% or less at the age of 45 y *Achieved standard (hypothetical):* Cumulative incidence of clinical heart failure in survivors treated with chest radiation ≥35 Gy is 6% at the age of 45 y[54]

volume exposing the heart who have received an echocardiogram within 2 years after completion of therapy. Structure indicators relate to the presence or amount of staff, clients, money, beds, supplies, and buildings. An example related to childhood cancer survivorship care may be the proportion of pediatric oncology centers with a long-term follow-up clinic to provide survivorship care. From the survivor or patient perspective, and that of the insurer or payer, the ultimate consideration is the desired outcome.[40] Outcome indicators are valid as performance indicators to the extent that outcomes, such as mortality, morbidity, or hospitalization, reflect the quality of specific care.[42] For instance, the proportion of survivors treated with greater than or equal to 35 Gy radiotherapy to a volume exposing the heart who have developed clinical heart failure before the age of 45 years. Quality indicators are operationalized with the support of review criteria and standards of care (ie, CPGs). A review criterion is a clearly defined statement referring to the actual provision of care to individuals or populations of patients from a case-to-case basis.[43] It should be precise and unambiguous, to allow for reliable and valid retrospective review. Reliability means that the indicator can be measured similarly in different situations and by different observers, whereas validity implies that the indicator is related to the outcome of interest. Some types of indicators, such as blood pressure or kidney function, are easier to quantify than others. In the transition from evidence-based to value-based health care, more emphasis has been put on patient-centered aspects of health care, such as health-related quality of life or patient satisfaction.

At present, there have been no efforts for the development of quality indicators in childhood cancer survivorship care. Several quality indicators have been developed for adult cancer care through combined evidence- and consensus-based processes.[44-48] One of the more extensive and comprehensive endeavors is the Quality Oncology Practice Initiative, launched by the American Society of Clinical Oncology in 1997, which currently encompasses 120 quality measures for cancer care. However, only seven of these indicators relate to survivorship, of which only four are applicable to childhood cancer survivors: (1) completion of a chemotherapy treatment summary within 3 months of the end of chemotherapy, (2) discussion of infertility risks before chemotherapy, (3) discussion of fertility preservation options, and (4) queries about smoking status including appropriate interventions.[49] A wide range of relevant topics for childhood cancer survivors are therefore not addressed and assessed systematically. Nevertheless, it is promising that the use of quality indicators in adult cancer care has a positive effect on provided care.[50,51] For example, clinics that have adopted the Quality Oncology Practice Initiative measures for cancer care improved their performance over time. Specifically, those measures that address new clinical methods, such as giving antinausea and antivomiting medication when administering highly emetogenic chemotherapy, demonstrated rapidly increasing performance rates. However, for other clinically relevant measures, such as assessing smoking status and counseling for infertility risks and fertility preservation, the participating centers consistently performed poorly, indicating that measurement itself is not sufficient for improving clinical care.[50] In a different study, compliance to a quality measure for removal of 12 regional lymph nodes at colon cancer resection showed improvement after introduction of a reporting program, and better risk-adjusted survival.[51]

Because the evidence base for long-term follow-up recommendations in survivorship care is expanding, the evaluation of actual clinical quality of care becomes more important. Although there are currently no systematic quality evaluations in childhood cancer survivorship care, nor have there been efforts for development of quality indicator sets, it would be useful to initiate such collaborations, to encourage further improvement within clinics and enable benchmarking between clinics and countries. The shift from paper to electronic medical records and the increase in cancer and survivor registries will greatly increase their feasibility and cost-effectiveness. Survivor participation should be central to these initiatives, because their experiences are pivotal in the concept of value-based health care. However, it should be emphasized that single-center evaluations of care quality and multistakeholder approaches can identify gaps in the current quality of provided care and might spark new research initiatives, thereby initiating a new cycle in the quality of care improvement process.

SUMMARY

Physicians involved in the care of childhood cancer survivors, and survivors, should be aware of the health problems that survivors may experience and provide high-quality, long-term follow-up care based on CPGs. The cyclical pattern of evidence generation, implementation, and evaluation drives current health care practices and systems. CPGs are essential for health care providers to translate research findings into clinical practice, and for patients to make well-informed health care decisions. The development and use of quality indicators are important to evaluate the impact of CPGs on the quality of care and survivor health outcomes. International collaboration among clinicians, researchers, guideline developers, patients, and survivors is essential in bridging the gap between research and clinical practice and evaluation of the quality of care. In this way we can optimize care and thereby the health and quality of life of childhood cancer survivors.

DISCLOSURE

The authors have no conflicts of interest relevant to this article to disclose.

REFERENCES

1. Phillips SM, Padgett LS, Leisenring WM, et al. Survivors of childhood cancer in the United States: prevalence and burden of morbidity. Cancer Epidemiol Biomarkers Prev 2015;24(4):653–63.
2. Trama A, Botta L, Foschi R, et al. Survival of European adolescents and young adults diagnosed with cancer in 2000-07: population-based data from EUROCARE-5. Lancet Oncol 2016;17(7):896–906.
3. Geenen MM, Cardous-Ubbink MC, Kremer LCM, et al. Medical assessment of adverse health outcomes in long-term survivors of childhood cancer. JAMA 2007;297(24):2705–15.
4. Oeffinger KC, Mertens AC, Sklar CA, et al. Chronic health conditions in adult survivors of childhood cancer. N Engl J Med 2006;355(15):1572–82.
5. Yeh JM, Nekhlyudov L, Goldie SJ, et al. A model-based estimate of cumulative excess mortality in survivors of childhood cancer. Ann Intern Med 2010;152(7): 409–17. W131-408.
6. Harrop JP, Dean JA, Paskett ED. Cancer survivorship research: a review of the literature and summary of current NCI-designated cancer center projects. Cancer Epidemiol Biomarkers Prev 2011;20(10):2042–7.
7. Evidence-Based Medicine Working Group. Evidence-based medicine. A new approach to teaching the practice of medicine. JAMA 1992;268(17):2420–5.
8. Guyatt GH, Haynes RB, Jaeschke RZ, et al. Users' Guides to the Medical Literature: XXV. Evidence-based medicine: principles for applying the Users' Guides to patient care. Evidence-Based Medicine Working Group. JAMA 2000;284(10): 1290–6.

9. Haynes RB, Sackett DL, Gray JM, et al. Transferring evidence from research into practice: 1. The role of clinical care research evidence in clinical decisions. ACP J Club 1996;125(3):A14–6.
10. Kremer LC, Sieswerda E, van Dalen EC. Tips and tricks for understanding and using SR results – no 15: clinical practice guidelines. Evid Based Child Health 2009;4:1333–5.
11. Woolf SH, Grol R, Hutchinson A, et al. Clinical guidelines: potential benefits, limitations, and harms of clinical guidelines. BMJ 1999;318(7182):527–30.
12. Institute of Medicine (IOM). Clinical practice guidelines we can trust. Washington, DC: The National Academies Press; 2011.
13. Ansari S, Rashidian A. Guidelines for guidelines: are they up to the task? A comparative assessment of clinical practice guideline development handbooks. PLoS One 2012;7(11):e49864.
14. Grimshaw JM, Russell IT. Effect of clinical guidelines on medical practice: a systematic review of rigorous evaluations. Lancet 1993;342(8883):1317–22.
15. Grimshaw JM, Thomas RE, MacLennan G, et al. Effectiveness and efficiency of guideline dissemination and implementation strategies. Health Technol Assess 2004;8(6):iii–iv, 1-72.
16. Inwald EC, Ortmann O, Zeman F, et al. Guideline concordant therapy prolongs survival in HER2-positive breast cancer patients: results from a large population-based cohort of a cancer registry. Biomed Res Int 2014;2014:137304.
17. Lugtenberg M, Burgers JS, Westert GP. Effects of evidence-based clinical practice guidelines on quality of care: a systematic review. Qual Saf Health Care 2009; 18(5):385–92.
18. Smith TJ, Hillner BE. Ensuring quality cancer care by the use of clinical practice guidelines and critical pathways. J Clin Oncol 2001;19(11):2886–97.
19. Jacoby I. The Consensus Development Program of the National Institutes of Health. Int J Technol Assess Health Care 1985;1(2):420–32.
20. Children's Oncology Group. Long-term follow-up guidelines for survivors of childhood, adolescent and young adult cancers. Version 5.0. 2019. Available at: http://www.survivorshipguidelines.org/pdf/2018/COG_LTFU_Guidelines_v5.pdf. Accessed November 13, 2019.
21. Dutch Childhood Oncology Group. Guidelines for follow-up in survivors of childhood cancer 5 years after diagnosis. 2010. Available at: https://www.skion.nl/workspace/uploads/richtlijn_follow-up_na_kinderkanker_deel_1_1.pdf. Accessed November 13, 2019.
22. Therapy based on long-term follow up practice statement. UK Children's Cancer Study Group Late Effects Group. In: Skinner R, Wallace WHB, Levitt GA, editors 2005. Available at: https://www.uhb.nhs.uk/Downloads/pdf/CancerPbTherapyBasedLongTermFollowUp.pdf. Accessed November 13, 2019.
23. Scottish Intercollegiate Guidelines Network. Long term follow up of survivors of childhood cancer. A national clinical guideline. 2013. Available at: https://www.sign.ac.uk/assets/sign132.pdf. Accessed November 13, 2019.
24. Germino JC, Elmore JG, Carlos RC, et al. Imaging-based screening: maximizing benefits and minimizing harms. Clin Imaging 2016;40(2):339–43.
25. Kremer LCM, Mulder RL, Oeffinger KC, et al. A worldwide collaboration to harmonize guidelines for the long-term follow-up of childhood and young adult cancer survivors: a report from the International Late Effects of Childhood Cancer Guideline Harmonization Group. Pediatr Blood Cancer 2013;60(4):543–9.

26. Mulder RL, Kremer LCM, Hudson MM, et al. Recommendations for breast cancer surveillance for female survivors of childhood, adolescent, and young adult cancer given chest radiation: a report from the International Late Effects of Childhood Cancer Guideline Harmonization Group. Lancet Oncol 2013;14(13):e621–9.

27. Armenian SH, Hudson MM, Mulder RL, et al. Recommendations for cardiomyopathy surveillance for survivors of childhood cancer: a report from the International Late Effects of Childhood Cancer Guideline Harmonization Group. Lancet Oncol 2015;16(3):e123–36.

28. van Dorp W, Mulder RL, Kremer LCM, et al. Recommendations for premature ovarian insufficiency surveillance for female survivors of childhood, adolescent, and young adult cancer: a report from the international late effects of childhood cancer guideline Harmonization Group in Collaboration With the PanCareSurFup Consortium. J Clin Oncol 2016;34(28):3440–50.

29. Skinner R, Mulder RL, Kremer LC, et al. Recommendations for gonadotoxicity surveillance in male childhood, adolescent, and young adult cancer survivors: a report from the International Late Effects of Childhood Cancer Guideline Harmonization Group in collaboration with the PanCareSurFup Consortium. Lancet Oncol 2017;18(2):e75–90.

30. Clement SC, Kremer LCM, Verburg FA, et al. Balancing the benefits and harms of thyroid cancer surveillance in survivors of childhood, adolescent and young adult cancer: recommendations from the International Late Effects of Childhood Cancer Guideline Harmonization Group in collaboration with the PanCareSurFup Consortium. Cancer Treat Rev 2018;63:28–39.

31. Clemens E, van den Heuvel-Eibrink MM, Mulder RL, et al. Recommendations for ototoxicity surveillance for childhood, adolescent, and young adult cancer survivors: a report from the International Late Effects of Childhood Cancer Guideline Harmonization Group in collaboration with the PanCare Consortium. Lancet Oncol 2019;20(1):e29–41.

32. Grol R, Grimshaw J. From best evidence to best practice: effective implementation of change in patients' care. Lancet 2003;362(9391):1225–30.

33. Landier W, Bhatia S, Eshelman DA, et al. Development of risk-based guidelines for pediatric cancer survivors: the children's oncology group long-term follow-up guidelines from the Children's Oncology Group Late Effects Committee and Nursing Discipline. J Clin Oncol 2004;22(24):4979–90.

34. Poplack DG, Fordis M, Landier W, et al. Childhood cancer survivor care: development of the Passport for Care. Nat Rev Clin Oncol 2014;11(12):740–50.

35. Hjorth L, Haupt R, Skinner R, et al. Survivorship after childhood cancer: PanCare: a European Network to promote optimal long-term care. Eur J Cancer 2015; 51(10):1203–11.

36. Campbell SM, Roland MO, Buetow SA. Defining quality of care. Soc Sci Med 2000;51(11):1611–25.

37. Institute of Medicine Committee on Quality Health Care in America. Crossing the quality chasm: a new health system for the 21st century. Washington, DC: National Academy Press; 2001.

38. Lawrence M. Indicators of quality in health care. Eur J Gen Pract 1997;3(3): 103–8.

39. Donabedian A. Evaluating the quality of medical care. Milbank Q 2005;83(4): 691–729.

40. McGlynn EA, Asch SM. Developing a clinical performance measure. Am J Prev Med 1998;14(3 Suppl):14–21.

41. Rubin HR, Pronovost P, Diette GB. From a process of care to a measure: the development and testing of a quality indicator. Int J Qual Health Care 2001; 13(6):489–96.
42. Rubin HR, Pronovost P, Diette GB. The advantages and disadvantages of process-based measures of health care quality. Int J Qual Health Care 2001; 13(6):469–74.
43. Campbell SM, Braspenning J, Hutchinson A, et al. Research methods used in developing and applying quality indicators in primary care. Qual Saf Health Care 2002;11(4):358–64.
44. Hermens RP, Ouwens MM, Vonk-Okhuijsen SY, et al. Development of quality indicators for diagnosis and treatment of patients with non-small cell lung cancer: a first step toward implementing a multidisciplinary, evidence-based guideline. Lung Cancer 2006;54(1):117–24.
45. Malafa MP, Corman MM, Shibata D, et al. The Florida Initiative for Quality Cancer Care: a regional project to measure and improve cancer care. Cancer Control 2009;16(4):318–27.
46. Rauscher GH, Murphy AM, Orsi JM, et al. Beyond the mammography quality standards act: measuring the quality of breast cancer screening programs. AJR Am J Roentgenol 2014;202(1):145–51.
47. Woodhouse B, Pattison S, Segelov E, et al. Consensus-derived quality performance indicators for neuroendocrine tumour care. J Clin Med 2019;8(9):E1455.
48. Neuss MN, Desch CE, McNiff KK, et al. A process for measuring the quality of cancer care: the quality oncology practice initiative. J Clin Oncol 2005;23(25): 6233–9.
49. Mayer DK, Shapiro CL, Jacobson P, et al. Assuring quality cancer survivorship care: we've only just begun. Am Soc Clin Oncol Educ Book 2015;e583–91. https://doi.org/10.14694/EdBook_AM.2015.35.e583.
50. Neuss MN, Malin JL, Chan S, et al. Measuring the improving quality of outpatient care in medical oncology practices in the United States. J Clin Oncol 2013; 31(11):1471–7.
51. Shulman LN, Browner AE, Palis BE, et al. Compliance with cancer quality measures over time and their association with survival outcomes: the Commission on Cancer's experience with the quality measure requiring at least 12 regional lymph nodes to be removed and analyzed with colon cancer resections. Ann Surg Oncol 2019;26(6):1613–21.
52. Michel G, Mulder RL, van der Pal HJH, et al. Evidence-based recommendations for the organization of long-term follow-up care for childhood and adolescent cancer survivors: a report from the PanCareSurFup Guidelines Working Group. J Cancer Surviv 2019;13(5):759–72.
53. Essig S, Skinner R, von der Weid NX, et al. Follow-up programs for childhood cancer survivors in Europe: a questionnaire survey. PLoS One 2012;7(12): e53201.
54. Mulrooney DA, Yeazel MW, Kawashima T, et al. Cardiac outcomes in a cohort of adult survivors of childhood and adolescent cancer: retrospective analysis of the Childhood Cancer Survivor Study cohort. BMJ 2009;339:b4606.
55. van der Kooi ALF, Mulder RL, Hudson MM, et al. Counseling and surveillance of obstetrical risks for female childhood, adolescent, and young adult cancer survivors: recommendations from the international late effects of childhood cancer guideline harmonization group. Am J Obstet Gynecol 2020;S0002-9378(20): 30614-1.

Childhood Cancer Survivorship: Daily Challenges

Fiona Schulte, PhD[a,b],*, Caitlin Forbes, MSc[c,d],
Amanda Wurz, PhD[c], Michaela Patton, BA[c],
K. Brooke Russell, MSc[c], Saskia Pluijm, PhD[e], Kevin R. Krull, PhD[f]

KEYWORDS

- Fatigue • Pain • Physical activity • Health behaviors • Social adjustment
- Survivorship

KEY POINTS

- Survivors of childhood cancer are at elevated risk of experiencing fatigue, pain, decreased physical activity, engagement in risky health behavior, and poor social adjustment.
- Risks are more pronounced for survivors of specific diagnoses or those receiving specific treatment protocols (eg, survivors of central nervous system (CNS) tumors or receiving CNS-directed therapies).
- Interventions to address these outcomes are in their infancy.
- Future research should focus on exploring the antecedents and consequences of these outcomes.

BACKGROUND

Survivors of childhood cancer have an elevated lifelong risk of developing chronic health problems or late effects. These negative effects encompass physical, psychological, social, and cognitive domains and include fatigue, pain, lifestyle (ie, decreased physical activity, engagement in risky health behaviors), and poor social adjustment.[1–4] The prevalence of late effects among survivors of childhood cancer is

Funding information: Alberta Children's Hospital Research Institute; Charbonneau Cancer Research Institute; The Daniel Family Chair in Psychosocial Oncology
[a] Department of Oncology, Division of Psychosocial Oncology, Cumming School of Medicine, University of Calgary, Calgary, Alberta, Canada; [b] Hematology, Oncology and Transplant Program, Alberta Children's Hospital, Calgary, Alberta, Canada; [c] University of Calgary, Calgary, Alberta, Canada; [d] Alberta Children's Hospital, Calgary, Alberta, Canada; [e] Princess Maxima Center for Pediatric Oncology, Utrecht, Netherlands; [f] St. Jude Children's Research Hospital, Memphis, TN, USA
* Corresponding author. Department of Oncology, Division of Psychosocial Oncology, Cumming School of Medicine, University of Calgary, 2202 2 St SW, Calgary, Alberta T2S 3C3, Canada.
E-mail address: Fiona.schulte@albertahealthservices.ca
Twitter: @schultefiona (F.S.)

Pediatr Clin N Am 67 (2020) 1083–1101
https://doi.org/10.1016/j.pcl.2020.07.004
0031-3955/20/© 2020 Elsevier Inc. All rights reserved.

staggering: 95% will be diagnosed with at least one chronic health condition by the age of 45 years; 80.5% will be diagnosed with a disabling or life-threatening condition.[5] Many of these late effects have severe consequences that can lead to premature mortality and long-term morbidity.[6] The adoption of a variety of health behaviors may attenuate or exacerbate some of the health problems.

Knowledge related to the late effects in survivors of childhood cancer is also evolving, as research dedicated to this field becomes more sophisticated in its methodology. Specifically, research related to outcomes including fatigue, pain, lifestyle behaviors, and social adjustment after treatment have benefited from studies that have included larger sample sizes, more robust approaches to measurement, and greater specificity with respect to populations sampled (eg, focus on specific diagnosis or treatment protocol).

The goal of this review is to examine the state of the recent literature with respect to fatigue, pain, lifestyle behaviors, and social adjustment among survivors of childhood cancer and identify directions for future research. For each outcome the following questions were asked: what is the problem, who is at risk, and what can be done about it? Specifically, the authors sought to determine the prevalence of each outcome, the risk factors associated with each outcome, and finally whether there are interventions that exist to help remediate problems.

METHODS

A comprehensive literature search was completed using the following databases: PubMed, PsycINFO, SPORTDiscus, and EMBASE, using search terms listed in **Table 1**. Articles were reviewed independently by study authors (FS, CF, AW, MP) using the following inclusion criteria: (1) published in English; (2) included children diagnosed with cancer between 0 and 21 years of age; (3) described survivors 5 years from diagnosis and/or 2 years from therapy completion; and (4) were original studies. In addition, articles had to be published between 2014 and December 3, 2019. Separate reviews were conducted for each outcome examined (ie, fatigue, pain, physical activity, lifestyle behaviors, social adjustment).

RESULTS

Across the 5 different outcomes examined, a total of 11,545 articles were retrieved (Fatigue $n = 705$; Pain $n = 429$; Physical Activity $n = 1730$; Lifestyle Behaviors $n = 3032$; Social adjustment $n = 5649$). Articles were scanned at the title/abstract level and ultimately 333 were retained for inclusion in the current review (Fatigue $n = 30$; Pain $n = 21$; Physical Activity $n = 150$; Lifestyle behaviors $n = 45$; Social adjustment $n = 87$). What follows is a narrative summary of the state of the literature with regard to fatigue, pain, physical activity, lifestyle behaviors, and social adjustment.

Fatigue

The Canadian Cancer Society defines fatigue as "a general lack of energy, tiredness or exhaustion. It is different from the tiredness a person usually feels at the end of the day. Fatigue is not necessarily related to activity and may not go away with additional rest or sleep".[7] Fatigue is conceptualized to be a multifactorial product of physiologic (eg, circadian rhythms, metabolic status), physical (eg, physical activity level, disease and treatment factors, comorbid symptoms and conditions), and psychosocial (eg, behavior, mental-health variables, demographic variables) determinants.[8,9] Although limited, there is conflicting evidence regarding the prevalence of fatigue between survivors of childhood cancers and controls, with recent reports indicating a prevalence

Table 1
Search terms used

Search Category	Terms Used
Outcome	
Fatigue	Fatigue[ti]
Pain	Pain[ti]
Physical Activity	"physical activity"[ti] OR exercise[mh]
Lifestyle	alcohol OR smoking OR sun protection OR tobacco OR Marijuana OR illicit [Title/Abstract]))
Social Adjustment	"social behavior"[mh:noexp] OR "social skills"[mh] OR "social skills"[tiab] OR relationship*[tiab] OR social[ti])) relations[ti] OR relationship*[ti] OR conflict*[ti])) OR "independent living"[mh] OR "independent living"[tiab] OR income OR marital[ti] OR marriage[ti] OR unmarried[tiab] OR (social[ti] AND support[ti]) OR job[ti] OR vocation[ti]
Population	child[mh] OR child[ti] OR children*[ti] OR kids[ti] OR youth[ti] OR juvenile[ti] OR pediatric*[ti] OR pediatric*[ti] OR infant[mh] OR infant*[ti] OR infancy[ti] OR schoolchildren[ti] OR childhood[ti] OR preschooler*[ti] OR girls[ti] OR boys[ti] OR adolescen*[ti] OR adolescent[mh] OR teen[ti] OR teens[ti] OR teenager*[ti]
Problem	neoplasms[mh] OR neoplas*[tiab] OR cancer*[tw] OR tumor*[tiab] OR tumor*[tiab] OR carcinoma*[tiab] OR malignan*[tiab] OR oncolog*[tiab] OR oncolog*[jour] OR metasta*[tiab] OR leukemia*[tiab] OR lymphoma* [tiab] OR hodgkin[tiab] OR hodgkin*[tiab] OR T-cell[tiab] OR B-cell[tiab] OR non-hodgkin[tiab] OR sarcoma[tiab] OR sarcom*[tiab] OR sarcoma [tiab] Ewing's[tiab] OR Ewing*[tiab] OR osteosarcoma[tiab] OR osteosarcom*[tiab] OR "wilms tumor"[tiab] OR wilms*[tiab] OR nephroblastom*[tiab] OR neuroblastoma[tiab] OR neuroblastom*[tiab] OR rhabdomyosarcoma[tiab] OR rhabdomyosarcom*[tiab] OR teratoma [tiab] OR teratom*[tiab] OR hepatoma[tiab] OR hepatom*[tiab] OR hepatoblastoma[tiab] OR hepatoblastom*[tiab] OR PNET[tiab] OR medulloblastoma[tiab] OR medulloblastom*[tiab] OR PNET*[tiab] OR "neuroectodermal tumors"[tiab] OR retinoblastoma[tiab] OR retinoblastom*[tiab] OR meningioma[tiab] OR meningiom*[tiab] OR glioma[tiab] OR gliom* OR "brain cancer"[tiab] OR (brain[ti] AND (cancer* [ti] OR neoplasm*[ti])) OR brain tumor*[tiab] OR brain tumor*[tiab] OR "posterior fossa syndrome"[tiab]

ranging from 13.8%, an average of 13.1 years, posttreatment to 48.4%.[10,11] Although some studies suggest that survivors of any childhood cancer have significantly worse fatigue than controls or population norms,[11–14] others have found no significant differences across heterogeneous samples of cancer survivors or among specific diagnoses.[10,15] One possible explanation for these disjointed findings is that this literature continues to be plagued by widely differing methodologies. Fatigue scales used within the literature vary widely or have simply determined the presence of fatigue based on a single yes/no question.[12,16] Moreover, this literature has almost exclusively included samples of survivors of childhood cancers with heterogeneous diagnoses, complicated by varying treatment protocols. Further, research in this area has evaluated survivors of childhood cancers aged anywhere from 10 to greater than 30 years posttreatment together in analyses, potentially clouding findings.

There is consistency within the literature with respect to the factors related to increased fatigue among survivors of childhood cancer. Specifically, fatigue has been found to be related to greater emotional distress, including depression, and lower quality of life. Emerging research also links fatigue to pain.[10,14,15,17,18] Limited evidence also suggests that fatigue in survivors of childhood cancer is related to neurocognitive functioning, particularly among female survivors.[19] Unfortunately, given the largely observational nature of these studies, directionality of these relationships cannot be determined. More longitudinal research exploring fatigue over time would help clarify potential mechanisms and associations.

Interventions

The last 5 years has seen a growth in the development of interventions to combat fatigue in survivors of childhood cancer. One innovative study examined the use of cognitive behavior therapy for treatment of fatigue with moderately successful findings.[20] Physical activity interventions have also been identified as successful therapies for fatigue.[21] These interventions are discussed later in greater detail.

Pain

Pain has become of increased interest in more recent literature related to survivors of childhood cancer. Among the few studies that investigated chronic pain, the prevalence is estimated to be between 11% and 56%.[22,23] Although, only one study[22] explored chronic pain using a valid definition of pain lasting 3 months or longer. Similar to the methodological limitations that plague the research on fatigue, pain is typically measured using items derived from health-related quality-of-life questionnaires or created by the investigators. Both options only use 1 or 2 items to capture pain, which is a cause for concern because pain is a complex, multidimensional construct that includes intensity, frequency, duration, chronicity, interference, and affect, all of which cannot be captured in 1 or 2 items. Future research should reference the chronic noncancer pain literature to better capture multiple dimensions of pain in this unique population using validated, theoretically grounded measures of pain. Moreover, longitudinal are needed to reliably assess the chronicity and duration of pain.

Certain disease and treatment factors may put individuals at risk for experiencing pain in survivorship. Evidence suggests that survivors of high-risk acute lymphoblastic leukemia,[24] bone tumors,[13,24] and soft tissue sarcomas[13] may experience more pain than those of children with other cancer diagnoses. Survivors may be at increased risk of experiencing pain if they have a history of total knee replacement surgery,[25] radiation,[26] disease recurrence,[26] or posttreatment meningioma.[27] Finally, there is evidence to suggest that high-risk neuroblastoma survivors who underwent hematopoietic stem cell transplantation also experience pain in survivorship.[27] There is consistent evidence to suggest that female survivors report more pain than male survivors,[23,26,28] but there is conflicting evidence for the relationship between age at diagnosis and pain as well as current age and pain.

Pain in survivors of childhood cancer is associated with a myriad of poor psychosocial outcomes. Survivors with pain are more likely to report increased fatigue,[13,15,23,29] daytime sleepiness,[15] psychological distress,[30,31] anxiety,[31] and depression.[31] Pain in survivors of childhood cancer is also generally related to diminished health-related quality of life.[26,32,33] In terms of social factors, there is evidence to suggest that pain is related to lower socioeconomic status.[31] Based on the current literature, the directionality of the association between pain and psychosocial outcomes is unclear in that there is not enough evidence to suggest causal relationships. More longitudinal research exploring pain over time would help clarify this.

Interventions

To date, no pain management interventions exist for survivors of childhood cancer, despite the literature suggesting that many survivors experience pain after their treatment has completed. Psychological treatment of the management of chronic pain in noncancer populations aims to reduce disability due to pain, but research on these treatments has not been extended to survivors of childhood cancer. Researchers are encouraged to draw from the chronic noncancer pain intervention literature to test the feasibility, acceptability, and efficacy of these interventions on survivors.

Lifestyle After Treatment

Protective behavior

Physical activity One lifestyle behavior that can improve health among survivors of childhood cancer is physical activity. Physical activity has been defined as any bodily movement resulting in increased energy expenditure above resting level, whereas exercise is a subset of physical activity that is planned, structured, and repetitive.[34] For the purpose of this overview of the literature, the broader term "physical activity" is used throughout.

Research has demonstrated that physical activity levels typically decrease during treatment and often remain low thereafter.[35] As a result, childhood cancer survivors engage in physical activity at similar or lower rates than their peers without a history of cancer.[36–41] The reason for the low rates of physical activity among childhood cancer survivors may be related to a range of influencing factors. Indeed, physical activity among childhood cancer survivors may be influenced by personal (eg, past experience, competing demands), physical (eg, fatigue, fitness levels), psychological (eg, fear of injury, self-confidence, and self-esteem), medical (eg, physical limitations), social (eg, parental attitudes toward physical activity), cognitive (eg, developmental status), and environmental factors (eg, lack of programs/opportunities).[42–44]

Benefits of physical activity There are numerous observational studies examining beneficial relationships between participating in physical activity and greater physical, psychological, social, and cognitive outcomes in survivors of childhood cancer.[37,45–47] Further, researchers have found that physical activity is positively associated with improved cardiopulmonary functioning[48] and better cardiovascular profiles (ie, lower fat mass and greater lean muscle mass).[49,50] This is seen even among childhood cancer survivors who were treated with cardiotoxic agents[51] such as anthracyclines.[52] Higher levels of rigorous-intensity physical activity has also been associated with a lower risk of cardiovascular events in a dose-dependent manner among survivors of Hodgkin lymphoma[53] and lower all-cause mortality in a sample composed of mixed cancer survivors.[54]

The evidence linking physical activity to health benefits in survivors is primarily from cross-sectional studies with leukemia and lymphoma survivors or mixed samples with limited representation from other types of cancer (eg, brain tumor, bone tumor). Thus, evidence for whether higher levels of physical activity improves physical, psychological, social, and cognitive outcomes over time, and the ways in which these relationships may differ across subgroups, remains unclear. In addition, a relatively narrow range of psychological and social outcomes (eg, self-esteem, social support) have been explored across studies and interactions between studied variables have rarely been examined. This gap in knowledge leaves questions regarding potential mediators and moderators and the processes through which physical activity exerts its beneficial effects unanswered. For those seeking to understand the relationships between physical activity and physical, psychological, social, and cognitive outcomes, biobehavioral models may be a useful starting place to guide variable selection. Although several avenues for future research remain, collectively, the published evidence suggests that higher physical activity is associated with a range of positive effects.

Interventions Experimental studies show that physical activity interventions are safe, feasible, and beneficial in children after treatment of cancer.[55-60] Among childhood cancer survivors, a range of benefits have been documented covering behavioral, physical, psychological, and social outcomes.[21,61-69] Specifically, researchers have reported improved physical health (eg, reduced cancer-related fatigue, improved body composition, physical fitness, and coordination), psychological health (eg, greater self-efficacy, positive mood, and quality of life), and social well-being (eg, fostering feelings of social support).[21,61-69] Although there is some variability in these effects, positive outcomes are observed across interventions that range in duration and intensity from giving childhood cancer survivors physical activity equipment (eg, bike,[61] Fitbit[64]), to a 4-day adventure training program,[21,62] to a 12-week physical activity intervention, composed of 2 to 3 weekly supervised sessions, lasting for 30 to 90 minutes.[66] There is also early evidence to suggest that physical activity has a positive impact on some of the common cancer-related complications children face following treatment. Specifically, physical activity may improve neurocognitive function (eg, cortical thickness, reaction time)[70-72] and alleviate symptoms of cardiac toxicity.[73,74] Bone mineral density has also been shown to improve with low-magnitude, high-frequency mechanical stimulation (which may mimic some aspects of physical activity).[75]

Notwithstanding the benefits reported and contributions made by the studies described earlier, there remain important gaps in knowledge. There is variability in terms of intervention designs and measures used. This precludes the ability to pool data and draw robust conclusions. More research is needed to provide insight into the effects of physical activity on a broader range of outcomes relevant to childhood cancer survivors (eg, self-esteem). Adherence to physical activity interventions can also be challenging, with some researchers reporting adherence as low as 25%.[60] Delineating whether nonsignificant and/or mixed effects are due to poor adherence, inadequate physical activity doses, or other reasons is therefore difficult. Although adherence is typically highest within supervised interventions, home-based intervention techniques are often preferable with this population due to pragmatic considerations (eg, small, geographically spread out population). Exploring strategies to promote behavior change outside of a supervised intervention by incorporating behavior change techniques (eg, goal setting, action planning)[76] may be one way to facilitate adherence within home-based interventions in this population.

Risky behavior
Smoking Recent evidence suggests that survivors of childhood cancer smoke at rates ranging from 9.1% to 34.6%.[77,78] Although most of the studies found that survivors smoke at rates lower than the general population or control groups,[79-82] some find survivors smoke at the same rate,[36,83] or even higher rates than controls.[78,84,85] Among large cohort studies, the St. Jude Lifetime Cohort Study (SJLIFE) found that 24.9% of survivors of childhood cancer smoked compared with 28.3% in control group,[86] whereas the Childhood Cancer Survivor Study (CCSS) reported 14.3% of survivors of childhood cancer smoked versus 21.3% in sibling controls,[87] and the British Childhood Cancer Survivor Survey (BCCSS) found that survivors of childhood cancer smoked less frequently than British population norms.[79,88] A meta-analysis by Marjerrison and colleagues[82] found the frequency of survivors of childhood cancer

who smoke was 22% and survivors of childhood cancer were less likely to smoke compared with siblings and healthy controls.

It is of course encouraging that survivors generally smoke less frequently than the general population. However, it remains concerning that any survivors smoke given the additive health risks associated with smoking in this population. Smoking in the general population has been linked to significant health problems including pulmonary dysfunction and cancer. In fact, cardiac and pulmonary dysfunction are among the most common late effects experienced by survivors of childhood cancer (56.4% and 65.2%, respectively).[89] Smoking in this medically vulnerable population has been associated with poorer mental health and physical health[90] including peripheral neuropathy[86] and decreased bone marrow density (BMD), which may put survivors at risk of osteoporosis and bone fractures.[91,92] Oancea and colleagues[93] found decline in pulmonary function in a young cohort of survivors of childhood cancer (median age 35 years) with a history of smoking. Former smokers (median 10 years from quitting) who reported smoking approximately 4.5 packs of cigarettes per day mirrored the pulmonary function of individuals in the general population who smoked 10 packs per day. This study shows that young survivors of childhood cancer are at risk of lung disease even with moderate levels of smoking. Treatment factors such as radiation makes survivors with a history of smoking particularly vulnerable for adverse health outcomes such as lung cancer[82] and increased risk of miscarriage.[94]

Perhaps equally concerning is evidence that survivors of childhood cancer underreport their smoking status in research studies. Huang and colleagues found that 37% of survivors of childhood cancer who reported that they were former smokers were currently smoking when their status was verified by bioanalysis. In addition, 7% of those who reported never smoking were found to be smokers. Misclassification of smoking status was related to younger age, male sex, and current marijuana use.[95]

Longitudinal data from the CCSS found that older age at diagnosis was associated with increased risk of any history of smoking.[80] Treatment factors such as receiving therapy toxic to the lungs or heart was not associated with smoking. Survivors who currently had one or more chronic health problem were also equally likely to smoke. Rates of smoking increased with age[96] and having peers who smoke[81]; however, survivors were more likely to delay initiation of smoking compared with peers.[36]

Alcohol use Rates of alcohol consumption in survivors of childhood cancer are difficult to characterize because of the various reporting methods. Some studies report on percentage of survivors who currently drink alcohol, whereas others report on the number of alcoholic units or drinks per week. Other studies classify drinking habits as being risky or binge drinking. Many studies indicate a similar percentage of drinking or binge drinking among survivors of childhood cancer,[36,84,97,98] whereas other studies report a lower percentage compared with siblings and healthy controls.[79,86,88,99] A meta-analysis by Marjerrison and colleagues[82] found 20% of survivors were binge drinking, which was lower compared with siblings but similar to healthy controls.

Young adult survivors may be particularly prone to risky drinking. Among leukemia survivors in the SJLIFE cohort, 43% reported risky drinking behavior classified as men taking more than 4 drinks per day or more than 14 drinks per week or women who take more than 3 drinks per day or more than 7 drinks per week. Cantrel and Posner[84] also reported more young adult survivors of childhood cancer binge drinking (43.3%) among the National Longitudinal Study of Adolescent Health. Using criteria from the *Diagnostic and Statistical Manual of Mental Disorders, 4th Edition*, 72.2% had at least one alcohol abuse symptom, whereas 51.1% were classified as having severe alcohol abuse symptoms. A French study by Bagur and colleagues[100] similarly found a high level of risky drinking in young adult male survivors who were more likely to have an alcohol dependence or abuse problem compared with men in the general French population (19.6% vs 9.4%).

Despite high levels of problem drinking in young adult survivors, it seems that survivors of childhood cancer begin drinking later than their peers.[36,77,101] This delayed onset of alcohol use may be attributed to delayed socialization or parent protectiveness following cancer treatment[77] but it may provide health care providers with an opportunity to engage young patients in conversations about alcohol use and healthy lifestyle choices.

Drinking alcohol before 18 years of age was related to a 30% increase in memory impairment, 30% increase in risk of depression, and 60% increase in risk of anxiety.[101] Risky drinking has been associated with frailty in survivors of leukemia,[92] and binge drinking has been associated with increased emotional distress.[101] Even a moderate level of alcohol consumption has been linked to decreased BMD.[92]

Drug use Street drug use in survivors of childhood cancer has not been well characterized. A meta-analysis by Marjerrison and colleagues[82] found only 7 articles reporting rates of drug use in survivors of childhood cancer. Overall, drug use was 15% in survivors of childhood cancer, which was less than that in matched controls. Several studies have attempted to capture cannabis use in this population. The reported use of cannabis in survivors of childhood cancer varies widely from 8%[97] to 53%.[100]

In adolescent and young adult survivors of childhood cancer, risk of cannabis use increased with age.[96,100] In a cohort of young survivors of childhood cancer in the United States, increased depressive symptoms, male sex, and higher socioeconomic status were associated with increased marijuana use.[96]

Multiple substance use Nearly 50% of the general population engages in multiple risky health behaviors such as alcohol use, smoking cigarettes, and drug use.[99] Co-occurring risky health behaviors can compound health problems that put survivors of childhood cancer at particularly high risk.[99] For example, adolescents from the CCSS who reported binge drinking, marijuana use, and smoking cigarettes were more likely to engage in risky sexual behavior including unsafe sex and early initiation of sexual activity.[102] Milam and colleagues[96] found that 16% of adolescent and young adult (AYA) survivors of childhood cancer used multiple risky substances (drinking, smoking, and/or marijuana), whereas Lowe and colleagues[103] reported that 24% of AYA survivors engaged in multiple risky behaviors. In a study by Huang and colleagues[95] examining smoking habits in adult survivors of childhood cancer, 81% of self-identified smokers also reported using marijuana.

Clinical factors such as age at diagnosis and cancer type are not related to substance use[96]; however, increased age for AYAs[104] and psychological distress[96,99,103] predict multiple substance use.

Interventions Given the serious health impacts of risky health behaviors in survivors of childhood cancer, early and continuous psychosocial support and education is required. Unfortunately, very few intervention studies have been conducted in the last 5 years and their success is limited. Survivors of childhood cancer from the St. Jude Lifetime Cohort were enrolled in a randomized control trial for a smoking quitline.[89] Quitlines are a commonly used intervention in the general population with reports showing a 40% increase in cessation rates. All participants received free nicotine replacement products and received a cognitive behavior intervention targeted for survivors of childhood cancer. Following bioverification of smoking status at the

12-month follow-up, the success of this study was only 2%. In fact, 80% of those who reported they had successfully quit smoking at the end of the intervention were found to be using tobacco products when tested for cotinine. The high rate of falsifying smoking status may be linked to survivors of childhood cancer feeling pressure to report that they have quit smoking, especially in the context of a randomized control trial designed to assist smoking cessation.

Nagler and colleagues[105] investigated the use of health information media for informing healthy lifestyle choices in survivors of childhood cancer. Adult survivors who access health media are more likely to engage in healthy behaviors. Among a population of survivors of childhood cancer who were previously enrolled in a smoking cessation intervention, 34.2% accessed health information on television (ie, news reports) weekly, whereas 20.1% sought out information in print media and 16.7% used online sources.

Social Adjustment

Social adjustment has been broadly defined as the extent to which one attains socially desirable and developmentally appropriate goals.[106] Research overwhelmingly continues to identify survivors of childhood cancer at risk of social adjustment difficulties. Specifically, survivors of childhood cancer tend to be more withdrawn compared with their peers and are less likely to have reciprocated best friend nominations.[107] As adults, survivors are identified as at risk of having poorer outcomes including not being married, not living independently, and using social benefits compared with the general population.[108–110] Importantly, one of the most significant contributions to this literature over the last 5 years is the recommendation that opportunities for social interaction should be provided as a standard of care in pediatric oncology.[111] Although the recommendation itself is focused more on children during active cancer treatment it acknowledges that social interactions are a critical unmet need.

Evidence continues to acknowledge that survivors of central nervous system (CNS) tumors and survivors receiving CNS-directed therapies are particularly vulnerable to the development of social difficulties following cancer treatment.[112] Large cohort studies examining potential risk factors for social difficulties have revealed that radiotherapy to head and/or neck and an original CNS tumor diagnosis negatively influenced all social outcomes examined in childhood cancer survivors.[108] Using data from the Childhood Cancer survivor study, Schulte and colleagues[113] reported that survivors of CNS tumors were more likely to have 0 friends (15.3%) and to interact with friends less than once per week (41.0%) in comparison with survivors of solid tumors (2.9% and 13.6%, respectively) and siblings (2.3% and 8.7%, respectively). Desjardins and colleagues[114] reported that approximately half of survivors of pediatric brain tumors did not have any reciprocated best friend nominations and 25% were not nominated by any peer as a best friend. Social difficulties among survivors of CNS tumors may also persist into adulthood and affect relationship status.[115]

Previous reviews focused on social adjustment among survivors of cancer have highlighted the need to move away from superficial assessment of social outcomes that lack a conceptual framework for greater depth in investigation.[116] The research related to social adjustment in survivors of childhood cancer has advanced significantly in the last several years due in large part to the increased application of theoretic frameworks related to the social development in children with acquired brain injury.[117] Specifically, consideration of a theoretic framework has facilitated more comprehensive approaches to operationalizing social adjustment, which considers the need for multileveled, multiinformant assessments and also acknowledges the important role of insult-related (eg, diagnosis, treatment) and noninsult-related (eg, family functioning) risk and resilience factors. Subsequently, the literature has gained greater specificity with respect to the components of social adjustment that might be affected as a result of cancer diagnosis and treatment, identification of those who may be at risk, and consideration of some of the potential moderating and mediating factors.

Accordingly, the last 5 years has witnessed greater homogeneity in investigation of social adjustment difficulties by diagnosis including specific considerations of retinoblastoma,[118] astrocytoma,[119] medulloblastoma,[120,121] and Wilms tumor.[88] In addition, there has been greater consideration of specific treatment effects such as hyperfractioned versus conventionally fractionated radiation therapy, revealing that long-term social outcomes were better among ALL survivors who received hyperfractioned radiation.[122]

Other factors that have been explored in the context of social outcomes include treatment-induced hearing loss, which was found to be associated with reduced social attainment.[123] In addition, more consistently, cognitive functions including attention and executive functioning are being considered in conjunction with social adjustment. Not surprisingly, there is a strong association between the 2, whereby greater cognitive dysfunction has been linked to increased social difficulties.[109,115,120,124–126]

Interventions

Over the last 5 years there has been increased attention to the development of interventions to improve social interactions with a specific focus on especially vulnerable populations, namely, survivors of pediatric brain tumor. For example, Barrera and colleagues[127] conducted a multisite randomized control trial of a group social skills intervention program designed to remediate social difficulties among survivors of CNS tumors. The results of this work revealed a statistically significant effect compared with a placebo control group for self-reported social skills that persisted after 6-month follow-up. No differences were found however, for parent-proxy or teacher reports.

Devine and colleagues[128] reported on the feasibility and preliminary outcomes of a peer-mediated intervention. The focus of this intervention was to train peer leaders to engage classmates. Although the intervention was deemed acceptable and feasible to implement in schools, no changes in peer-reported measures were noted with the exception of friendship nominations.

Most recently, consistent with efforts to improve cognitive function using computerized training and literature linking cognitive function with social outcomes, Mendoza and colleagues[129] sought to determine whether the benefits observed using computerized training generalized to social outcomes across all survivors of childhood cancer. Unfortunately results of this study did not find cognitive gains from a computerized rehabilitation program translated to an improvement in social skills.

DISCUSSION

The goal of the current review was to examine the state of the literature with respect to late effect outcomes including fatigue, pain, lifestyle after cancer treatment, and social adjustment among survivors of childhood cancer. Specifically, the authors sought to determine the prevalence of and risk factors associated with each outcome and to explore interventions that have attempted to target each outcome. With respect to each outcome examined, there is evidence to suggest survivors are at elevated risk of experiencing fatigue, pain, decreased physical activity, engagement in risky health behavior, and poor social adjustment. Risks are more pronounced for survivors of specific diagnoses or receiving specific treatment protocols (eg, survivors of CNS tumors or receiving CNS-directed therapies). However, findings remain inconclusive as to whether prevalence is greater than or equivalent to that observed among the general population. Regardless, given survivors of childhood cancer are at significant risk for late effects of their diagnoses and treatments, there is a critical need to acknowledge these risks.

Examination of variables that may be related to the outcomes reviewed reveals critical clinical or medical risk factors including the diagnosis of a CNS tumor or treatment with CNS directed therapy.[112] Overwhelmingly, for survivors experiencing fatigue, pain, lower physical activity, engagement in risky health behaviors, or poor social adjustment, there is a strong association with poorer psychological functioning. Unfortunately, given the fact that most of the studies are observational in nature, the direction of these associations cannot be established. Longitudinal research is needed to determine the significant pathways and identify targets for intervention. Perhaps most interesting from the current review was the interrelations between the outcomes of study. Specifically, fatigue, pain, and physical activity are highly interrelated. Cognitive performance also seems to be a pervasive mediating or moderating factor. Future research should aim to study these pieces simultaneously, rather than in isolation, to gather a more comprehensive understanding of how they might be related to one another.

It was encouraging to see the implementation of interventions across the outcomes examined, with the exception of pain. However, intervention work to date has focused primarily on the management of these outcomes during active treatment. More research is needed in the management of fatigue, pain, and engagement in physical activity in the survivorship stage. For those interventions that do exist, most remain in the pilot stages of development, and more research is needed to determine efficacy. Moreover, for those that do exist, few incorporate long-term follow-up assessments, which limits the ability to draw conclusions regarding the sustained effects of the intervention on a range of outcomes. More effort is needed in the development of interventions and given the comorbidities noted earlier, interventions might benefit from multipronged targets. Once these steps have been taken, greater efforts to ensure successful implementation of interventions must be taken.

Across studies, limitations related to the existing research continue to exist. First, childhood cancer is relatively rare, and so small sample sizes are common. Published studies have typically included small sample sizes, without control groups, with participants varying in lengths of survivorship, primarily representing leukemia, lymphoma, and brain cancer survivors. This challenge is exacerbated during survivorship due to the geographic spread of survivors. Second, most outcomes reviewed (ie, fatigue, pain, physical activity, social adjustment) are complex behaviors that necessitate considering factors at varying levels (eg, individual, social, institutional). Examination of these outcomes using single-item measures are not enough. Researchers are encouraged to capture multiple dimensions of these outcomes in order to capture a deeper understanding of how survivors of childhood might be affected.

Future research in this area should focus on exploring the antecedents and consequences of these outcomes. This research would benefit from the following: including larger and more diverse groups of survivors across different cancer types and at varying stages of survivorship to ensure adequate power to detect main and subgroup effects, using/linking to existing databases and/or being multisite, including a wider range of outcomes that are important to childhood cancer survivors, consistent measures (so as to facilitate meta-analyses and enable data pooling), and longer-term interventions and follow-up. In the meantime, researchers and cancer centers should attempt to provide high-quality and accessible health information to survivors through various media outlets to encourage healthy behaviors. Providing survivors with adequate mental health resources and appropriate education will assist them in making healthy choices.

DISCLOSURE

The authors have no conflicts of interest to declare.

REFERENCES

1. Phillips SM, Padgett LS, Leisenring WM, et al. Survivors of childhood cancer in the United States: prevalence and burden of morbidity. Cancer Epidemiol Biomarkers Prev 2015;24(4):653–63.
2. Chemaitilly W, Sklar CA. Childhood cancer treatments and associated endocrine late effects: a concise guide for the pediatric endocrinologist. Horm Res Paediatr 2019;91(2):74–82.
3. Bitsko MJ, Cohen D, Dillon R, et al. Psychosocial late effects in pediatric cancer survivors: a report from the children's oncology group. Pediatr Blood Cancer 2016;63(2):337–43.
4. Friend AJ, Feltbower RG, Hughes EJ, et al. Mental health of long-term survivors of childhood and young adult cancer: A systematic review. Int J Cancer 2018; 143(6):1279–86.
5. Hudson MM, Ness KK, Gurney JG, et al. Clinical ascertainment of health outcomes among adults treated for childhood cancer. JAMA 2013;309(22): 2371–81.
6. Hudson MM, Oeffinger KC, Jones K, et al. Age-dependent changes in health status in the Childhood Cancer Survivor cohort. J Clin Oncol 2015;33(5):479–91.
7. Canadian CS. Managing Side Effects. Available at: http://www.cancer.ca/en/cancer-information/diagnosis-and-treatment/managing-side-effects/fatigue/?region=on. Accessed July 9, 2018.
8. Glaus A. Fatigue in patients with cancer: analysis and assessment, vol. 145. Berlin: Springer Science & Business Media; 2012.
9. Barsevick AM, Irwin MR, Hinds P, et al. Recomendations for high-priority research on cancer-related fatigue in children and adults. J Natl Cancer Inst 2013;105(19):1432–40.
10. Frederick NN, Kenney L, Vrooman L, et al. Fatigue in adolescent and adult survivors of non-CNS childhood cancer: a report from project REACH. Support Care Cancer 2016;24(9):3951–9.
11. Ho KY, Li WHC, Lam KWK, et al. Relationships among fatigue, physical activity, depressive symptoms, and quality of life in Chinese children and adolescents surviving cancer. Eur J Oncol Nurs 2019;38:21–7.
12. Daniel L, Kazak AE, Li Y, et al. Relationship between sleep problems and psychological outcomes in adolescent and young adult cancer survivors and controls. Support Care Cancer 2016;24(2):539–46.
13. Kelada L, Wakefield CE, Heathcote LC, et al. Perceived cancer-related pain and fatigue, information needs, and fear of cancer recurrence among adult survivors of childhood cancer. Patient Educ Couns 2019;102(12):2270–8.
14. Ho KY, Li WH, Lam KW, et al. The psychometric properties of the chinese version of the fatigue scale for children. Cancer Nurs 2016;39(5):341–8.

15. Rach AM, Crabtree VM, Brinkman TM, et al. Predictors of fatigue and poor sleep in adult survivors of childhood Hodgkin's lymphoma: a report from the Childhood Cancer Survivor Study. J Cancer Surviv 2017;11(2):256–63.
16. Brand SR, Chordas C, Liptak C, et al. Screening for fatigue in adolescent and young adult pediatric brain tumor survivors: accuracy of a single-item screening measure. Support Care Cancer 2016;24(8):3581–7.
17. Karimi M, Cox AD, White SV, et al. Fatigue, physical and functional mobility, and obesity in pediatric cancer survivors. Cancer Nurs 2019;43(4):E239–45.
18. Zeller B, Ruud E, Havard Loge J, et al. Chronic fatigue in adult survivors of childhood cancer: associated symptoms, neuroendocrine markers, and autonomic cardiovascular responses. Psychosomatics 2014;55(6):621–9.
19. Cheung YT, Brinkman TM, Mulrooney DA, et al. Impact of sleep, fatigue, and systemic inflammation on neurocognitive and behavioral outcomes in long-term survivors of childhood acute lymphoblastic leukemia. Cancer 2017; 123(17):3410–9.
20. Boonstra A, Gielissen M, van Dulmen-den Broeder E, et al. Cognitive behavior therapy for persistent severe fatigue in childhood cancer survivors: a pilot study. J Pediatr Hematol Oncol 2019;41(4):313–8.
21. Li WH, Ho K, Lam K, et al. Adventure-based training to promote physical activity and reduce fatigue among childhood cancer survivors: A randomized controlled trial. Int J Nurs Stud 2018;83:65–74.
22. Johannsdottir IMR, Hamre H, Fossa SD, et al. Adverse health outcomes and associations with self-reported general health in childhood lymphoma survivors. J Adolesc Young Adult Oncol 2017;6(3):470–6.
23. Sadighi ZS, Ness KK, Hudson MM, et al. Headache types, related morbidity, and quality of life in survivors of childhood acute lymphoblastic leukemia: a prospective cross sectional study. Eur J Paediatr Neurol 2014;18(6):722–9.
24. Hsiao CC, Chiou SS, Hsu HT, et al. Adverse health outcomes and health concerns among survivors of various childhood cancers: Perspectives from mothers. Eur J Cancer Care 2016;27(6):e12661.
25. Katsumoto S, Maru M, Yonemoto T, et al. Uncertainty in young adult survivors of childhood and adolescent cancer with lower-extremity bone tumors in Japan. J Adolesc Young Adult Oncol 2019;8(3):291–6.
26. Recklitis CJ, Liptak C, Footer D, et al. Prevalence and correlates of pain in adolescent and young adult survivors of pediatric brain tumors. J Adolesc Young Adult Oncol 2019;8(6):641–8.
27. Bowers DC, Moskowitz CS, Chou JF, et al. Morbidity and mortality associated with meningioma after cranial radiotherapy: a report from the childhood cancer survivor study. J Clin Oncol 2017;35(14):1570–6.
28. Arpaci T, Kilicarslan Toruner E. Assessment of problems and symptoms in survivors of childhood acute lymphoblastic leukaemia. Eur J Cancer Care 2016; 25(6):1034–43.
29. Zeller B, Loge JH, Kanellopoulos A, et al. Chronic fatigue in long-term survivors of childhood lymphomas and leukemia: Persistence and associated clinical factors. J Pediatr Hematol Oncol 2014;36(6):438–44.
30. D'Agostino NM, Edelstein K, Zhang N, et al. Comorbid symptoms of emotional distress in adult survivors of childhood cancer. Cancer 2016;122(20):3215–24.
31. Oancea SC, Brinkman TM, Ness KK, et al. Emotional distress among adult survivors of childhood cancer. J Cancer Surviv 2014;8(2):293–303.
32. Schultz KA, Chen L, Chen Z, et al. Health conditions and quality of life in survivors of childhood acute myeloid leukemia comparing post remission

chemotherapy to BMT: a report from the children's oncology group. Pediatr Blood Cancer 2014;61(4):729–36.

33. Macartney G, VanDenKerkhof E, Harrison MB, et al. Symptom experience and quality of life in pediatric brain tumor survivors: a cross-sectional study. J Pain Symptom Manage 2014;48(5):957–67.

34. American Council on Exercise. Physical activity vs. exercise: what's the difference? 2015. Available at: https://http://www.acefitness.org/education-and-resources/lifestyle/blog/5460/physical-activity-vs-exercise-what-s-the-difference. Accessed December 6, 2016.

35. Kowaluk A, Wozniewski M, Malicka I. Physical activity and quality of life of healthy children and patients with hematological cancers. Int J Environ Res Public Health 2019;16(15):03.

36. Aguero G, Sanz C. Assessment of cardiometabolic risk factors among adolescent survivors of childhood cancer. Arch Argent Pediatr 2015;113(2):119–25.

37. Antwi GO, Jayawardene W, Lohrmann DK, et al. Physical activity and fitness among pediatric cancer survivors: a meta-analysis of observational studies. Support Care Cancer 2019;27(9):3183–94.

38. Bogg TF, Shaw PJ, Cohn RJ, et al. Physical activity and screen-time of childhood haematopoietic stem cell transplant survivors. Acta Paediatr 2015;104(10):e455–9.

39. Carretier J, Boyle H, Duval S, et al. A review of health behaviors in childhood and adolescent cancer survivors: toward prevention of second primary cancer. J Adolesc Young Adult Oncol 2016;5(2):78–90.

40. Chung O, Li HCW, Chiu SY, et al. The impact of cancer and its treatment on physical activity levels and behavior in Hong Kong Chinese childhood cancer survivors. Cancer Nurs 2014;37(3):E43–51.

41. Schindera C, Weiss A, Hagenbuch N, et al. Physical activity and screen time in children who survived cancer: A report from the Swiss Childhood Cancer Survivor Study. Pediatr Blood Cancer 2019;67:e28046.

42. Yelton L, Forbis S. Influences and barriers on physical activity in pediatric oncology patients. Front 2016;4:131.

43. Gotte M, Kesting S, Winter C, et al. Experience of barriers and motivations for physical activities and exercise during treatment of pediatric patients with cancer. Pediatr Blood Cancer 2014;61(9):1632–7.

44. Ross WL, Le A, Zheng DJ, et al. Physical activity barriers, preferences, and beliefs in childhood cancer patients. Support Care Cancer 2018;26(7):2177–84.

45. Hooke MC, Rodgers C, Taylor O, et al. Physical activity, the childhood cancer symptom cluster-leukemia, and cognitive function: A longitudinal mediation analysis. Cancer Nurs 2018;41(6):434–40.

46. Tonorezos ES, Ford JS, Wang L, et al. Impact of exercise on psychological burden in adult survivors of childhood cancer: A report from the Childhood Cancer Survivor Study. Cancer 2019;125(17):3059–67.

47. Zhang FF, Hudson MM, Huang IC, et al. Lifestyle factors and health-related quality of life in adult survivors of childhood cancer: A report from the St. Jude Lifetime Cohort Study. Cancer 2018;124(19):3918–23.

48. Lemay V, Caru M, Samoilenko M, et al. Physical activity and sedentary behaviors in childhood acute lymphoblastic leukemia survivors. J Pediatr Hematol Oncol 2019;42(1):53–60.

49. Slater ME, Ross JA, Kelly AS, et al. Physical activity and cardiovascular risk factors in childhood cancer survivors. Pediatr Blood Cancer 2015;62(2):305–10.

50. Slater ME, Steinberger J, Ross JA, et al. Physical activity, fitness, and cardiometabolic risk factors in adult survivors of childhood cancer with a history of hematopoietic cell transplantation. Biol Blood Marrow Transplant 2015;21(7): 1278–83.

51. Bourdon A, Grandy SA, Keats MR. Aerobic exercise and cardiopulmonary fitness in childhood cancer survivors treated with a cardiotoxic agent: a meta-analysis. Support Care Cancer 2018;26(7):2113–23.

52. Christiansen JR, Kanellopoulos A, Lund MB, et al. Impaired exercise capacity and left ventricular function in long-term adult survivors of childhood acute lymphoblastic leukemia. Pediatr Blood Cancer 2015;62(8):1437–43.

53. Jones LW, Liu Q, Armstrong GT, et al. Exercise and risk of major cardiovascular events in adult survivors of childhood hodgkin lymphoma: a report from the childhood cancer survivor study. J Clin Oncol 2014;32(32):3643–50.

54. Scott JM, Li N, Liu Q, et al. Association of exercise with mortality in adult survivors of childhood cancer. JAMA Oncol 2018;4(10):1352–8.

55. Grimshaw SL, Taylor NF, Shields N. The feasibility of physical activity interventions during the intense treatment phase for children and adolescents with cancer: a systematic review. Pediatr Blood Cancer 2016;63(9):1586–93.

56. Morales JS, Valenzuela PL, Rincon-Castanedo C, et al. Exercise training in childhood cancer: a systematic review and meta-analysis of randomized controlled trials. Cancer Treat Rev 2018;70:154–67.

57. Baumann FT, Bloch W, Beulertz J. Clinical exercise interventions in pediatric oncology: a systematic review. Pediatr Res 2013;74(4):366–74.

58. Braam KI, van der Torre P, Takken T, et al. Physical exercise training interventions for children and young adults during and after treatment for childhood cancer: an update. Cochrane Database Syst Rev 2016;(3):CD008796.

59. Klika R, Tamburini A, Galanti G, et al. The role of exercise in pediatric and adolescent cancer: a review of assessments and suggestions for clinical implementation. J Func Morph Kin 2018;3(7):1–19.

60. Esbenshade AJ, Ness KK. Dietary and exercise interventions for pediatric oncology patients: the way forward. J Natl Cancer Inst Monogr 2019; 2019(54):157–62.

61. Burke SM, Brunet J, Wurz A, et al. Cycling through cancer: exploring childhood cancer survivors' experiences of well- and ill-being. Adapt Phys Activ Q 2017; 34(4):345–61.

62. Chung OK, Li HC, Chiu SY, et al. Sustainability of an integrated adventure-based training and health education program to enhance quality of life among chinese childhood cancer survivors: a randomized controlled trial. Cancer Nurs 2015;38(5):366–74.

63. Huang JS, Dillon L, Terrones L, et al. Fit4Life: a weight loss intervention for children who have survived childhood leukemia. Pediatr Blood Cancer 2014;61(5): 894–900.

64. Le A, Mitchell HR, Zheng DJ, et al. A home-based physical activity intervention using activity trackers in survivors of childhood cancer: A pilot study. Pediatr Blood Cancer 2017;64(2):387–94.

65. Manchola-Gonzalez JD, Bagur-Calafat C, Girabent-Farres M, et al. Effects of a home-exercise programme in childhood survivors of acute lymphoblastic leukaemia on physical fitness and physical functioning: results of a randomised clinical trial. Support Care Cancer 2019;10:10.

66. Piscione PJ, Bouffet E, Timmons B, et al. Exercise training improves physical function and fitness in long-term paediatric brain tumour survivors treated with cranial irradiation. Eur J Cancer 2017;80:63–72.

67. Muller C, Krauth KA, Gerss J, et al. Physical activity and health-related quality of life in pediatric cancer patients following a 4-week inpatient rehabilitation program. Support Care Cancer 2016;24(9):3793–802.

68. Howell CR, Krull KR, Partin RE, et al. Randomized web-based physical activity intervention in adolescent survivors of childhood cancer. Pediatr Blood Cancer 2018;65(8):e27216.

69. Sabel M, Sjolund A, Broeren J, et al. Active video gaming improves body coordination in survivors of childhood brain tumours. Disabil Rehabil 2016;38(21): 2073–84.

70. Sabel M, Sjolund A, Broeren J, et al. Effects of physically active video gaming on cognition and activities of daily living in childhood brain tumor survivors: a randomized pilot study. Neurooncol Pract 2017;4(2):98–110.

71. Riggs L, Piscione J, Laughlin S, et al. Exercise training for neural recovery in a restricted sample of pediatric brain tumor survivors: a controlled clinical trial with crossover of training versus no training. Neuro-oncol. 2017;19(3):440–50.

72. Szulc-Lerch KU, Timmons BW, Bouffet E, et al. Repairing the brain with physical exercise: Cortical thickness and brain volume increases in long-term pediatric brain tumor survivors in response to a structured exercise intervention. Neuroimage Clin 2018;18:972–85.

73. Long TM, Rath SR, Wallman KE, et al. Exercise training improves vascular function and secondary health measures in survivors of pediatric oncology related cerebral insult. PLoS One 2018;13(8):e0201449.

74. Jarvela LS, Saraste M, Niinikoski H, et al. Home-based exercise training improves left ventricle diastolic function in survivors of childhood ALL: a tissue doppler and velocity vector imaging study. Pediatr Blood Cancer 2016;63(9): 1629–35.

75. Mogil RJ, Kaste SC, Ferry RJ Jr, et al. Effect of low-magnitude, high-frequency mechanical stimulation on BMD among young childhood cancer survivors: a randomized clinical trial. JAMA Oncol 2016;2(7):908–14.

76. Michie S, Richardson M, Johnston M, et al. The behavior change technique taxonomy (v1) of 93 hierarchically clustered techniques: building an international consensus for the reporting of behavior change interventions. Ann Behav Med 2013;46(1):81–95.

77. Milam J, Slaughter R, Tobin JL, et al. Childhood cancer survivorship and substance use behaviors: a matched case-control study among hispanic adolescents and young adults. J Adolesc Health 2018;63(1):115–7.

78. Asfar T, Dietz NA, Arheart KL, et al. Smoking behavior among adult childhood cancer survivors: what are we missing? J Cancer Surviv 2016;10(1):131–41.

79. Fidler MM, Frobisher C, Guha J, et al. Long-term adverse outcomes in survivors of childhood bone sarcoma: the British Childhood Cancer Survivor Study. Br J Cancer 2015;112(12):1857–65.

80. Gibson TM, Liu W, Armstrong GT, et al. Longitudinal smoking patterns in survivors of childhood cancer: An update from the Childhood Cancer Survivor Study. Cancer 2015;121(22):4035–43.

81. Kasteler R, Belle F, Schindera C, et al. Prevalence and reasons for smoking in adolescent Swiss childhood cancer survivors. Pediatr Blood Cancer 2019; 66(1):e27438.

82. Marjerrison S, Hendershot E, Empringham B, et al. Smoking, Binge Drinking, and Drug Use Among Childhood Cancer Survivors: A Meta-Analysis. Pediatr Blood Cancer 2016;63(7):1254–63.

83. Howell CR, Wilson CL, Yasui Y, et al. Neighborhood effect and obesity in adult survivors of pediatric cancer: A report from the St. Jude lifetime cohort study. Int J Cancer 2019;147(2):338–49.

84. Cantrell MA, Posner MA. Engagement in high-risk behaviors among young adult survivors of childhood cancer compared to healthy same-age peers surveyed in the national longitudinal study of adolescent health. J Adolesc Young Adult Oncol 2016;5(2):146–51.

85. Myrdal OH, Kanellopoulos A, Christensen JR, et al. Risk factors for impaired pulmonary function and cardiorespiratory fitness in very long-term adult survivors of childhood acute lymphoblastic leukemia after treatment with chemotherapy only. Acta Oncol 2018;57(5):658–64.

86. Ness KK, DeLany JP, Kaste SC, et al. Energy balance and fitness in adult survivors of childhood acute lymphoblastic leukemia. Blood 2015;125(22):3411–9.

87. Dietz AC, Chen Y, Yasui Y, et al. Risk and impact of pulmonary complications in survivors of childhood cancer: A report from the Childhood Cancer Survivor Study. Cancer 2016;122(23):3687–96.

88. Wong KF, Reulen RC, Winter DL, et al. Risk of adverse health and social outcomes up to 50 years after wilms tumor: the British childhood cancer survivor study. J Clin Oncol 2016;34(15):1772–9.

89. Klesges RC, Krukowski RA, Klosky JL, et al. Efficacy of a tobacco quitline among adult survivors of childhood cancer. Nicotine Tob Res 2015;17(6):710–8.

90. Ness KK, Hudson MM, Jones KE, et al. Effect of temporal changes in therapeutic exposure on self-reported health status in childhood cancer survivors. Ann Intern Med 2017;166(2):89–98.

91. van Atteveld JE, Pluijm SMF, Ness KK, et al. Prediction of low and very low bone mineral density among adult survivors of childhood cancer. J Clin Oncol 2019; 37(25):2217–25.

92. Wilson CL, Chemaitilly W, Jones KE, et al. Modifiable factors associated with aging phenotypes among adult survivors of childhood acute lymphoblastic leukemia. J Clin Oncol 2016;34(21):2509–15.

93. Oancea SC, Gurney JG, Ness KK, et al. Cigarette smoking and pulmonary function in adult survivors of childhood cancer exposed to pulmonary-toxic therapy: results from the St. Jude lifetime cohort study. Cancer Epidemiol Biomarkers Prev 2014;23(9):1938–43.

94. Gawade PL, Oeffinger KC, Sklar CA, et al. Lifestyle, distress, and pregnancy outcomes in the Childhood Cancer Survivor Study cohort. Am J Obstet Gynecol 2015;212(1):47.e1-10.

95. Huang IC, Klosky JL, Young CM, et al. Misclassification of self-reported smoking in adult survivors of childhood cancer. Pediatr Blood Cancer 2018;65(9): e27240.

96. Milam J, Slaughter R, Meeske K, et al. Substance use among adolescent and young adult cancer survivors. Psychooncology 2016;25(11):1357–62.

97. Berger C, Casagranda L, Pichot V, et al. Dysautonomia in childhood cancer survivors: a widely underestimated risk. J Adolesc Young Adult Oncol 2019; 8(1):9–17.

98. Stolley MR, Sharp LK, Tangney CC, et al. Health behaviors of minority childhood cancer survivors. Cancer 2015;121(10):1671–80.

99. Lown EA, Hijiya N, Zhang N, et al. Patterns and predictors of clustered risky health behaviors among adult survivors of childhood cancer: A report from the Childhood Cancer Survivor Study. Cancer 2016;122(17):2747–56.

100. Bagur J, Massoubre C, Casagranda L, et al. Psychiatric disorders in 130 survivors of childhood cancer: preliminary results of a semi-standardized interview. Pediatr Blood Cancer 2015;62(5):847–53.

101. Brinkman TM, Lown EA, Li C, et al. Alcohol consumption behaviors and neurocognitive dysfunction and emotional distress in adult survivors of childhood cancer: a report from the Childhood Cancer Survivor Study. Addiction 2019;114(2): 226–35.

102. Klosky JL, Foster RH, Li Z, et al. Risky sexual behavior in adolescent survivors of childhood cancer: a report from the Childhood Cancer Survivor Study. Health Psychol 2014;33(8):868–77.

103. Lowe K, Escoffery C, Mertens AC, et al. Distinct health behavior and psychosocial profiles of young adult survivors of childhood cancers: a mixed methods study. J Cancer Surviv 2016;10(4):619–32.

104. Hollen PJ, O'Laughlen MC, Hellems MA, et al. Comparison of two cohorts of medically at-risk adolescents engaging in substance use (cancer survivors and asthmatics): Clinical predictors for monitoring care. J Am Assoc Nurse Pract 2019;31(9):513–21.

105. Nagler RH, Puleo E, Sprunck-Harrild K, et al. Health media use among childhood and young adult cancer survivors who smoke. Support Care Cancer 2014;22(9):2497–507.

106. Yeates KO, Bigler ED, Dennis M, et al. Social outcomes in childhood brain disorder: A heuristic integration of social neuroscience and developmental psychology. Psychol Bull 2007;133:535–56.

107. Brinkman TM, Li C, Vannatta K, et al. Behavioral, social, and emotional symptom comorbidities and profiles in adolescent survivors of childhood cancer: a report from the childhood cancer survivor study. J Clin Oncol 2016;34(28):3417–25.

108. Font-Gonzalez A, Feijen EL, Sieswerda E, et al. Social outcomes in adult survivors of childhood cancer compared to the general population: linkage of a cohort with population registers. Psychooncology 2016;25(8):933–41.

109. Brinkman TM, Krasin MJ, Liu W, et al. Long-term neurocognitive functioning and social attainment in adult survivors of pediatric cns tumors: results from the st jude lifetime cohort study. J Clin Oncol 2016;34(12):1358–67.

110. Brinkman TM, Ness KK, Li Z, et al. Attainment of functional and social independence in adult survivors of pediatric CNS tumors: a report from the St Jude Lifetime Cohort Study. J Clin Oncol 2018;36(27):2762–9.

111. Christiansen HL, Bingen K, Hoag JA, et al. Providing children and adolescents opportunities for social interaction as a standard of care in pediatric oncology. Pediatr Blood Cancer 2015;62(Suppl 5):S724–49.

112. Brinkman TM, Recklitis CJ, Michel G, et al. Psychological symptoms, social outcomes, socioeconomic attainment, and health behaviors among survivors of childhood cancer: current state of the literature. J Clin Oncol 2018;36(21): 2190–7.

113. Schulte F, Brinkman TM, Li C, et al. Social adjustment in adolescent survivors of pediatric central nervous system tumors: A report from the Childhood Cancer Survivor Study. Cancer 2018;124(17):3596–608.

114. Desjardins L, Barrera M, Chung J, et al. Are we friends? Best friend nominations in pediatric brain tumor survivors and associated factors. Support Care Cancer 2019;27(11):4237–44.

115. Schulte F, Kunin-Batson AS, Olson-Bullis BA, et al. Social attainment in survivors of pediatric central nervous system tumors: a systematic review and meta-analysis from the Children's Oncology Group. J Cancer Surviv 2019;13(6): 921–31.

116. Schulte F. Social competence in pediatric brain tumor survivors: breadth versus depth. Curr Opin Oncol 2015;27(4):306–10.

117. Hocking MC, McCurdy M, Turner E, et al. Social competence in pediatric brain tumor survivors: application of a model from social neuroscience and developmental psychology. Pediatr Blood Cancer 2015;62(3):375–84.

118. Brinkman TM, Merchant TE, Li Z, et al. Cognitive function and social attainment in adult survivors of retinoblastoma: a report from the St. Jude Lifetime Cohort Study. Cancer 2015;121(1):123–31.

119. Effinger KE, Stratton KL, Fisher PG, et al. Long-term health and social function in adult survivors of paediatric astrocytoma: A report from the Childhood Cancer Survivor Study. Eur J Cancer 2019;106:171–80.

120. Holland AA, Colaluca B, Bailey L, et al. Impact of attention on social functioning in pediatric medulloblastoma survivors. Pediatr Hematol Oncol 2018;35(1): 76–89.

121. Kieffer V, Chevignard MP, Dellatolas G, et al. Intellectual, educational, and situation-based social outcome in adult survivors of childhood medulloblastoma. Dev Neurorehabil 2019;22(1):19–26.

122. Tang A, Alyman C, Anderson L, et al. Long-Term Social Outcomes of Hyperfractionated Radiation on Childhood ALL Survivors. Pediatr Blood Cancer 2016; 63(8):1445–50.

123. Brinkman TM, Bass JK, Li Z, et al. Treatment-induced hearing loss and adult social outcomes in survivors of childhood CNS and non-CNS solid tumors: Results from the St. Jude Lifetime Cohort Study. Cancer 2015;121(22):4053–61.

124. Hocking MC, Quast LF, Brodsky C, et al. Caregiver perspectives on the social competence of pediatric brain tumor survivors. Support Care Cancer 2017; 25(12):3749–57.

125. Puhr A, Ruud E, Anderson V, et al. Social attainment in physically well-functioning long-term survivors of pediatric brain tumour; the role of executive dysfunction, fatigue, and psychological and emotional symptoms. Neuropsychol Rehabil 2019;1–25. https://doi.org/10.1080/09602011.2019.1677480.

126. Desjardins L, Solomon A, Janzen L, et al. Executive functions and social skills in pediatric brain tumor survivors. Appl Neuropsychol Child 2018;9(1):83–91.

127. Barrera M, Atenafu EG, Sung L, et al. A randomized control intervention trial to improve social skills and quality of life in pediatric brain tumor survivors. Psychooncology 2018;27(1):91–8.

128. Devine KA, Bukowski WM, Sahler OJ, et al. Social competence in childhood brain tumor survivors: feasibility and preliminary outcomes of a peer-mediated intervention. J Dev Behav Pediatr 2016;37(6):475–82.

129. Mendoza LK, Ashford JM, Willard VW, et al. Social functioning of childhood cancer survivors after computerized cognitive training: a randomized controlled trial. Children (Basel) 2019;6(10):105.

Psychological Outcomes, Health-Related Quality of Life, and Neurocognitive Functioning in Survivors of Childhood Cancer and Their Parents

Gisela Michel, PhD[a],*, Tara M. Brinkman, PhD[b,c],
Claire E. Wakefield, PhD[d,e], Martha Grootenhuis, PhD[f]

KEYWORDS

- Distress • Depression • Anxiety • Neuropsychological • Parent • Intervention
- Health-related quality of life • Posttraumatic stress

KEY POINTS

- Many childhood cancer survivors do well after treatment, but a substantial subgroup experiences psychological distress and reduced health-related quality of life. This subgroup may benefit from supportive interventions.
- Many parents report psychological distress after completion of their child's cancer treatment and years into their child's long-term survivorship. Parents experiencing distress should be offered support.

Continued

All authors contributed equally to the article.

[a] Department of Health Sciences and Medicine, University of Lucerne, Frohburgstrasse 3, PO Box 4466, Lucerne 6002, Switzerland; [b] Department of Epidemiology and Cancer Control, St. Jude Children's Research Hospital, 262 Danny Thomas Place, MS 735, Memphis, TN 38105, USA; [c] Department of Psychology, St. Jude Children's Research Hospital, 262 Danny Thomas Place, MS 740, Memphis, TN 38105, USA; [d] School of Women's and Children's Health, UNSW Medicine, UNSW Sydney, Sydney, Australia; [e] Behavioural Sciences Unit, Kids Cancer Centre, Sydney Children's Hospital, Level 1 South, High Street, Randwick, New South Wales 2031, Australia; [f] Princess Máxima Center for Pediatric Oncology, PO Box 85090, Utrecht 3508 AB, the Netherlands
* Corresponding author.
E-mail address: Gisela.michel@unilu.ch
Twitter: @MichelUnilu (G.M.); @tara_brinkman (T.M.B.); @CEwakefield (C.E.W.); @marthagroo-tenhu (M.G.)

Pediatr Clin N Am 67 (2020) 1103–1134
https://doi.org/10.1016/j.pcl.2020.07.005   **pediatric.theclinics.com**
0031-3955/20/© 2020 The Author(s). Published by Elsevier Inc. This is an open access article under the CC BY license (http://creativecommons.org/licenses/by/4.0/).

Continued

- Neurocognitive problems are highly prevalent, particularly among survivors who received central nervous system–directed therapies. Pharmacologic and nonpharmacologic treatment approaches should be considered.
- Various interventions to help survivors and their families to cope with and adapt to the cancer experience have been developed, but there is a lack of rigorous evidence on their effectiveness and few are implemented into routine care.

INTRODUCTION

Childhood cancer is a severe disease striking children and their families unexpectedly. In developed countries, 5-year survival currently exceeds 80%[1]; however, cancer remains the most common disease-related cause of death among children.[2] Treatment of childhood cancer can last several years and often disrupts normal developmental experiences and family home-life routines. These disruptions, in the context of disease-related events and experiences, may leave survivors and family members vulnerable to psychological distress both during and after treatment. Moreover, the effects of cancer-directed therapies may affect survivors' neurocognitive health and health-related quality of life (HRQOL) many years following the completion of treatment.

This article reviews potential psychological and neurocognitive consequences of young survivors (through 21 years of age, and who were diagnosed with cancer before the age of 18 years) and their families, as well as interventions developed to address these late effects. The authors searched PubMed for reviews on the topics of psychological distress, HRQOL, neurocognitive functioning, family/parents, and interventions in survivors of childhood cancer, and complemented these findings with studies identified by experts in the field.

PSYCHOLOGICAL HEALTH AND HEALTH-RELATED QUALITY OF LIFE
Psychological Health in Survivors

Psychological health problems in survivors of childhood cancer encompass a variety of outcomes, including depression, anxiety, externalizing behavioral problems, and posttraumatic stress symptoms (PTSS). Psychological health also includes reference to positive outcomes such as benefit finding and posttraumatic growth (PTG; benefit finding and PTG reflect positive outcomes that can be experienced after highly stressful events, such as closer relationships and greater appreciation of life).

Two early reviews showed few psychological difficulties in young survivors of childhood cancer,[3,4] and reported similar outcomes for childhood cancer survivors and children from the general population.[4] Overall, these findings were confirmed in a later review showing that up to 80% to 90% of survivors are psychologically well.[5] However, many survivors do report both negative and positive outcomes after cancer treatment.[6] A considerable number of survivors report psychological problems, and, even if symptoms are not severe enough to warrant a clinical diagnosis, they might impair HRQOL, and many survivors benefit from support or interventions. An overview of included reviews is provided in **Table 1** and summarized here.

General distress: overall, reviews show that around 6% to 30% of young survivors report symptoms of psychological distress.[5,7] Survivors report decreased positive mood and self-esteem and increased sleeping difficulties and problem behaviors,

Table 1
Reviews on psychological outcomes in survivors of childhood cancer

Study	Aim	Number of Included Studies, Type of Review	Included Survivors	Outcome Measured	Results
Bruce,[13] 2006	Estimate prevalence and risk factors of PTSD and PTSS in survivors of childhood cancer	• 7 studies on survivors • 9 studies on survivors and their parents • Narrative synthesis	Sample sizes: • 23–500 survivors Inclusion criteria • 5 wk to 11 y after diagnosis	PTSS and PTSD	• Prevalence of current PTSD ranging from 4.7%–21% • Lifetime prevalence ranging from 20.5%–35% • Prevalence of PTSS: from 0%–12.5% • Overall, prevalence of cancer-related PTSD and PTSS in childhood survivors seems higher than in the general population
Duran,[16] 2013	Examine the existing literature on PTG and the perception of benefit finding among childhood cancer survivors and their families	• 20 quantitative studies • 12 qualitative studies • 3 mixed studies • Narrative synthesis	Sample size: • Total of 2087 childhood cancer survivors • Diagnosis of cancer at <19 y of age	Positive effects of childhood cancer experiences	Five main themes of positive outcomes: 1. Making sense of cancer experience (meaning-making) 2. Appreciation of life 3. Greater self-knowledge 4. Positive attitudes toward family 5. Desire to pay back society

(continued on next page)

Table 1
(continued)

Study	Aim	Number of Included Studies, Type of Review	Included Survivors	Outcome Measured	Results
Eiser et al,[3] 2000	Determine psychological consequences of surviving childhood cancer	• 14 studies with survivors aged ≤21 y • Narrative synthesis	Sample sizes: • 17–130 survivors	General mental health issues	• 12 studies report at least for part of outcomes similar or better (less anxious and depressed; school status, behavior, overall happiness, and satisfaction more positively rated) • 8 studies reported at least in some parts poorer outcomes in survivors (adjustment problems, poorer body image; social competence and so forth). One study reported severe PTSD symptoms in 12.5% of survivors
McDonnell et al,[9] 2017	Synthesize current knowledge about anxiety among adolescent survivors of pediatric cancer	• 24 articles • 20 quantitative studies • 1 qualitative study • 3 mixed methods • Narrative synthesis and effect sizes	Sample sizes: • 18–407 survivors	• Posttraumatic stress • Anxiety • Worry	• Overall finding: adolescent survivors are at risk for anxiety-related distress • PTSS were common among adolescent survivors; PTSD was more likely in survivors compared with general population but less likely than in adolescents with other trauma

Source	Purpose	Methods	Sample	Outcomes	Findings
Mertens & Gilleland Marchak,[5] 2015	Systematic review of the reported mental health outcomes in adolescent childhood cancer survivors	• 17 articles • Narrative synthesis	Sample size: • 29–2979 survivors Inclusion criteria: • 11–20 y at the time of study • Diagnosed with cancer before 18 y of age • At least 1 y off therapy	• Psychosocial functioning • Emotional concerns and distress • Depression • Anxiety • Posttraumatic stress	• Anxiety: mixed results with some samples reporting more, others comparable levels with comparison peers • Worry: less worry about general symptoms such as headaches, tiredness, minor illnesses, but worries about fertility, cancer risk for their children, and disclosing illness to peers or romantic partner • Most adolescent survivors are fine • 10%–20% of survivors consistently report various psychological difficulties • Global problems with distress and general emotional functioning were reported by 13%–29% of adolescent survivors • PTSD ranged from 8.0%–13.8%, with PTSS being higher
Michel & Vetsch,[7] 2015	Review the available evidence on screening for psychological distress in childhood cancer survivors	• 8 articles (4 articles included survivors aged <20 y only) • Narrative synthesis	Sample sizes: • 32–202 survivors	Distress measured with: • HUI 2 system • BYI-II • BDI-Y • SDQ	• Depending on measure and outcome, between 6.2% (HUI 2, Mobility) and 22.0% (HUI 2, sensation) of adolescent survivors reported psychological distress

(continued on next page)

Table 1
(continued)

Study	Aim	Number of Included Studies, Type of Review	Included Survivors	Outcome Measured	Results
Taieb et al,[12] 2003	• Estimate the prevalence of PTSS and/or PTSD in childhood cancer survivors • Search for predictors of posttraumatic stress response	• 8 studies on childhood cancer survivors only • 5 studies both survivors and their parents • Narrative synthesis	Sample size: • 6–300 survivors • Mean age at study 8–16 y	PTSS and PTSD	• Prevalence of PTSS of moderate to severe intensity or PTSD: 2%–20% of survivors • Lifetime prevalence of PTSD: 20.5%-35% • Two controlled studies with the largest sample sizes (N = 309 and N = 130 showed no significant differences between childhood cancer survivors and healthy control children) Predictors: • Subjective beliefs about past and present life threat, general level of anxiety, unsatisfactory or chaotic family functioning/poor social or family support
Stam et al,[4] 2001	Describe emotional adjustment, including self-esteem, anxiety, depression, and posttraumatic stress	• 40 articles • Narrative synthesis	Sample size: • 20–309 survivors Inclusion criteria: • Survivors aged up to 18 y	Emotional adjustment measured with standardized instruments including: • Self-esteem • Anxiety • Depression • Posttraumatic stress	• Prevalence of psychosocial problems experienced by survivors is similar to that found in children in the general population • Overall, emotional adjustment of the survivors as a group was within normal limits, not differing from that in their healthy peers

Study	Objective	Methods	Sample size	Outcome	Predictors
					Predictors: • Survivors' adjustment associated with older age at diagnosis, longer time off treatment, irradiation therapy, severe medical late effects, parents and family functioning
Turner et al,[17] 2018	Review the relationship between PTG and demographic, medical, and psychosocial correlates in individuals of any age who were affected by cancer in childhood or adolescence	• 18 studies • Narrative synthesis and meta-analysis	Sample size: • 8730 participants in total • In 10 studies all participants aged <21 y • Average age at time of survey 17.92 y	PTG	Predictors: • Participants who were older when surveyed, or older when diagnosed with cancer, were more likely to experience PTG • Less time since diagnosis and treatment completion was associated with greater PTG • Small, significant, positive correlation between posttraumatic stress and PTG • Greater social support and optimism were associated with greater PTG in individuals affected by childhood or adolescent cancer
Wakefield et al,[6] 2010	Review psychosocial functioning in children who have completed cancer treatment	• 19 studies • Narrative synthesis of quantitative studies • Metaethnography of qualitative studies	Sample sizes: • Qualitative studies: 1–51 survivors	Psychosocial outcomes	• Medium to large effects for decreased positive mood and self-esteem, and increased sleeping difficulties and problem behavior

(continued on next page)

Study	Aim	Number of Included Studies, Type of Review	Included Survivors	Outcome Measured	Results
			• Quantitative studies: 6–161 survivors Inclusion criteria: • Survivors diagnosed with cancer • Treatment completion <5 y previously at age <18 y		• More anxiety than healthy children (by 2–3 y posttreatment completion anxiety seems to normalize) • Smaller effects for depression, PTSD-like symptoms, learning difficulties, emotional stability, and HRQOL • Positive outcomes include high levels of global self-worth, good behavioral conduct, and psychosocial hardiness
Zada et al,[10] 2013	Characterize the prevalence and burden of emotional dysfunction in this population of patients/children with cranio-pharyngiomas	• 8 studies on emotional/affective dysfunction • Calculation of a combined prevalence	Sample size: • Total of 146 children with cranio-pharyngiomas	Emotional/affective disturbances	39.7% (58 out of 146) survivors reported emotional/affective dysfunction, mainly depressive symptoms

Abbreviations: ALL, acute lymphoblastic leukemia; BDI-Y, Beck Depression Inventory for Youth; BYI-II, Beck Youth Inventory-II; HUI 2, Health Utilities Index Mark 2 system; PTSD, posttraumatic stress disorder; SDQ, strength and difficulties questionnaire.

Table 1 (continued)

with overall generally small to medium effects.[6] A large study using data from almost 4000 adolescent survivors of childhood cancer participating in the Childhood Cancer Survivor Study (CCSS) showed that around two-third of survivors had no significant parent-reported behavioral, social, or emotional symptoms. However, around 16% showed increased externalizing behaviors (eg, aggressive or antisocial behavior), 9% showed increased internalizing behaviors (eg, symptoms of depression, anxiety, or social withdrawal), and 5% experienced increased global symptoms (both internalizing and externalizing) compared with siblings. Internalizing problems were especially prevalent among survivors who had been treated with cranial radiotherapy, with 31% showing these problems (although none showed externalizing problems only).[8] Survivors of leukemia or central nervous system (CNS) tumors, survivors who were older at diagnosis, women, those self-reporting late effects, and those whose parents experienced distress were shown to be at higher risk for psychological distress.[5,6]

Anxiety: There are mixed results regarding the experience of anxiety after childhood cancer.[9] This finding might be caused by changes in anxiety with increasing time posttreatment. Shortly after end of treatment, survivors report experiencing more anxiety, which then decreases by 2 to 3 years posttreatment.[6] Higher anxiety can be experienced when children are returning to school and might interfere with school- entry.[9] Studies have also shown that social anxiety might increase with time after treatment and can be particularly associated with perceived illness impact and poor body image.[9] Also, adolescent survivors are at particularly high risk for experiencing anxiety, rather than other forms of distress.[9]

Related to anxiety are worries. Survivors commonly report worries about relapse, disclosing their illness to peers and potential romantic partners, fertility, and potential cancer risk for their children.[9] Worries may increase the likelihood of risky behavior (eg, alcohol consumption) and decrease positive health behavior (eg, exercise).[9] However, many survivors also report feeling less worried about headaches, body image, being tired, minor illnesses, and dying.[9] Risk factors for reporting more worries depend on the type of worries but include older age, female sex, diagnosis (CNS tumor, lymphoma, Wilms tumor, other tumors), risk awareness, and perceiving the illness as not being caused by chance.[9]

Depression: similar to anxiety, results are mixed with respect to the experience of depression in young survivors of childhood cancer. Some studies indicate that survivors are less depressed than peers,[3] or show small effects for risk of increased depression and emotional instability.[6] However, subgroups of survivors do seem to be at increased risk of depression. For example, 1 review of 8 studies on children with craniopharyngioma indicated that 40% of these survivors reported affective dysfunction, mainly depression.[10] In addition, reports on antidepressant use among survivors generally suggest that survivors are more likely to be prescribed antidepressants than the general population, with survivors treated with stem-cell transplant and solid tumors in the extremities at highest risk.[11]

PTSS seem to be common among adolescent survivors of childhood cancer, with a current prevalence of 2% to 20% and a lifetime prevalence of 21% to 35%.[5,12,13] However, the prevalence is not as high as in adolescents who have experienced other forms of trauma.[13] In contrast with other traumas, there is some indication that PTSS do not decrease with increasing time following cancer diagnosis.[12,13] A recent study found that, although PTSS are common, posttraumatic stress disorder (PTSD) is rare in young survivors.[14] Risk factors for PTSS among cancer survivors include female sex, poor family functioning, parental PTSS, experiencing late effects of treatment, relapse, anxiety, perceived life threat, and greater treatment intensity.[9,13]

However, other studies have found that objective disease and treatment severity are not associated with experience of PTSS.[12,13]

Many survivors also report positive outcomes such as increased sense of self-worth, good behavioral conduct, and psychosocial hardiness after childhood cancer.[6]

Posttraumatic growth (PTG)[15] is a frequently reported positive outcome of childhood cancer, not only in survivors but in the family as a whole. Childhood cancer survivors often report positive outcomes related to making sense of the cancer experience (meaning making), appreciation of life, greater self-knowledge, positive attitudes toward the family, and desire to give back to society.[16] In childhood cancer survivors, PTG seems to be associated with older age at diagnosis and at measurement.[17] It seems that a certain developmental stage (and cognitive capacity) is necessary to experience PTG; however, with increasing time following diagnosis, there may be a decrease in the experience of PTG.[17] More social support and higher optimism have been shown to be associated with higher levels of PTG.[17]

Psychological Outcomes in Parents of Childhood Cancer Survivors

Parents experience high levels of distress when their child is diagnosed with cancer,[18] which remain increased throughout treatment.[19] With increasing time after diagnosis, overall parents' distress tends to decrease, although there is a substantial subgroup of parents who experience persistent psychological distress in the long term. Reviews summarizing psychological outcomes in parents are shown in **Table 2**.[18,20,21] At particular risk are mothers[19] and parents who experienced high levels of distress, problematic coping, and adjustment difficulties shortly after diagnosis and in early treatment.[20,21] With end of treatment, positive feelings such as relief predominate, but at the same time uncertainty can increase.[20] Parents become aware about the possibility of relapse and worry about the child's health, social life, and possible infertility.[20,21] Some report high levels of anxiety, anger, guilt, or self-blame.[20,21]

A subgroup of parents also experience posttraumatic stress. Concurrent prevalence of PTSD is estimated at 6% to 30% and lifetime prevalence at 27% to 54%, which is higher than among parents in the general population.[12,13,21] PTSS also seem to be more frequent in parents than in survivors[13] and are more prevalent in mothers than in fathers.[18] Additional risk factors are low social support, problems with family functioning, and prior stressful life events. Parents' subjectively experienced severity of the cancer diagnosis and treatment is associated with PTSS, whereas the objective severity is not.[13] Also, the presence of PTSS in one partner is associated with PTSS in the other parent.[12]

Similar to survivors, parents also report psychological growth.[22] Mothers report positive experiences, such as improved relationships and a change in values, whereas fathers tend not to report these experiences.[16,21]

One recent review indicated that social support and access to psychological counseling starting after diagnosis of cancer in the child and continuing during treatment can help parents in the long term.[21] Nonetheless, psychosocial support systems should also be available to parents in need after their child's cancer treatment completion.[23]

Health-Related Quality of Life

The World Health Organization defines childhood HRQOL as "a child's goals, expectations, standards or concerns about their overall health and health-related domains."[24,25] With a growing number of children with cancer surviving, HRQOL has gained increasing attention in pediatric oncology research. When measuring HRQOL, it is important to take into account generic versus disease-specific questionnaires,

Table 2
Reviews on psychological outcomes in parents of childhood cancer survivors

Study	Aim	Number of Included Studies, Type of Review	Included Survivors	Outcomes Measured	Results
Bruce,[13] 2006	Estimate prevalence and risk factors of PTSD and PTSS in survivors of childhood cancer and parents	• 8 studies on parents of survivors • 9 studies on survivors and their parents • Narrative synthesis	Sample sizes: • 23–500 survivors • 5 wk to 11 y after diagnosis	PTSS and PTSD	• Incidences of current cancer-related PTSD in parents 6.2%–25% • Lifetime prevalence of PTSD in parents: 27%–54% • Prevalence of PTSS: 9.8%–44% • Rates of PTSD and PTSS are higher than those found in the general population and also exceed those in survivors Predictors of PTSD and PTSS • Female gender, reduced social support and family functioning, prior stressful life events, subjective severity of event (but not objective severity)
Duran,[16] 2013	Examine the existing literature on PTG and the perception of benefit finding among childhood cancer survivors and their families	• 20 quantitative studies • 12 qualitative studies • 3 mixed studies • Narrative synthesis	Sample size: • Total of 115 childhood cancer survivor parents (689 mothers, 341 fathers, and 85 listed only as parents) Inclusion criteria: • Diagnosis of cancer at <19 y of age	• Positive effects of childhood cancer experiences • Positive psychological outcome or personal growth	• Mothers report PTG • Fathers did not say anything about positive experiences

(continued on next page)

Table 2
(continued)

Study	Aim	Number of Included Studies, Type of Review	Included Survivors	Outcomes Measured	Results
Ljungman et al,[21] 2014	Describe the nature and prevalence of the long-term psychological late effects of childhood cancer for parents of childhood cancer survivors and summarize factors associated with late effects	• 15 articles • Narrative synthesis	Sample size: • 1045 in total (624 mothers and 289 fathers, some gender unknown) • Survivors 8–20 y at study (plus 1 study 25.6 y)	Diverse measures of psychological distress: • General symptoms and distress • PTSS • Worry • Disease-related thoughts and feelings • Adjustment and coping • Family functioning/marital adjustment • Positive outcomes	• Psychological distress, family functioning, and coping in normal range • PTSS 21%–44% at severe level • Feelings of anger, guilt, self-blame, and fear of relapse • Worries and concerns regarding the child's health, social life, and possible infertility • Mostly no negative effects on marital relationship • Improved relationships and changed values caused by the cancer experience Predictors: • Coping and adjustment stronger predictors of emotional function than children's medical and disease-related variables • Childs late effect associated with parents' level of PTSS • Access to social support systems during cancer treatment may help parents emotional well-being in the long term
Pai et al,[19] 2007	Summarize and examine the impact of pediatric cancer on parent and family functioning	• 29 studies (13 on survivors) • Meta-analysis	Sample sizes: • 10–309 participants • Average ages of children: 4–19 y	• Depression • Anxiety • PTSS • Global measure of distress • Family functioning	• Parental distress decreased with increasing since the diagnosis Predictors: • Mothers reported slightly more psychological distress than fathers up to 1 y postdiagnosis

| Taieb et al,[12] 2003 | • Estimate the prevalence of PTSS and/or PTSD in parents of childhood cancer survivors
• Search for predictors of posttraumatic stress response | • 6 studies on parents only
• 5 studies both survivors and their parents
• Narrative synthesis | Sample sizes:
• 30–320 parents/families
• Mean age at study 10–14 y | PTSS and PTSD | • Prevalence of PTSS of moderate to severe intensity or PTSD: 10%–30% of parents
• Lifetime prevalence of PTSD: 54% (only 1 study)
• In 2 controlled studies with the largest sample sizes, both mothers and fathers of survivors reported significantly higher levels of PTSS than comparison parents
Predictors:
• Subjective beliefs about past and present life threat, general level of anxiety, unsatisfactory or chaotic family functioning/ poor social or family support
• Presence of posttraumatic stress in one parent is associated with presence of symptoms in the other parent |
| Vrijmoet-Wiersma et al,[18] 2008 | Estimate prevalence and nature of parental strain | • 26 studies on parents of survivors
• Narrative synthesis | • Survivors 6 mo to 10 y after completion of treatment
• 15 mo to 13 y since diagnosis | • Parental strain
• Parental stress reactions
• Adaptation related to caring for a child with cancer | • Levels of strain decreased to almost normal levels over time in most parents, but remain persistently high in a substantial subgroup
Predictors:
• Depression might persist in parents who initially react with moderate to high levels of depressive symptoms
• PTSS symptoms in mothers remain high; fathers' PTSS symptoms decrease
• Parents with high levels of emotional strain at diagnosis |

(continued on next page)

Table 2
(continued)

Study	Aim	Number of Included Studies, Type of Review	Included Survivors	Outcomes Measured	Results
Wakefield et al,[20] 2011	Examine the positive and negative psychosocial impacts of completing childhood cancer treatment on parents	• 15 articles • Narrative synthesis	Sample size: • 2 families to 122 mothers and 109 fathers • Average 9 mo to 5 y after diagnosis • Survivors 8–14 y at study	Positive and negative feelings	• Treatment completion entails both positive and negative feelings • Parents are generally resilient at treatment completion • Anxiety about risk of relapse can be high at end of treatment but tends to decrease with time

Abbreviations: PTG post-traumatic growth, PTSS post-traumatic stress symptoms, PTSD post-traumatic stress disorder age-specific questionnaires with a narrow versus a wide age range, self-report versus proxy report, and paper-pencil versus online questionnaires.[26] The number of questionnaires being used is large, with the Pediatric Quality of Life Inventory (PedsQL) among the most often used in children,[27,28] and questionnaires such as the Short Form-36 (SF-36)[29] in adults. HRQOL of survivors has mostly been examined in comparison with healthy peers or siblings.

Although results of single studies are mixed, the overall picture indicates that children experience reduced HRQOL during treatment, which then returns to normal or even improves after completion of therapy and into survivorship.[30,31] Pediatric CNS tumor survivors experience worse HRQOL compared with both general population norms as well as survivors of other types of cancer.[32–34] Acute lymphoblastic leukemia (ALL) survivors tend to report lower HRQOL compared with healthy controls, but better HRQOL than survivors of other cancer types.[35] However, some studies have shown that survivors may report better quality of life than their peers,[30,31] which may be caused by response shift (being able to compare with a time in life when HRQOL was worse) or PTG.[30] It is important to monitor and discuss HRQOL, symptoms, and psychosocial functioning in daily clinical practice, which can be facilitated by portals such as the evidence-based KLIK PROM portal.[36]

Medical factors are the most frequently studied risk factors and include characteristics of the disease (diagnosis) and treatment (intensity). Results have been mixed, but fairly consistent risk factors associated with low HRQOL in survivors include certain cancer and treatment types[30] and presence of medical late effects.[27,31,35] CNS tumor survivors are at risk for poor HRQOL if they had an infratentorial tumor, cranial radiation therapy, or hydrocephalus.[34] CNS tumor survivors with lower intelligence quotient and behavioral problems are also at increased risk of poor HRQOL.[34] Among bone tumor survivors, meta-analyses showed no differences in HRQOL between patients who underwent limb-sparing surgery versus amputation.[37]

Many determinants have been studied in relation to HRQOL, but these show conflicting results, likely because of the small number of studies per determinant and different HRQOL questionnaires used.[27] Just as with healthy peers, women are at higher risk for reduced HRQOL.[27,30,37] Other risk factors include older age at diagnosis[27,30,31,33,37] and socioeconomic disadvantage.[27,30]

Studies have thus far rarely focused on more personal protective family and child factors,[27] although some positive results have been shown for positive coping or social support.[31]

Psychological Interventions for Young Childhood Cancer Survivors and Their Parents

There is an increasing focus on developing interventions to attempt to improve outcomes for families affected by childhood cancer.[38] **Table 3** summarizes interventions that have been trialed for young childhood cancer survivors and/or their parents.

The Surviving Cancer Competently Intervention Program (SCCIP) is the intervention that has been trialed most extensively to date. SCCIP is a family-focused intervention underpinned by cognitive-behavioral principles and family systems approaches, aiming to reduce PTSS in survivors, parents, and siblings.[39] The 1-day manualized SCCIP program is delivered via 4 sessions to 6 to 8 families together. One randomized trial reported that survivors who participated in SCCIP had fewer arousal symptoms than controls, whereas fathers in SCCIP experienced fewer intrusive thoughts than control fathers.[40] There were no significant effects of SCCIP on mothers or siblings, and the program did not affect anxiety for any group. A subsequent trial including families at the time of cancer diagnosis (SCCIP newly diagnosed) did not result in

Table 3
Summary of key interventions developed to support young survivors of childhood cancer and their families

Study	Intervention Details	Participants	Study Design	Main Outcome Measures	Findings
Families					
Kazak et al,[40] 2004, United States SCCIP	1-d face-to-face family group intervention that combines CBT and family therapy approaches to enhance coping skills, reduce stress, encourage cohesion	150 families: 150 survivors (10–19 y; 51% female), 146 mothers, 106 fathers, 99 siblings (10–21 y). Survivors had completed treatment 1–12 y prior	RCT with waiting-list control. Follow-up data collected 3–5 mo after intervention	Impact of Events Scale Revised. Posttraumatic Stress Disorder Reaction Index. State-Trait Anxiety Inventory. Revised Children's Manifest Anxiety Scale	Survivors: significantly greater reduction in PTSS (especially arousal symptoms) for intervention group compared with controls. No significant differences in anxiety between conditions Family: significantly greater reduction for fathers' PTSS (particularly intrusive thoughts) scores for intervention group compared with controls. There were no significant treatment effects for PTSS in mothers or siblings. There were no significant differences in family members' anxiety between conditions.

					Note: there were higher dropout rates in the intervention condition, differentially affecting participants with higher PTSS at baseline. An electronic version of SCCIP (eSCCIP) has recently been piloted
Salem et al,[43] 2017, Denmark FAMOS	6 sessions grounded in family systems theory and CBT delivered in participants' homes to support families to adopt healthy coping strategies after childhood cancer	68 families: 68 survivors (mean age 3.8 y, 50% female), 68 mothers, 60 fathers, 73 siblings (mean age 6 y). Families participated after the end of intensive cancer treatment	RCT with usual care control group. Data collected at baseline, and 6 and 12 mo postintervention	Retention and attrition in the RCT. Participation and retention in the intervention Acceptability of the intervention (20 items administered 6 mo postintervention) Psychosocial outcomes data will be reported in a future article	The FAMOS intervention was considered highly feasible and acceptable. The RCT participation rate was 62%. The study achieved a high participation rate for fathers. 93% of families allocated to FAMOS completed all the parent sessions. Parents reported moderate-high satisfaction with parent and child sessions, and appreciated receiving the intervention at home. 73% of parents reported learning useful cognitive skills and 47% reported using the CBT skills postintervention

(continued on next page)

Table 3
(continued)

Study	Intervention Details	Participants	Study Design	Main Outcome Measures	Findings
Survivors					
Maurice- Stam et al,[44] 2009, Netherlands OK Onco program	6 session, face-to-face psychoeducational group intervention Aims to improve: • Information seeking about cancer • Relaxation • Social competence • Positive thinking	11 children (5 female, aged 8–12 y) and their parents. Survivors had completed treatment 1–6 y prior	Pre-post pilot study. Data collected from survivors and parents. Follow-up data collected 0–4 wk after intervention	QOK- child, QOK parent Cognitive Control Strategies Scale Intervention also discussed qualitatively in focus groups	Information seeking/ giving (5-items): 6 children reported improvement on at least 1 item from baseline to postintervention. During focus groups, parents reported that seeking information seemed irrelevant to their children because treatment completed years prior (wanted to focus on current life) Relaxation (5-items): 5 children improved on at least 1 item. 5 children still found it difficult to relax during a visit to the doctor. 2 parents reported that the relaxation component was not effective

Social competence (7-items): results varied by item, with 6 children reporting improvement in the item "I know what I am capable of doing." However, 6 children had negative outcomes or showed no improvement for some items (eg, "With my friends I talk about disease")

Positive thinking (5-items): 5 children reported improvements on the items "I think my future looks positive" and "If I have gloomy thoughts about my disease, I know what to do to feel better." During focus groups, some parents noted that their children seemed more open after the intervention. Note: an online version of this program (Onco OK Online) has recently been piloted

(continued on next page)

Table 3
(continued)

Study	Intervention Details	Participants	Study Design	Main Outcome Measures	Findings
Sansom-Daly et al,[48] 2019, Australia Recapture Life	6 × 90-min online group sessions (plus 1 booster), based on CBT principles Recapture Life goals: improve quality of life, reduce distress, and facilitate healthy coping Study goals: assess acceptability, feasibility, and safety of intervention	45 AYAs aged 15–25 y (23 female, mean age = 21 y). Survivors had completed treatment within last 12 mo 19 support people (parent, partner or friend)	RCT with 3 arms: Recapture Life vs online peer-support group vs waiting list. Follow-up data collected 6 wk from beginning of intervention, 5 wk after booster, and 12 mo after last session	Feasibility: technological difficulties Acceptability: opt-in/ retention rates. Perceived benefit and burden Safety: clinically concerning distress cases	Recapture Life seemed to be feasible, acceptable, and safe. Feasibility data were positive; however, technological difficulties were common (at least once in 71% of sessions). Acceptability data included a 30% opt-in rate and 87% enrollment rate. 75% of participants attended ≥5 of 6 sessions. High perceived benefit, low perceived burden. 54% of AYAs returned a clinically concerning distress screen during the program; however, none reflected acute mental health risks

Study	Intervention	Sample	Design	Measures	Results
Santacroce et al,[46] 2010, United States, Heros Plus	Participants received usual care plus telephone-delivered coping skills training. One-on-one 7-session telephone-delivered program covering cognitive reframing, relaxation, managing uncertainty, communication skills, and problem solving	21 AYAs aged 15–25 y (53% female, mean age 21 y) and 20 parents. Survivors were diagnosed >5 y ago and completed treatment >2 y ago	RCT (usual care control) Follow-up data collected 4 wk after intervention and 12 wk after study enrollment	Mishel Uncertainty in Illness Scale State-Trait Anxiety Inventory. Posttraumatic Stress Disorder Reaction Index Posttraumatic Growth Inventory Growth Through Uncertainty Scale	Results suggested telephone delivery was feasible. Small sample size precluded inferential statistics. Investigators suggested generally positive effects, particularly in benefit finding
Parents					
Bragadottir,[49] 2008, Iceland	Computer-mediated support group intervention (via email so that participants can remain anonymous) to improve coping through mutual support Aimed to decrease parental anxiety, depression, somatization, and stress. Also assessed the extent to which participants received mutual support	21 parents (11 mothers and 10 fathers) of children <5 y after completing cancer treatment (mean age not reported; however, most children were <5 y old at diagnosis)	Pre-post pilot Data collected before intervention (T1), 2 mo after intervention (T2), and 4 mo later (T3)	Symptom Checklist-90 Perceived Stress Scale Perceived Mutual Support Scale	For mothers, there was a significant improvement in depression from T2 to T3. For fathers, there was a significant improvement in anxiety from T1 to T3. For fathers, there was a significant improvement in perceived stress from T2 to T3 For mothers, helpfulness, altruism, instillation of hope, and universality were the strongest indicators of mutual support. For fathers, instillation of hope, universality, helpfulness, and group cohesion were strongest indicators of mutual support

(continued on next page)

Table 3
(continued)

Study	Intervention Details	Participants	Study Design	Main Outcome Measures	Findings
					Mothers used the intervention more than fathers. Most fathers did not write messages for other parents during the intervention
Wakefield et al,[50] 2016, Australia Cascade	3 × 120-min online group sessions delivered online. Grounded in CBT principles, as well as family systems approaches. Cascade goals: improve quality of life, reduce distress and facilitate healthy coping. Trial assessed feasibility and acceptability of Cascade and early efficacy	47 parents (39 mothers) of children aged 2–16 y were randomized to Cascade (n = 25) or a 6-mo waiting list (n = 22). Survivors had completed cancer treatment within the last 5 y	Randomized controlled trial (waiting-list control). Parents completed questionnaire at baseline, 1–2 wk, and 6 mo after intervention	Feasibility: response and attrition rates Acceptability: California Psychotherapy Alliance Scale Youth Satisfaction Questionnaire Outcomes: Quality of Life Family Caregiver Tool. Depression Anxiety Stress Scale. McMaster Family Assessment Device	Cascade seemed feasible and acceptable. Response rate was 54%, 96% of parents remained engaged across sessions, 80% completed every questionnaire. 40% of parents thought the number of sessions was appropriate, 37% desired more sessions. 70% of parents indicated that Cascade was quite or very beneficial, no parent rated Cascade as very or quite burdensome.

6 parents noted that Cascade was time consuming but the benefits outweighed the costs. There was no significant main effect of group (waiting list vs intervention) or time (baseline vs 1–2 wk postintervention vs 6 mo follow-up) on quality of life, psychological functioning, or family functioning

Fear of cancer recurrence was significantly lower at follow-up for both groups

Abbreviations: AYA, adolescent and young adult; Cascade, Cope, adapt, survive, life after cancer; CBT, cognitive behavior therapy; FAMOS, Family-oriented Support; QOK, Questionnaire Op Koers; RCT, randomized controlled trial; SCCIP, Surviving Cancer Competently Intervention Program.

significant differences in the measured outcomes.[41] An e-health version of SCCIP has recently been piloted, suggesting that eSCCIP may be acceptable, feasible, and usable.[42]

Also focused on provision of psychosocial support to whole families is the more recent Family-oriented Support (FAMOS) intervention.[43] The 6-module intervention is delivered in families' homes, which may have enabled a large number of fathers (60 fathers from 68 families) to participate in a randomized controlled trial (RCT). The FAMOS feasibility and acceptability data are promising, with most invited families agreeing to participate and 93% of parents completing all FAMOS sessions. Evaluation revealed largely positive acceptability data, with parents also reporting that they learnt useful cognitive skills (73%) and that they used cognitive behavior therapy (CBT) skills since completing the intervention (47%).[43] Psychosocial outcomes data are forthcoming.

Three interventions have focused on survivors directly, rather than whole families. The 6-session OK Onco program is designed to improve information seeking, relaxation, social competence, and positive thinking.[44] The pilot reported positive outcomes, particularly on social competence and positive thinking. Qualitative focus group data suggested that the intervention was appropriate for young survivors. A pilot of an online version (OK Onco Online) reported high levels of satisfaction and low dropout rate.[45] Focusing on survivors in the adolescent and young adult (AYA) age range, Heros Plus[46] offered AYAs 7 30-minute telephone sessions to develop skills to cope with uncertainty in illness. An RCT reported promising findings (particularly for benefit finding), although the small sample size precluded significance testing. A recent 3-arm randomized trial[47] of the online Recapture Life program reported that Recapture Life was acceptable to survivors, feasible to deliver, and did not increase participants' distress across the 6-week program.[48]

In addition, 2 interventions have focused on delivering psychological support directly to parents to improve coping skills and reduce distress. In Iceland, Bragadottir[49] offered a 4-month computer-mediated support group intervention, reporting declines over time in mothers' depression and fathers' anxiety symptoms. Fathers also experienced an improvement in perceived stress over time. In Australia, Wakefield and colleagues[50] offered parents an online group videoconferencing intervention (Cascade [cope, adapt, survive, life after cancer]), reporting that the intervention was feasible to deliver and acceptable to parents. However, there were no significant differences in quality of life between parents who participated in Cascade compared with wait-listed parents immediately postintervention or after 6 months. An enhanced version of Cascade is currently being assessed in a 3-arm RCT.[51]

Although the data discussed earlier seem promising, they are not conclusive with regard to effectiveness. Reported effect sizes are typically small and several interventions have not reported significant effects on any measured outcomes. There may be several factors driving the modest findings reported to date. Most trials recruited small samples[44,46,48–50] or did not use a control group.[44,49] Interventions included heterogeneous groups (eg, survivors with all types of tumors) and did not prescreen participants for existing distress. Given the emerging evidence that tailored interventions for more distressed participants can yield stronger effects than standardized interventions,[52] there is a clear need to evaluate tailored interventions for patients most at risk. It is also possible that current trials have not selected the most appropriate outcome variables, suggesting a need to adopt measures that sensitively assess clinically important outcomes.[52] There are also several other trials, not included in this review, that used marginally different eligibility criteria,[53,54] related domains such as social skills,[55,56] health knowledge/perceptions,[57] or sleep,[58,59] or included families of children with chronic illness.[60–62]

There are multiple opportunities to improve future intervention trials. Conducting larger studies using more standardized intervention approaches and research designs would enable pooling of results to test effectiveness more rigorously.[63] There is a lack of evidence regarding whether psychological interventions can achieve long-term change for this population, with most studies to date focusing on short-term impacts (with the exception of FAMOS[43] and Recapture Life[50]). There is also a need to consider how best to provide support for men, especially fathers, who are currently underrepresented in research studies.[40,50] As e-health interventions become increasingly prevalent, future studies need to carefully consider the potential benefits and challenges of delivering on-line psychological support to families of childhood cancer survivors.[63] In addition, to date, few (if any) interventions have been successfully integrated into routine clinical care. An ongoing challenge will be to identify sustainable strategies to enable interventions to continue to be offered to families into the long term.

NEUROCOGNITIVE FUNCTIONING
Neurocognitive Problems

Survivors of childhood cancer are at risk for developing neurocognitive impairments secondary to their disease and treatment. Although prevalence estimates vary across studies, more than 35% of survivors may experience neurocognitive late effects.[64] Survivors of CNS tumors are at the greatest risk of developing neurocognitive impairments.[65] Beyond deficits in general intelligence, impairments are often observed in processing speed, executive functions (eg, verbal fluency, cognitive flexibility), memory, and attention.[64,66,67] The most salient risk factors for impairment in CNS tumor survivors include higher dose of cranial radiation therapy (CRT), larger brain volume irradiated, and younger age at diagnosis.[65] In addition, female sex, obstructive hydrocephalus, posterior fossa syndrome, and seizures have been identified as risk factors for neurocognitive impairment.[64,65] The risk of impairment following CRT often increases in a dose-dependent manner; however, younger age at CRT remains the most important risk factor even at a lower CRT dose.[67] Importantly, advances in CRT techniques have resulted in significant dose and target volume reductions to healthy brain tissue and have been shown to reduce neurocognitive morbidities.[66,68,69] Proton CRT minimizes dose exposure to normal brain tissue, and early studies suggest improved outcomes following treatment with proton CRT,[70–73] although long-term follow-up data are needed.

Increased rates of neurocognitive impairment also have been reported in survivors of childhood leukemia.[65,74] Historically, CRT prophylaxis was a critical component of curative therapy for ALL and was strongly associated with neurocognitive impairment, with higher doses of CRT conferring greater risk for poorer outcomes.[74] Contemporary treatment protocols, which consist of intensified intravenous and intrathecal chemotherapies (ie, methotrexate, cytarabine) for standard-risk patients, have resulted in reduced neurocognitive morbidities.[65,75,76] However, survivors of ALL remain at heightened risk for neurocognitive impairment compared with population norms and healthy controls.[75,77] Risk factors include female sex, younger age at diagnosis, and longer time since diagnosis.[65] Among survivors treated with chemotherapy only, longitudinal data suggest that many ALL survivors develop attention problems by the end of therapy[78,79] and present with executive dysfunction and processing speed deficits more than 5 years after diagnosis.[78]

Neurocognitive impairments can have a significant impact on educational and functional outcomes for survivors.[80] A recent meta-analysis reported that childhood cancer survivors are significantly less likely to complete secondary or tertiary level education compared with their classmates without cancer and more likely to require special education services.[81] Moreover, among survivors of ALL and CNS tumors, neurocognitive deficits have been associated with reduced rates of college graduation, employment, and independent living in adulthood.[66,75]

Interventions for Neurocognitive Problems

Educational accommodations are among the most routinely provided interventions to survivors of childhood cancer. Common accommodations provided in the classroom include shortened or modified assignments, extended test-taking time, copies of class notes, modified seating within the classroom, and specialized instruction.[65] Researchers have investigated several targeted treatment approaches focused on the remediation of specific neurocognitive deficits. Early pharmacologic studies investigated the short-term and long-term efficacy of the psychostimulant methylphenidate in survivors of CNS tumors and ALL.[82,83] In 1 study, methylphenidate was associated with improved attention and social skills in survivors, but similar gains in academic performance were not observed.[82] A 24-week trial of the acetylcholinesterase inhibitor donepezil was associated with improvements in executive functioning and visual memory in brain tumor survivors.[84] Promising nonpharmacologic intervention approaches have included home-based computerized cognitive training such as Cogmed.[85–87] Improvements have been observed in the cognitive skills targeted by the interventions (eg, working memory), with maintenance of gains observed at 6-months after the intervention.[87] More recently, investigators have examined the impact of physical activity interventions on neurocognitive functioning in childhood cancer survivors. A 12-week group-based exercise intervention was associated with improved reaction time and increased white matter and hippocampal volume in brain tumor survivors,[88] whereas a 24-week Web-based physical activity intervention was associated with improved inhibitory control in a heterogeneous group of survivors; however, the observed improvement was not maintained at a 6-month follow-up.[89] In contrast, a recent examination of neurofeedback in brain tumor survivors did not show positive effects on attention, memory, processing speed, or executive function.[90]

SUMMARY

Despite largely positive outcomes for survivors of childhood cancer and their families, there remains a substantial group who have psychological, HRQOL-related, and neurocognitive problems. If untreated, these problems can persist into adulthood and very-long-term survivorship.[91] Several interventions have been developed and tested, with promising findings reported in pilot studies and small-scale RCTs. There is a critical need to offer survivors and their families targeted support, starting with the diagnosis of cancer and continuing through treatment and into survivorship. Recently published psychosocial standards of care for childhood cancer survivors[92] can be used as a framework to implement and evaluate the efficacy of interventions in the future.

DISCLOSURE

The authors have nothing to disclose.

REFERENCES

1. Howlader N, Noone A, Krapcho M, et al. SEER cancer statistics review, 1975-2016. Bethesda (MD): National Cancer Institute; 2019.

2. National Vital Statistics System, Centers of Disease Control and Prevention. 10 leading causes of death by age group, United States – 2017. 2019. Available at: https://www.cdc.gov/injury/wisqars/leadingcauses.html. Accessed November 14, 2019.
3. Eiser C, Hill JJ, Vance YH. Examining the Psychological Consequences of Surviving Childhood Cancer: Systematic Review as a Research Method in Pediatric Psychology. J Pediatr Psychol 2000;25(6):449–60.
4. Stam H, Grootenhuis MA, Last BF. Social and emotional adjustment in young survivors of childhood cancer. Support Care Cancer 2001;9(7):489–513.
5. Mertens AC, Gilleland Marchak J. Mental health status of adolescent cancer survivors. Clin Oncol Adolesc Young Adults 2015;5:87–95.
6. Wakefield CE, McLoone J, Goodenough B, et al. The psychosocial impact of completing childhood cancer treatment: a systematic review of the literature. J Pediatr Psychol 2010;35(3):262–74.
7. Michel G, Vetsch J. Screening for psychological late effects in childhood, adolescent and young adult cancer survivors: a systematic review. Curr Opin Oncol 2015;27(4):297–305.
8. Brinkman TM, Li C, Vannatta K, et al. Behavioral, social, and emotional symptom comorbidities and profiles in adolescent survivors of childhood cancer: a report from the Childhood Cancer Survivor Study. J Clin Oncol 2016;34(28):3417–25.
9. McDonnell GA, Salley CG, Barnett M, et al. Anxiety Among Adolescent Survivors of Pediatric Cancer. J Adolesc Health 2017;61(4):409–23.
10. Zada G, Kintz N, Pulido M, et al. Prevalence of neurobehavioral, social, and emotional dysfunction in patients treated for childhood craniopharyngioma: a systematic literature review. PLoS One 2013;8(11):e76562.
11. Lund LW, Winther JF, Cederkvist L, et al. Increased risk of antidepressant use in childhood cancer survivors: a Danish population-based cohort study. Eur J Cancer 2015;51(5):675–84.
12. Taieb O, Moro MR, Baubet T, et al. Posttraumatic stress symptoms after childhood cancer. Eur Child Adolesc Psychiatry 2003;12(6):255–64.
13. Bruce M. A systematic and conceptual review of posttraumatic stress in childhood cancer survivors and their parents. Clin Psychol Rev 2006;26(3):233–56.
14. Tillery R, Willard VW, Long A, et al. Posttraumatic stress in young children with cancer: Risk factors and comparison with healthy peers. Pediatr Blood Cancer 2019;66(8):e27775.
15. Tedeschi RG, Calhoun LG. The Posttraumatic Growth Inventory: measuring the positive legacy of trauma. J Trauma Stress 1996;9(3):455–71.
16. Duran B. Posttraumatic growth as experienced by childhood cancer survivors and their families: a narrative synthesis of qualitative and quantitative research. J Pediatr Oncol Nurs 2013;30(4):179–97.
17. Turner JK, Hutchinson A, Wilson C. Correlates of post-traumatic growth following childhood and adolescent cancer: A systematic review and meta-analysis. Psychooncology 2018;27(4):1100–9.
18. Vrijmoet-Wiersma CM, van Klink JM, Kolk AM, et al. Assessment of Parental Psychological Stress in Pediatric Cancer: A Review. J Pediatr Psychol 2008;33(7):694–706.
19. Pai AL, Greenley RN, Lewandowski A, et al. A meta-analytic review of the influence of pediatric cancer on parent and family functioning. J Fam Psychol 2007;21(3):407–15.
20. Wakefield CE, McLoone JK, Butow P, et al. Parental adjustment to the completion of their child's cancer treatment. Pediatr Blood Cancer 2011;56(4):524–31.

21. Ljungman L, Cernvall M, Gronqvist H, et al. Long-Term Positive and Negative Psychological Late Effects for Parents of Childhood Cancer Survivors: A Systematic Review. PLoS One 2014;9(7):e103340.

22. Phipps S, Long A, Willard VW, et al. Parents of Children With Cancer: At-Risk or Resilient? J Pediatr Psychol 2015;40(9):914–25.

23. Christen S, Mader L, Baenziger J, et al. "I wish someone had once asked me how I'm doing": Disadvantages and support needs faced by parents of long-term childhood cancer survivors. Pediatr Blood Cancer 2019;66(8):e27767.

24. World Health Organization. WHOQOL-BREF: introduction, administration, scoring and generic version of the assessment. Geneva (Switzerland): World Health Organization; 1996.

25. Fayed N, de Camargo OK, Kerr E, et al. Generic patient-reported outcomes in child health research: a review of conceptual content using World Health Organization definitions. Dev Med Child Neurol 2012;54(12):1085–95.

26. Haverman L, Limperg PF, Young NL, et al. Paediatric health-related quality of life: what is it and why should we measure it? Arch Dis Child 2016;102(5):393–400.

27. Klassen AF, Anthony SJ, Khan A, et al. Identifying determinants of quality of life of children with cancer and childhood cancer survivors: a systematic review. Support Care Cancer 2011;19(9):1275–87.

28. Klassen AF, Strohm SJ, Maurice-Stam H, et al. Quality of life questionnaires for children with cancer and childhood cancer survivors: a review of the development of available measures. Support Care Cancer 2010;18(9):1207–17.

29. Ware JE Jr, Kosinski M, Bjorner JB, et al. SF-36v2® Health Survey: administration guide for clinical trial investigators. Lincoln (RI): Quality Metric Incorporated; 2008.

30. McDougall J, Tsonis M. Quality of life in survivors of childhood cancer: a systematic review of the literature (2001-2008). Support Care Cancer 2009;17(10): 1231–46.

31. Shin H, Bartlett R, De Gagne JC. Health-Related Quality of Life Among Survivors of Cancer in Adolescence: An Integrative Literature Review. J Pediatr Nurs 2019; 44:97–106.

32. Schulte F, Russell KB, Cullen P, et al. Systematic review and meta-analysis of health-related quality of life in pediatric CNS tumor survivors. Pediatr Blood Cancer 2017;64(8):e26442.

33. Macartney G, Harrison MB, VanDenKerkhof E, et al. Quality of life and symptoms in pediatric brain tumor survivors: a systematic review. J Pediatr Oncol Nurs 2014;31(2):65–77.

34. Bell H, Ownsworth T, Lloyd O, et al. A systematic review of factors related to children's quality of life and mental health after brain tumor. Psychooncology 2018; 27(10):2317–26.

35. Vetsch J, Wakefield CE, Robertson EG, et al. Health-related quality of life of survivors of childhood acute lymphoblastic leukemia: a systematic review. Qual Life Res 2018;27(6):1431–43.

36. Haverman L, van Oers HA, van Muilekom MM, et al. Options for the Interpretation of and Recommendations for Acting on Different PROMs in Daily Clinical Practice Using KLIK. Med Care 2019;57(Suppl 5):S52–8.

37. Stokke J, Sung L, Gupta A, et al. Systematic review and meta-analysis of objective and subjective quality of life among pediatric, adolescent, and young adult bone tumor survivors. Pediatr Blood Cancer 2015;62(9):1616–29.

38. Howells L, Hulbert-Williams NJ, Blagden SP. New challenges in psycho-oncology: Using drug development methodology to improve survivorship and supportive care intervention trials. Psychooncology 2019;28(7):1362–6.

39. Kazak AE, Simms S, Barakat L, et al. Surviving cancer competently intervention program (SCCIP): a cognitive-behavioral and family therapy intervention for adolescent survivors of childhood cancer and their families. Fam Process 1999;38(2):175–91.

40. Kazak AE, Alderfer MA, Streisand R, et al. Treatment of posttraumatic stress symptoms in adolescent survivors of childhood cancer and their families: a randomized clinical trial. J Fam Psychol 2004;18(3):493–504.

41. Stehl ML, Kazak AE, Alderfer MA, et al. Conducting a randomized clinical trial of an psychological intervention for parents/caregivers of children with cancer shortly after diagnosis. J Pediatr Psychol 2009;34(8):803–16.

42. Canter KS, Deatrick JA, Hilgart MM, et al. eSCCIP: A psychosocial ehealth intervention for parents of children with cancer. Clin Pract Pediatr Psychol 2019;7(1):44–56.

43. Salem H, Johansen C, Schmiegelow K, et al. FAMily-Oriented Support (FAMOS): development and feasibility of a psychosocial intervention for families of childhood cancer survivors. Acta Oncol 2017;56(2):367–74.

44. Maurice-Stam H, Silberbusch LM, Last BF, et al. Evaluation of a psycho-educational group intervention for children treated for cancer: a descriptive pilot study. Psychooncology 2009;18(7):762–6.

45. Maurice-Stam H, Scholten L, De Gee EA, et al. Feasibility of an Online Cognitive Behavioral-based Group Intervention for Adolescents Treated for Cancer: a Pilot Study. J Psychosoc Oncol 2014;32(3):310–21.

46. Santacroce SJ, Asmus K, Kadan-Lottick N, et al. Feasibility and preliminary outcomes from a pilot study of coping skills training for adolescent–young adult survivors of childhood cancer and their parents. J Pediatr Oncol Nurs 2010;27(1):10–20.

47. Sansom-Daly UM, Wakefield CE, Bryant RA, et al. Online group-based cognitive-behavioural therapy for adolescents and young adults after cancer treatment: A multicenter randomised controlled trial of Recapture Life-AYA. BMC Cancer 2012;12(1):339.

48. Sansom-Daly UM, Wakefield CE, Bryant RA, et al. Feasibility, acceptability, and safety of the Recapture Life videoconferencing intervention for adolescent and young adult cancer survivors. Psychooncology 2019;28(2):284–92.

49. Bragadottir H. Computer-mediated support group intervention for parents. J Nurs Scholarsh 2008;40(1):32–8.

50. Wakefield CE, Sansom-Daly UM, McGill BC, et al. Acceptability and feasibility of an e-mental health intervention for parents of childhood cancer survivors: "Cascade". Support Care Cancer 2016;24(6):2685–94.

51. Wakefield CE, Sansom-Daly UM, McGill BC, et al. Online parent-targeted cognitive-behavioural therapy intervention to improve quality of life in families of young cancer survivors: study protocol for a randomised controlled trial. Trials 2015;16:153.

52. Brier MJ, Schwartz LA, Kazak AE. Psychosocial, health-promotion, and neurocognitive interventions for survivors of childhood cancer: a systematic review. Health Psychol 2015;34(2):130–48.

53. Schwartz CE, Feinberg RG, Jilinskaia E, et al. An evaluation of a psychosocial intervention for survivors of childhood cancer: paradoxical effects of response shift over time. Psychooncology 1999;8(4):344–54.

54. van Dijk-Lokkart EM, Braam KI, van Dulmen-den Broeder E, et al. Effects of a combined physical and psychosocial intervention program for childhood cancer patients on quality of life and psychosocial functioning: results of the QLIM randomized clinical trial. Psychooncology 2016;25(7):815–22.

55. Schulte F, Bartels U, Barrera M. A pilot study evaluating the efficacy of a group social skills program for survivors of childhood central nervous system tumors using a comparison group and teacher reports. Psychooncology 2014;23(5): 597–600.

56. Barrera M, Schulte F. A group social skills intervention program for survivors of childhood brain tumors. J Pediatr Psychol 2009;34(10):1108–18.

57. Hudson MM, Tyc VL, Srivastava DK, et al. Multi-component behavioral intervention to promote health protective behaviors in childhood cancer survivors: the protect study. Med Pediatr Oncol 2002;39(1). 2-1. [discussion: 2].

58. Zupanec S, Jones H, McRae L, et al. A Sleep Hygiene and Relaxation Intervention for Children With Acute Lymphoblastic Leukemia: A Pilot Randomized Controlled Trial. Cancer Nurs 2017;40(6):488–96.

59. Braam KI, van Dijk-Lokkart EM, Kaspers GJL, et al. Effects of a combined physical and psychosocial training for children with cancer: a randomized controlled trial. BMC Cancer 2018;18(1):1289.

60. Scholten L, Willemen AM, Last BF, et al. Efficacy of psychosocial group intervention for children with chronic illness and their parents. Pediatrics 2013;131(4): e1196–203.

61. Daniel LC, van Litsenburg RRL, Rogers VE, et al. A call to action for expanded sleep research in pediatric oncology: A position paper on behalf of the International Psycho-Oncology Society Pediatrics Special Interest Group. Psychooncology 2019. https://doi.org/10.1002/pon.5242.

62. Rayner M, Muscara F, Dimovski A, et al. Take A Breath: study protocol for a randomized controlled trial of an online group intervention to reduce traumatic stress in parents of children with a life threatening illness or injury. BMC Psychiatry 2016; 16(1):169.

63. Ryan D, Chafe R, Hodgkinson K, et al. Interventions to improve the aftercare of survivors of childhood cancer: A systematic review. Pediatr Hematol Oncol J 2018;3(4):90–8.

64. Ullrich NJ, Embry L. Neurocognitive dysfunction in survivors of childhood brain tumors. Semin Pediatr Neurol 2012;19(1):35–42.

65. Krull KR, Hardy KK, Kahalley LS, et al. Neurocognitive Outcomes and Interventions in Long-Term Survivors of Childhood Cancer. J Clin Oncol 2018;36(21): 2181–9.

66. Brinkman TM, Krasin MJ, Liu W, et al. Long-term neurocognitive functioning and social attainment in adult survivors of pediatric CNS tumors: results from the St Jude Lifetime Cohort Study. J Clin Oncol 2016;34(12):1358–67.

67. Palmer SL, Armstrong C, Onar-Thomas A, et al. Processing speed, attention, and working memory after treatment for medulloblastoma: an international, prospective, and longitudinal study. J Clin Oncol 2013;31(28):3494–500.

68. Merchant TE, Kiehna EN, Kun LE, et al. Phase II trial of conformal radiation therapy for pediatric patients with craniopharyngioma and correlation of surgical factors and radiation dosimetry with change in cognitive function. J Neurosurg 2006; 104(2 Suppl):94–102.

69. Merchant TE, Kiehna EN, Li C, et al. Radiation dosimetry predicts IQ after conformal radiation therapy in pediatric patients with localized ependymoma. Int J Radiat Oncol Biol Phys 2005;63(5):1546–54.

70. Kahalley LS, Ris MD, Grosshans DR, et al. Comparing Intelligence Quotient Change After Treatment With Proton Versus Photon Radiation Therapy for Pediatric Brain Tumors. J Clin Oncol 2016;34(10):1043–9.

71. Antonini TN, Ris MD, Grosshans DR, et al. Attention, processing speed, and executive functioning in pediatric brain tumor survivors treated with proton beam radiation therapy. Radiother Oncol 2017;124(1):89–97.

72. Pulsifer MB, Duncanson H, Grieco J, et al. Cognitive and Adaptive Outcomes After Proton Radiation for Pediatric Patients With Brain Tumors. Int J Radiat Oncol Biol Phys 2018;102(2):391–8.

73. Gross JP, Powell S, Zelko F, et al. Improved neuropsychological outcomes following proton therapy relative to x-ray therapy for pediatric brain tumor patients. Neuro Oncol 2019;21(7):934–43.

74. Cheung YT, Krull KR. Neurocognitive outcomes in long-term survivors of childhood acute lymphoblastic leukemia treated on contemporary treatment protocols: A systematic review. Neurosci Biobehav Rev 2015;53:108–20.

75. Krull KR, Brinkman TM, Li C, et al. Neurocognitive outcomes decades after treatment for childhood acute lymphoblastic leukemia: a report from the St Jude lifetime cohort study. J Clin Oncol 2013;31(35):4407–15.

76. Conklin HM, Krull KR, Reddick WE, et al. Cognitive outcomes following contemporary treatment without cranial irradiation for childhood acute lymphoblastic leukemia. J Natl Cancer Inst 2012;104(18):1386–95.

77. Kadan-Lottick NS, Zeltzer LK, Liu Q, et al. Neurocognitive functioning in adult survivors of childhood non-central nervous system cancers. J Natl Cancer Inst 2010; 102(12):881–93.

78. Liu W, Cheung YT, Conklin HM, et al. Evolution of neurocognitive function in long-term survivors of childhood acute lymphoblastic leukemia treated with chemotherapy only. J Cancer Surviv 2018;12(3):398–406.

79. Jacola LM, Krull KR, Pui CH, et al. Longitudinal Assessment of Neurocognitive Outcomes in Survivors of Childhood Acute Lymphoblastic Leukemia Treated on a Contemporary Chemotherapy Protocol. J Clin Oncol 2016;34(11):1239–47.

80. Fardell JE, Patterson P, Wakefield CE, et al. A Narrative Review of Models of Care for Adolescents and Young Adults with Cancer: Barriers and Recommendations. J Adolesc Young Adult Oncol 2018;7(2):148–52.

81. Saatci D, Thomas A, Botting B, et al. Educational attainment in childhood cancer survivors: a meta-analysis. Arch Dis Child 2019;105(4):339–46.

82. Conklin HM, Reddick WE, Ashford J, et al. Long-term efficacy of methylphenidate in enhancing attention regulation, social skills, and academic abilities of childhood cancer survivors. J Clin Oncol 2010;28(9):4465–72.

83. Mulhern RK, Khan RB, Kaplan S, et al. Short-term efficacy of methylphenidate: a randomized, double-blind, placebo-controlled trial among survivors of childhood cancer. J Clin Oncol 2004;22(23):4795–803.

84. Castellino SM, Tooze JA, Flowers L, et al. Toxicity and efficacy of the acetylcholinesterase (AChe) inhibitor donepezil in childhood brain tumor survivors: a pilot study. Pediatr Blood Cancer 2012;59(3):540–7.

85. Kesler SR, Lacayo NJ, Jo B. A pilot study of an online cognitive rehabilitation program for executive function skills in children with cancer-related brain injury. Brain Inj 2011;25(1):101–12.

86. Hardy KK, Willard VW, Bonner MJ. Computerized cognitive training in survivors of childhood cancer: a pilot study. J Pediatr Oncol Nurs 2011;28(1):27–33.

87. Conklin HM, Ashford JM, Clark KN, et al. Long-Term Efficacy of Computerized Cognitive Training Among Survivors of Childhood Cancer: A Single-Blind Randomized Controlled Trial. J Pediatr Psychol 2017;42(2):220–31.

88. Riggs L, Piscione J, Laughlin S, et al. Exercise training for neural recovery in a restricted sample of pediatric brain tumor survivors: a controlled clinical trial with crossover of training versus no training. Neuro Oncol 2017;19(3):440–50.

89. Howell CR, Krull KR, Partin RE, et al. Randomized web-based physical activity intervention in adolescent survivors of childhood cancer. Pediatr Blood Cancer 2018;65(8):e27216.

90. de Ruiter MA, Oosterlaan J, Schouten-van Meeteren AY, et al. Neurofeedback ineffective in paediatric brain tumour survivors: Results of a double-blind randomised placebo-controlled trial. Eur J Cancer 2016;64:62–73.

91. Brinkman TM, Recklitis CJ, Michel G, et al. Psychological Symptoms, Social Outcomes, Socioeconomic Attainment, and Health Behaviors Among Survivors of Childhood Cancer: Current State of the Literature. J Clin Oncol 2018;36(21): 2190–7.

92. Wiener L, Kazak AE, Noll RB, et al. Standards for the Psychosocial Care of Children With Cancer and Their Families: An Introduction to the Special Issue. Pediatr Blood Cancer 2015;62(S5):S419–24.

Subsequent Primary Neoplasms

Risks, Risk Factors, Surveillance, and Future Research

Michael Hawkins, DPhil[a],*, Smita Bhatia, MD, MPH[b],
Tara O. Henderson, MD, MPH[c], Paul C. Nathan, MD, MSc[d],
Adam Yan, MD[d], Jop C. Teepen, PhD[e], Lindsay M. Morton, PhD[f]

KEYWORDS

- Subsequent primary neoplasms • Second malignant neoplasms
- Second primary cancers • Secondary cancers • Radiotherapy • Chemotherapy
- Genetic variation • Genetic susceptibility • Surveillance • Screening
- Follow-up guidelines

KEY POINTS

- Risks of subsequent primary neoplasms after childhood, teenage, and young adult cancer are provided from large-scale cohorts which yield the most reliable estimates.
- Radiotherapy and chemotherapy for childhood cancer are each evaluated as a risk factor for subsequent primary neoplasms.
- New investigations are evaluating whether genomic variants modify treatment-related subsequent neoplasm risk among childhood cancer survivors.

Continued

Prof MM Hawkins - Children with Cancer (Project ID: 562799), The Brain Tumour Charity (Project ID; 594034), Public Health England (Project ID: 581678). Prof PC Nathan - no funders to acknowledge. Dr A Yan - no funders to acknowledge. Dr J C Teepen - Dutch Cancer Society (Grant no. 11388), Children Cancer Free Foundation (KiKa, Grant no.: 325). Prof S Bhatia - no funders to acknowledge. Prof TO Henderson - no funders to acknowledge. Dr LM Morton - no funders to acknowledge.
 a Epidemiology & Director of Centre, Centre for Childhood Cancer Survivor Studies, Institute of Applied Health Research, University of Birmingham, Robert Aitken Building, Birmingham B15 2TY, UK; b Institute for Cancer Outcomes and Survivorship, University of Alabama at Birmingham, Birmingham, AL, USA; c University of Chicago Comer Children's Hospital, Chicago, USA; d Division of Haematology/Oncology, The Hospital for Sick Children, Toronto, Canada; e Princess Maxima Centre for Paediatric Oncology, Utrecht, The Netherlands; f Division of Cancer Epidemiology and Genetics, National Cancer Institute, National Institutes of Health, USA
* Corresponding author.
E-mail address: m.m.hawkins@bham.ac.uk

Continued

- Surveillance, screening, and clinical follow-up guidelines for subsequent primary neoplasms after childhood cancer are each considered.
- Priorities for future research concerning subsequent primary neoplasms after childhood cancer are briefly summarized.

RISKS OF SUBSEQUENT PRIMARY NEOPLASMS AFTER CHILDHOOD, ADOLESCENT, AND YOUNG ADULT CANCER

Survivors of childhood cancer experience substantial premature mortality; in the British Childhood Cancer Survivor Study (BCCSS) cohort, by 50 years from diagnosis 30% of 5-year survivors had died when 6% were expected to have died from mortality rates in the general population.[1] Analysis of the same cohort revealed that among survivors at least 45 years from diagnosis 51% of excess number of deaths were caused by subsequent primary neoplasm (SPN).[1] However, efforts to reduce therapeutic exposures in more recent decades has contributed to a decline in late mortality in general and from SPN in particular, among 5-year survivors of childhood cancer.[2]

In this article the authors consider the risks of SPN after childhood cancer and compare these risks with those observed after adolescent and young adult (AYA) cancer; the carcinogenic impact of treatment of childhood cancer with radiotherapy and chemotherapy; the influence of inherited genetic susceptibility on the development of SPNs; and the role of surveillance, screening, and clinical follow-up guidelines.

Risks of Subsequent Primary Neoplasms After Childhood Cancer

The most reliable estimates of risk of SPN result from large-scale cohort studies with systematic long-term follow-up. Two large-scale population-based registry ascertained cohorts of childhood cancer survivors have been established: one in the United Kingdom, the BCCSS,[3–5] and another including all of the Nordic countries.[6] Three large-scale hospital-based cohorts of childhood cancer survivors have also been established: the North American Childhood Cancer Survivor Study (CCSS),[7–9] the Dutch Childhood Cancer Oncology Group—Long-Term Effects After Childhood Cancer (DCOG-LATER) cohort,[10,11] and the French Childhood Cancer Survivor Study (FCCSS).[12,13] A recent review of risk estimates resulting from the initial 4 of these cohorts concluded that beyond age 40 years the standardized incidence ratio (SIR) was consistently at least 2-fold that expected and the absolute excess risk (AER) increased with attained age.[14] Both SIRs and AERs were similar across cohorts younger than 40 years.[14]

Types of SPN observed in excess of that expected from the general population varies substantially by both attained age and interval from diagnosis. For example, within the BCCSS brain tumors and sarcomas, as an SPN accounted for 63% of the excess number of SPNs observed among survivors aged 5 to 19 years; in contrast 52% of the excess number of SPNs observed among survivors older than 40 years were carcinomas of digestive, genitourinary, respiratory, and breast sites.[3]

A pan-European collaboration has been initiated to exploit the advantages that Europe has relating to the establishment of population-based cancer registration in the Nordic countries and United Kingdom during the 1940s, 1950s, and 1960s, depending on the country. In the PanCare Childhood and Adolescent Cancer Survivor Care and Follow-up Studies (PanCareSurFup) SPN cohort comprises the largest ever assembled SPN cohort comprising 69,460 5-year survivors of cancer diagnosed before age 20 years in 12 European countries within which there was systematic ascertainment of all SPNs diagnosed.[15,16]

There was particular focus on subsequent primary bone, soft tissue sarcoma, digestive and genitourinary cancers because these 4 cancer types account for a substantial proportion of the excess number of SPNs observed in the short and long term. Approximately 300 subsequent primary cancers of each of these 4 types have been included in 4 nested case-control studies (1200 cases in total) to investigate the extent to which cumulative dose of radiation from radiotherapy, cumulative dose of specific cytotoxics, and particular genomic factors extracted from saliva are related to risk of developing specific types of SPN. So far the authors have published the cohort studies relating to bone[17] and soft tissue sarcoma.[18]

Risks of Subsequent Primary Neoplasms After Adolescent and Young Adult Cancer

Large-scale studies of survivors of AYA cancer have tended to focus on risks of SPNs after specific common cancers such as lymphoma, testes, or breast cancer. Only 2 studies have investigated the risks of developing any SPN after each type of AYA cancer. One study was based on Surveillance, Epidemiology and End Results (SEER) registry data and the main finding from this study was that AYA cancer survivors had a higher absolute risk of developing an SPN compared with childhood or mature adult cancer survivors.[19] This study did not investigate the risks of specific SPNs after each AYA cancer.[19] Recently published is the largest ever study to investigate the risks of SPNs after each specific AYA cancer and the first to provide excess risks of specific types of SPN after each of 16 types of AYA cancer, the Teenage and Young Adult Cancer Survivor Study.[20] The Teenage and Young Adult Cancer Survivor Study is a population-based cohort of 200,945 5-year survivors of cancer diagnosed when aged 15 to 39 years in England and Wales from January 1971 to December 2006. During 2,631,326 person-years of follow-up 12,321 SPNs were diagnosed in 11,565 survivors.[20]

The recent publication relating to the Teenage and Young Adult Cancer Survivor Study illustrates 2 key new findings.[20] Firstly, in individuals who survived at least 30 years from diagnosis of cervical cancer, testicular cancer, Hodgkin lymphoma in women, breast cancer, and Hodgkin lymphoma in men, the authors identified a small number of specific SPNs that account for 82%, 61%, 58%, 45%, and 41% of the total excess number of neoplasms, respectively, and provides an evidence base to inform priorities for clinical long-term follow-up.[20] Secondly, lung cancer accounted for a substantial proportion of the excess number of neoplasms across all AYA groups investigated and indicates need for further work aimed at preventing and reducing the risk of this cancer among current and future survivors. This latter finding is in marked contrast to survivors of childhood cancer who do not experience such substantial excess risks of lung cancer, and this may relate to the evidence that survivors of AYA cancer smoke notably in excess of that expected from the general population, and in contrast survivors of childhood cancer smoke much less than that expected from the general population.[20]

SUBSEQUENT PRIMARY NEOPLASM RISK RELATED TO RADIOTHERAPY

Radiotherapy exposure has been recognized as a risk factor for SPNs among childhood cancer survivors for decades. One of the first comprehensive reports on SPNs among childhood cancer survivors demonstrated that most of the SPNs developed in previously irradiated sites.[21]

Breast Cancer

Radiotherapy exposure to the chest is an important risk factor for female breast cancer.[22–25] Recent studies suggest that even at lower absorbed doses to the breast (<20 Gy), breast cancer risk can be substantially elevated,[24,26] especially among survivors who were exposed to a large volume of the breast, such as whole lung irradiation for pulmonary metastases in Wilms tumor or Ewing sarcoma survivors.[24] A linear dose-response relation has been observed in several studies.[22,24,26] Hormonal exposure can modify the radiation-related risk of breast cancer. Survivors who also received radiation to the ovaries were reported to have lower radiation-related breast cancer risks.[22,26] Furthermore, the effect of radiation has been suggested to be stronger when administered near menarche.[8] In addition, there is some recent evidence for a stronger effect of radiation among those who also received anthracyclines.[26]

Sarcoma

Sarcoma risk is increased in childhood cancer survivors and both radiotherapy and chemotherapy have been implicated to contribute to this excess risk.[4,25,27–29] A nested case-control study within the CCSS cohort found a linear dose-response for any sarcoma.[27] Several reports evaluated the radiation dose-response for *bone* sarcoma or *soft tissue* sarcoma specifically. For *bone* sarcoma, an increased risk with increasing dose has been observed.[4,29–31] However, some of these reports suggested a decline in relative risk at doses above 40 Gy.[4,30] Among the studies on *soft tissue* sarcoma, results were consistent with a linear dose-response relationship between radiation dose and risk.[12,28,32] In general, the dose-related risk seemed somewhat higher for *bone* sarcoma than for *soft tissue* sarcoma.[33]

Thyroid Cancer

A pooled analysis, consisting of data from 2 cohort studies and 2 case-control studies among childhood cancer survivors, showed that the relative risk of thyroid cancer increased linearly with radiation dose up to 10 Gy, after which the risk plateaued.[34] At doses higher than 30 Gy, the risk seems to decline, possibly because of cell-killing effects. The dose-response relationship was stronger among those exposed to radiotherapy at a younger age.

Colorectal Cancer

Risk of colorectal cancer has been shown to be elevated among childhood cancer survivors, and abdominal radiotherapy has been implicated as a risk factor.[3,13,35,36] Researchers from the French Childhood Cancer Survivor Cohort and the St Jude Lifetime Cohort (SJL) found a radiation dose-dependent effect on colorectal cancer risk,[13,36] and the results of the SJL study also suggested an effect of radiation volume, as the risk increased with an increasing number of colonic segments irradiated.[36] Cumulative incidence of colorectal cancer was shown to be similar to that among individuals with 2 or more first-degree relatives with colorectal cancer in the British Childhood Cancer Survivor Study.[3]

Central Nervous System Tumors

Central nervous system (CNS) tumors occur in excess among childhood cancer survivors.[10,37,38] Nearly all meningiomas and most of the gliomas present in survivors treated with cranial or craniospinal irradiation for brain tumors or acute lymphoblastic leukemia.[10,37,38] For both gliomas and meningiomas, a linear dose-response relation has been observed, which seems to be stronger for meningioma (range of excess relative risks (ERRs): 0.30–5.1 per Gy)[10,37,38] than for gliomas (range of ERRs: 0.079–0.33 per Gy).[37,38]

Nonmelanoma Skin Cancer

Nonmelanoma skin cancer, particularly basal cell carcinoma, is the most frequently observed SPN among childhood cancer survivors. Most of the basal cell carcinomas occur among previously irradiated patients.[11,39,40] A study in the Dutch LATER cohort observed that basal cell carcinoma risks increased with increasing skin surface area exposed.[11] A nested case-control study in the CCSS cohort demonstrated a linear radiation dose-response relation, with an ERR of 1.09 per Gy.[40]

Salivary Gland Tumors

Salivary gland tumor risks are elevated among childhood cancer survivors and a linear radiation dose-response relation was observed in a study in the CCSS cohort (ERR = 0.36 per Gy).[41]

Leukemia

In addition to the strong effects of chemotherapy on leukemia risk among childhood cancer survivors,[5,42–47] there is some evidence that radiotherapy exposure might add to the increased risk of subsequent leukemia.[5,44]

The results presented earlier mainly represent data from patients with childhood cancer treated decades ago, because those patients have sufficient follow-up time to evaluate risk of SPNs. In recent decades, radiotherapy practices have changed. Where possible, radiotherapy has been avoided or fields and doses have been reduced. For example, technological advances have led to the introduction of new techniques such as intensity-modulated radiotherapy (IMRT) and proton radiotherapy. These techniques aim to reduce the radiotherapy dose to the surrounding tissue, which might reduce the risk of SPNs.[48,49] However, with IMRT, the larger volume exposed to radiation (although at lower dose) can potentially increase SPN risk.[50,51] Proton therapy leads to an improvement in dose distribution by reducing the entrance dose and having virtually no exit dose.[52] However, there are some concerns regarding the secondary dose from neutron scatter with proton therapy, which might lead to an increased SPN risk compared with photon therapy.[53,54] It is important to carefully monitor patients with childhood cancer treated with those modern radiotherapy techniques and evaluate SPN risks in this population.

SUBSEQUENT PRIMARY NEOPLASM RISK RELATED TO CHEMOTHERAPY

Recent work has continued to highlight the independent influence of chemotherapy on the risk of SPNs in childhood cancer survivors. In the CCSS, among survivors exposed to only chemotherapy there was a 2.8-fold increased SPN risk compared with the general population (95% confidence interval [CI]: 2.5–3.2).[55] Chemotherapy increases the risk of both hematologic and solid SPN, depending on type and cumulative dose.

Chemotherapy and Subsequent Hematologic Malignancy

The most well-established association between chemotherapy and SPN relates to therapy-related acute myeloid leukemia (t-AML) and myelodysplastic syndrome (t-MDS).[5] Dose-dependent risks for t-AML/t-MDS are high (>10-fold increased) after almost all alkylating agents and topoisomerase II inhibitors.[5,45,56] Notably, the leukemogenicity of different agents in these chemotherapy families varies substantially, and the absolute excess risk is low due to the low background risk in the age-matched general population. Development of t-AML after alkylating agent exposure typically arises after a latency of 5 to 8 years, is frequently preceded by MDS, and often has a complex karyotype with chromosome 5/7 abnormalities.[5] In contrast, t-AML after topoisomerase II inhibitor exposure typically arises less than 3 years following therapy, is rarely preceded by MDS, and is most frequently characterized by 11q23 rearrangements.[57]

Chemotherapy and Subsequent Solid Tumors

Chemotherapy increases risk for solid SPN, which often occur at least 10 years after exposure.[14] Several classes of chemotherapy directly or indirectly affect the risk of development of these SPNs.

Alkylating agents

Alkylating agent exposures increase risk for gastrointestinal, thyroid, lung, breast, and bladder cancers; melanomas; and sarcomas.[4,29,35,36,55,58–62] Specifically, cyclophosphamide increases sarcoma risk in a dose-dependent manner.[4,25,27,29] Likewise, cyclophosphamide equivalent doses of greater than 18,000 mg/m^2 increase breast cancer risk by 3-fold (SIR, 3.0; 95% CI, 1.2–7.7).[60] Procarbazine and platinum have been associated with 3.2 (95% CI, 1.1–9.4) and 7.6-fold (95% CI, 2.3–25.5) increased risks, respectively, of gastrointestinal SPNs.[35] Procarbazine-related risks for the gastrointestinal tract may be related to direct exposure of the mucosa,[27,36,58] whereas the mechanisms of carcinogenesis for agents administered intravenously are unknown.

Anthracyclines

Risk for breast cancer and other solid malignancies, including sarcoma, are increased after anthracycline exposure.[25,27,60,63] In the CCSS cohort, risk for breast cancer in survivors treated with greater than 250 mg/m^2 of anthracycline and without chest radiotherapy exposure was increased by nearly 4-fold compared with the general population (SIR, 3.8; 95% CI 1.7–8.3).[60] Both the DCOG-LATER cohort and the SJL cohorts reported similar findings. The DCOG-LATER cohort reported a dose-dependent relationship between breast cancer risk and doxorubicin (P_{trend} <0.001).[25] The SJL cohort reported an increasing breast cancer risk in both those exposed to 1 to 249 mg/m^2 (hazard ratio [HR] = 2.6, 95% CI 1.1–6.2, P = .034) and those exposed to greater than 250 mg/m^2 (HR = 13.4, 95% CI 5.5–32.5, P<.001) of anthracyclines.[25,63] In both the CCSS and DCOG-LATER reports, breast cancer risk was highest after Li Fraumeni syndrome–associated cancers, suggesting a possible interaction between chemotherapy and genetic predisposition.[25,60] However, with whole-exome sequencing available in the SJL cohort, the risk of breast cancer remained elevated in survivors exposed to greater than 250 mg/m^2 excluding those survivors with an identified cancer predisposition gene.[63]

Indirect associations of chemotherapy and subsequent primary neoplasm risk

Chemotherapy can indirectly affect SPN risk. In Hodgkin lymphoma survivors,[59,64,65] higher cumulative procarbazine exposure was associated with a greater reduction of breast cancer risk, with 30% and 67% risk reductions for regimens with less than 8.4 g/m^2 and greater than 8.4 g/m^2 procarbazine, respectively.[64,65] This risk reduction seems to reflect the higher frequency of premature menopause in more intensively chemotherapy-treated patients, and their resultant reduced exposure to ovarian hormones.[65–67] Similarly, high cumulative alkylator exposure significantly reduced breast cancer risk in the CCSS cohort,[8] in contrast to earlier CCSS results that did not show a reduced breast cancer risk after alkylator therapy.[23] Breast cancer risk also increases in women with more than 10 years of ovarian function after chest radiotherapy compared with those with less.[8,65,67]

RISK OF SUBSEQUENT PRIMARY NEOPLASM AND GENOMICS

Inherited genetic susceptibility has long been known to play a role in SPN risk based on familial syndromes that predispose individuals to developing multiple primary neoplasms. Indeed, the occurrence of multiple primary tumors in an individual, particularly at a young age, was one of the earliest clues to inherited cancer predisposition syndromes.[68] Key examples of these syndromes include Li Fraumeni syndrome and hereditary retinoblastoma, which are caused by rare, highly penetrant germline mutations in the tumor suppressor genes *TP53* and *RB1*, respectively. In Li Fraumeni syndrome, overall, half of the women develop a first cancer by age 31 years and more than half of the men by age 46 years; of these individuals, approximately half will develop an SPN after a median of 10 years.[69] In contrast, in hereditary retinoblastoma nearly all individuals who inherit a germline mutation develop retinoblastoma in early childhood, typically within the first year of life. More than one-third of individuals are estimated to develop an SPN by age 40 years, although this estimate has been shown to vary by treatment exposure, specific *RB1* mutation, and family history of retinoblastoma.[70–73]

The field of cancer genomics has expanded rapidly in the last decade. Advances in technology and reductions in laboratory costs have now made it possible to broadly interrogate the entire genome using high-throughput microarray genotyping or next-generation sequencing in increasingly larger study populations. These advances are essential for enabling sufficient sample size to identify new disease-associated genes. In the general population, large-scale, international collaborative efforts to study breast cancer exemplify the discoveries that are possible with these new approaches. Genome-wide association studies (GWAS) using microarray genotyping for common single nucleotide polymorphisms have identified greater than 170 loci associated with breast cancer risk.[74] Although each of these individual loci has a very weak effect on risk (relative risks typically <1.2), combining the loci into a polygenic score provides dramatic risk stratification.[75] Large-scale sequencing studies also are demonstrating substantial heterogeneity in breast cancer risk associated with specific, rare mutations in *BRCA1* and *BRCA2*.[76]

Although these advances are only now beginning to be applied to assess genetic susceptibility to SPNs, as reviewed recently,[68,77,78] the future holds tremendous promise for advancing this research area to provide biological insights into SPN development and potentially changing clinical practice through front-line therapy decision-making and risk stratification for long-term patient follow-up. Paralleling research in the general population, most of the earliest studies focused on single nucleotide polymorphisms in candidate genes. However, unlike the general population, where specific exposure-disease relationships rarely have been taken into account in genetic association studies, initial studies in cancer survivors focused on genes in pathways such as DNA repair that mediate response to treatment exposures, which are the primary drivers of SPN risk. Although some of these reports have been promising, few have been replicated in independent study populations, thus further research is needed to clarify the role of common variation in DNA repair genes in SPN risk.

More recently, several GWAS or large-scale genotyping studies have been conducted to identify loci involved in SPN risk after childhood cancer, including SPN overall, therapy-related acute myeloid leukemia, breast cancer, and basal cell carcinoma.[79–83] Those studies each have identified novel putative loci associated with SPN risk, with one study also suggesting that the genetic risk factors for breast cancer as an SPN overlap at least somewhat with those in the general population.[81] Although further replication of these findings will be essential before clinical translation because of the substantial risk of false-positive findings when broadly interrogating the genome, the common frequency of the risk allele for many of the identified variants (2% to >30% of the population) demonstrates the substantial potential for applying these results in clinical practice.

Broader understanding of the role of rare variants in SPN risk also is warranted because they may be associated with high risks, even if they account for a relatively small fraction of SPN. The first large-scale sequencing study of SPN after childhood cancer demonstrated that fewer than 10% of childhood cancer survivors harbor rare, damaging mutations in a known cancer predisposition gene.[84] Ongoing analyses of additional large-scale sequencing studies are expected in the coming years and promise to shed light on the role of rare variants in SPN risk.

ROLE OF SURVEILLANCE, SCREENING, AND CLINICAL FOLLOW-UP GUIDELINES
Rationale for Surveillance

As a consequence of past treatments, behavioral factors such as smoking and alcohol, and host factors such as genetics, specific groups of childhood cancer survivors have a 10-fold increased risk of developing an SPN.[85,86] Given the significant morbidity and risk for premature mortality resulting from SPNs, risk-adapted surveillance protocols have been developed with the goal of detecting SPNs at an earlier and more treatable stage. In other patient groups at high risk of malignancy, such as individuals with cancer predisposition syndromes, adherence to risk-adapted surveillance protocols have been shown to reduce mortality from SPNs.[85–87] The same is assumed to be true for childhood cancer survivors, but this has never been established in a clinical trial.[88] For survivors at elevated SPN risk, surveillance for a given neoplasm is warranted if surveillance modalities exist that do not cause significant morbidity, allow for earlier identification and intervention that might reduce the SPN's impact, and do not cause an excess of false-positive results that lead to unnecessary further testing or intervention.[89,90]

Surveillance Guidelines

Numerous organizations have developed recommendations for SPN surveillance in childhood cancer survivors.[91] Substantial variation exists between guidelines, but as a general principle, periodic follow-up by a physician that includes a history and physical examination focused on evaluation of irradiated structures is warranted for all survivors. There is also a general consensus that breast cancer surveillance is appropriate for female survivors who have received chest irradiation, but the specifics of the required surveillance vary. North American organizations (The Children's Oncology Group and The National Comprehensive Cancer Network) uniquely recommend colorectal cancer surveillance for survivors who have received abdominal and/or pelvic radiation.[92,93] In an attempt to create a common strategy for SPN surveillance, the International Guideline Harmonization Group (IGHG)[94] was formed. The IGHG has published recommendations for breast[95] and thyroid cancer[96] surveillance (available at http://www.ighg.org/) and is currently developing guidelines for CNS and colorectal cancer surveillance as well.

Current Guideline Adherence

Unfortunately, most adult survivors of childhood cancer are not adherent to the recommended SPN surveillance, potentially resulting in preventable morbidity and mortality. In one study of North American survivors enrolled in the CCSS, adherence to SPN surveillance was 12.6%, 37.0%, and 22.3% for breast, colorectal, and skin cancer surveillance, respectively (Yan A and Nathan P, unpublished data, 2019). Survivor reported barriers to surveillance include lack of time, forgetting, a perception that surveillance is not important, concerns about insurance coverage and cost, and lack of physician recommendation for surveillance.[97,98] Psychosocial barriers include poor mental health, lower socioeconomic status, and lower educational level.[99–101] In 2012, only 12% of US general internists[102] and 9% of US and Canadian family doctors[103] felt at least "somewhat familiar" with care guidelines for childhood cancer survivors. A lack of primary care provider comfort with care guidelines likely contributes to poor adherence as well. Regular engagement with the health care system, receipt of a treatment summary, and patient-provider communication discussing the need for surveillance have been associated with better adherence to surveillance guidelines.[104–108]

Mechanisms to Improve Adherence

To address barriers to receiving risk-adapted surveillance, the United States Institute of Medicine and the European collaboration PanCare have recommended that all childhood cancer survivors receive a treatment summary and survivorship care plan (SCP) that documents their cancer treatment–related health risks and the recommended surveillance.[109–111] The impact of SCPs on surveillance outcomes in childhood cancer survivors is unclear.[112] In fact, little is known about how best to increase the completion of recommended surveillance testing. A recent systematic review that evaluated interventions to improve surveillance adherence only identified one randomized trial where the intervention significantly increased SPN surveillance.[98,113] In this trial, mailed information coupled with motivational telephone interviewing increased adherence to mammography in women at risk for subsequent breast cancer.[98] Other interventions that have been tried with less success include motivational telephone counseling, SCP provision, web-based virtual information, and mailing of health risk information.[98,114–116]

Cancer Predisposition Syndromes

In addition to the risk of SPNs as a consequence of cancer therapy, a subset of survivors is at high risk of SPNs secondary to an underlying cancer predisposition syndrome. Nearly 10% of childhood cancer survivors have an actionable germline genetic mutation, making yearly review of family cancer history and subsequent referral to genetics when necessary imperative.[117] Specific guidelines have been created for the more common pediatric cancer predisposition syndromes, such as Li-Fraumeni syndrome[118] and Beckwith Wiedemann syndrome.[119] When no specific recommendations exist for a given syndrome, the American Association of Cancer Research recommends screening for malignancy if effective screening modalities exist and the overall risk exceeds 5% in the first 20 years of life. In addition, they recommend that when the overall risk is between 1% and 5%, screening can be considered on an individual basis.[120]

Summary

Despite the availability of numerous guidelines that guide health care providers in providing surveillance for SPNs in childhood cancer survivors, very few survivors are currently adherent to recommendations, and few interventions have been successful in increasing surveillance. Further studies that develop and test interventions to improve adherence are needed.

PRIORITIES FOR FUTURE RESEARCH
Observational Studies to Address Specific Gaps in Knowledge

Subsequent primary neoplasms in survivors of adolescent and young adult cancer
A large population-based study described the risk of SPN in survivors of AYA cancer, reporting that a small number of specific SPNs account for a large proportion of the overall excess, with a prominence of lung cancer.[20] However, the association between therapeutic exposures and the risk of SPNs after AYA cancer remains unstudied, as does the role of lifestyle factors, which could have greater impact among AYA survivors than among childhood cancer survivors.[20]

Subsequent primary neoplasm risk in patients treated with immunotherapy
Targeted immunotherapy has emerged as an effective treatment option especially in pediatric malignancies.[121,122] Although the early toxicities are clearly described, there remains a significant gap in knowledge regarding the development of delayed complications, especially SPNs. Systematic, long-term follow-up of patients treated with targeted immunotherapy is needed to address this gap.

Solid subsequent primary neoplasm risk in patients treated with chemotherapy
Although the association between radiation and solid SPNs (thyroid, breast, brain, colorectal) is well established,[22,37,123] as is the risk between specific chemotherapeutic agents and therapy-related leukemia, there is emerging evidence regarding the role of adjuvant chemotherapy.[55] For example, treatment with anthracyclines may be a risk factor for thyroid cancer[55,61] and breast cancer.[55] These findings are based on small numbers of SPNs developing after exposure to a specific chemotherapy class. This gap could be addressed by pooling large well-characterized cohorts and case-control studies of survivors.

Subsequent primary neoplasm risk: interaction of behavioral factors or infections with genotoxic exposures
The risk of lung cancer is significantly increased in patients treated for Hodgkin lymphoma. Both chemotherapy and radiation contribute to the risk. Cigarette smoking multiplies the risk associated with both chemotherapy and radiation.[124,125] However, interaction between smoking and therapeutic exposures has not been examined for other types of SPN, such as esophageal, oropharyngeal, and gastric carcinoma. Furthermore, behavioral factors such as excessive alcohol consumption or a diet rich in processed meats has not been examined in this population. Finally, the interaction between chronic viral infections (hepatitis B virus, hepatitis C virus, human papillomavirus, Epstein-Barr virus) and prolonged immune suppression due to genotoxic exposures in increasing the risk of SPNs remains unstudied.

Temporal Changes in Subsequent Primary Neoplasm Risk with Changes in Treatment Strategies

With the decrease in the proportion of patients receiving radiation as well as a progressive reduction in the dose and field of radiation, the relative rates of meningioma and nonmelanoma skin cancers have declined over the past several decades.[9] Additional follow-up using pooled data from other well-characterized cohorts is needed to understand whether the decline in SPNs is limited to just these 2 specific types of SPNs, or whether smaller samples precluded the ability to detect trends for other SPNs, such as breast cancer. Further, these trends need to be placed within the context of increasing use of chemotherapy and changes in surveillance practice. Most importantly, as the cancer survivor population ages, it is important to understand the lifelong risk of SPN and particularly the types of SPNs that account for most of the excess observed later in life.

Identification of Survivors at Highest Risk of Subsequent Primary Neoplasm and Potential for Targeted Interventions

Although the magnitude of association between radiation exposure and SPN risk is moderate-to-large (3.1-fold to 15.9-fold)[126] with clear evidence for a dose-response relationship,[22,37,123] there is wide variation in individual susceptibility, suggesting the role of genetic susceptibility in modifying this association.[32,127–136] Genetic variants may modify the association between radiation and SPN risk or increase the risk of SPNs even in the absence of radiation.[60] Indeed, cancer survivors who carry a deleterious, high-penetrance mutation are at increased risk for SPNs.[132–134,137,138] However, the low frequency of these mutations in the general population[139] suggests that the attributable risk is likely small. The interindividual variability in risk of SPNs is more likely related to common polymorphisms in low-penetrance genes that regulate drug metabolism or those responsible for DNA repair.[140,141] Although there is significant effort currently expended on identifying genetic variants and their association with SPNs, an equally important aspect of this discovery currently lagging involves understanding the functional relevance of the identified genetic variants. Although we can speculate about the relevance of a specific genetic variant, it is critical to delve into the functional aspects of the identified variant in order to understand the mechanistic basis of SPNs; this is critical in order to develop risk-reducing interventions. An equally important, yet underutilized opportunity is the use of demographic, clinical (therapeutic exposures), behavioral, and genetic information to determine the individual risk of SPN. An example is the risk prediction model developed for survivors at risk for radiation-related brain tumors,[142] where the sensitivity and specificity of predicting survivors of childhood cancer at highest or lowest risk of subsequent CNS tumors was 87.5% and 83.5%, respectively.

Radiation continues to serve as a critical backbone of treatment of childhood cancer, and although there may be options to use alternative treatments on a case-by-case basis (for patients at highest risk of SPN), the pediatric oncology community is reluctant to replace radiation with alternative treatments for *all patients*. In addition, among childhood cancer survivors already exposed to radiation, offering screening or behavioral/pharmacologic interventions based on personal risk could be cost-effective and better accepted by the survivor population. Finally, a deeper understanding of the mechanistic basis of radiation-related SPNs would lead us closer to developing targeted interventions.

Screening recommendations for early detection of subsequent primary neoplasms in childhood cancer survivors

The primary goal of risk-based surveillance is to facilitate early detection of treatment-related complications (including SPNs) in childhood cancer survivors.[89,94] However, there is an opportunity to examine the cost-effectiveness of screening recommendations[95,96] that tailor the intensity of screening based on personal SPN risk. Simulation, using Markov health states is currently being used to address cost-effectiveness of breast cancer screening recommendations.[143]

Interventions to reduce subsequent primary neoplasm risk in childhood cancer survivors

Breast cancer, brain tumors, sarcoma, thyroid cancer, and gastrointestinal malignancies constitute most of the non-skin cancer SPNs. All these SPNs are radiation related, with a clear dose-response relationship. Understanding the pathogenesis of each of these tumors could inform specific interventions, which when applied in those at highest risk would significantly improve the efficacy of such an intervention. As an example, Bhatia and colleagues[144] recently completed a pharmacologic intervention for reducing the risk of radiation-related breast SPN in childhood cancer survivors, using a randomized, double-blinded, placebo-controlled trial design. The biological premise is based on the fact that endogenous estrogens play a role in radiation-related breast carcinogenesis.

REFERENCES

1. Reulen RC, Winter DL, Frobisher C, et al. Long-term cause-specific mortality among survivors of childhood cancer. JAMA 2010;304(2):172–9.
2. Armstrong GT, Chen Y, Yasui Y, et al. Reduction in late mortality among 5-year survivors of childhood Cancer. N Engl J Med 2016;374:833–42.
3. Reulen RC, Frobisher C, Winter DL, et al. Long-Term Risks of Subsequent Primary Neoplasms Among Survivors of Childhood Cancer. JAMA 2011;305(22):2311–9.
4. Hawkins MM, Wilson LM, Burton HS, et al. Radiotherapy, alkylating agents, and risk of bone cancer after childhood cancer. J Natl Cancer Inst 1996;88:270–8.
5. Hawkins MM, Wilson LM, Stovall MA, et al. Epipodophyllotoxins, alkylating agents, and radiation and risk of secondary leukaemia after childhood cancer. BMJ 1992;304:951–8.
6. Olsen JH, Moller T, Anderson H, et al. Lifelong cancer incidence in 47,697 patients treated for childhood cancer in the Nordic countries. J Natl Cancer Inst 2009;101:806–13.
7. Turcotte LM, Whitton J, Friedman D, et al. Risk of subsequent neoplasms during the fifth and sixth decades of life in the Childhood Cancer Survivor Cohort. J Clin Oncol 2015;33:3568–75.
8. Moskowitz CS, Chou JF, Sklar CA, et al. Radiation-associated breast cancer and gonadal hormone exposure: a report from the Childhood Cancer Survivor Study. Br J Cancer 2017;117:290–9.
9. Turcotte LM, Liu Q, Yasui Y, et al. Temporal trends in treatment and subsequent neoplasm risk among 5-year survivors of childhood cancer, 1970-2015. JAMA 2017;317:814–24.
10. Kok JL, Teepen JC, van Leeuwen FE, et al. Risk of benign meningioma after childhood cancer in the DCOG-LATER cohort: contributions of radiation dose, exposed cranial volume, and age. Neuro Oncol 2019;21:392–403.
11. Teepen JC, Kok JL, Kremer LC, et al. Long-term risk of skin cancer among childhood cancer survivors: a DCOG-LATER cohort study. J Natl Cancer Inst 2019;111(8):845–53.
12. Menu-Branthomme A, Rubino C, Shamsaldin A, et al. Radiation dose, chemotherapy and risk of soft tissue sarcoma after solid tumours during childhood. Int J Cancer 2004;110:87–93.
13. Allodji RS, Haddy N, Vu-Bezin G, et al. Risk of subsequent colorectal cancers after a solid tumor in childhood: Effects of radiation therapy and chemotherapy. Pediatr Blood Cancer 2019;66:e27495.

14. Turcotte LM, Neglia JP, Reulen RC, et al. Risk, risk factors, and surveillance of subsequent malignant neoplasms in survivors of childhood cancer: a review. J Clin Oncol 2018;36(21):2145–52.

15. Grabow D, Kaiser M, Hjorth L, et al. The PanCareSurFup cohort of 83,333 5-year survivors of childhood cancer: a cohort from 12 European countries. Eur J Epidemiol 2018;33(3):335–49.

16. Byrne J, Alessi D, Allodji RS, et al. The PanCareSurFup consortium: research and guidelines to improve lives for survivors of childhood cancer. Eur J Cancer 2018;103:238–48.

17. Fidler MM, Reulen RC, Winter DL, et al. Risk of subsequent primary bone cancers among 69,460 5-year survivors of childhood and adolescent cancer in Europe. J Natl Cancer Inst 2017;110(2):183–94.

18. Bright CJ, Hawkins MM, Winter DL, et al. Risk of soft-tissue sarcoma among 69,460 5-year survivors of childhood cancer in Europe. J Natl Cancer Inst 2017;110(6):649–60.

19. Lee JS, DuBois SG, Coccia PF, et al. Increased risk of second malignant neoplasms in adolescents and young adults with cancer. Cancer 2016;122(1): 116–23.

20. Bright CJ, Reulen RC, Winter DL, et al. Risk of subsequent primary neoplasms in survivors of adolescent and young adult cancer (Teenage and Young Adult Cancer Survivor Study): a population-based cohort study. Lancet Oncol 2019;20(4): 531–45.

21. Meadows AT, Baum E, Fossati-Bellani F, et al. Second malignant neoplasms in children: an update from the late effects study group. J Clin Oncol 1985;3: 532–8.

22. Inskip PD, Robison LL, Stovall M, et al. Radiation dose and breast cancer risk in the childhood cancer survivor study. J Clin Oncol 2009;27:3901–7.

23. Kenney LB, Yasui Y, Inskip PD, et al. Breast cancer after childhood cancer: a report from the Childhood Cancer Survivor Study. Ann Intern Med 2004;141: 590–7.

24. Moskowitz CS, Chou JF, Wolden SL, et al. Breast cancer after chest radiation therapy for childhood cancer. J Clin Oncol 2014;32:2217–23.

25. Teepen JC, van Leeuwen FE, Tissing WJ, et al. Long-term risk of subsequent malignant neoplasms after treatment of childhood cancer in the DCOG LATER study cohort: role of chemotherapy. J Clin Oncol 2017;35:2288–98.

26. Veiga LH, Curtis RE, Morton LM, et al. Association of breast cancer risk after childhood cancer with radiation dose to the breast and anthracycline use: a report from the childhood cancer survivor study. JAMA Pediatr 2019;173(12): 1171–9.

27. Henderson TO, Rajaraman P, Stovall M, et al. Risk factors associated with secondary sarcomas in childhood cancer survivors: a report from the childhood cancer survivor study. Int J Radiat Oncol Biol Phys 2012;84:224–30.

28. Jenkinson HC, Winter DL, Marsden HB, et al. A study of soft tissue sarcomas after childhood cancer in Britain. Br J Cancer 2007;97:695–9.

29. Tucker MA, D'Angio GJ, Boice JD Jr, et al. Bone sarcomas linked to radiotherapy and chemotherapy in children. N Engl J Med 1987;317:588–93.

30. Le Vu B, de Vathaire F, Shamsaldin A, et al. Radiation dose, chemotherapy and risk of osteosarcoma after solid tumours during childhood. Int J Cancer 1998;77: 370–7.

31. Schwartz B, Benadjaoud MA, Clero E, et al. Risk of second bone sarcoma following childhood cancer: role of radiation therapy treatment. Radiat Environ Biophys 2014;53:381–90.

32. Wong FL, Boice JD Jr, Abramson DH, et al. Cancer incidence after retinoblastoma. Radiation dose and sarcoma risk. JAMA 1997;278:1262–7.

33. Berrington de Gonzalez A, Kutsenko A, Rajaraman P, et al. Sarcoma risk after radiation exposure. Clin Sarcoma Res 2012;2:18.

34. Veiga LH, Lubin JH, Anderson H, et al. A pooled analysis of thyroid cancer incidence following radiotherapy for childhood cancer. Radiat Res 2012;178: 365–76.

35. Henderson TO, Oeffinger KC, Whitton J, et al. Secondary gastrointestinal cancer in childhood cancer survivors: a cohort study. Ann Intern Med 2012;156: 757–66. W-260.

36. Nottage K, McFarlane J, Krasin MJ, et al. Secondary colorectal carcinoma after childhood cancer. J Clin Oncol 2012;30:2552–8.

37. Neglia JP, Robison LL, Stovall M, et al. New primary neoplasms of the central nervous system in survivors of childhood cancer: a report from the Childhood Cancer Survivor Study. J Natl Cancer Inst 2006;98:1528–37.

38. Taylor AJ, Little MP, Winter DL, et al. Population-based risks of CNS tumors in survivors of childhood cancer: the British Childhood Cancer Survivor Study. J Clin Oncol 2010;28:5287–93.

39. Perkins JL, Liu Y, Mitby PA, et al. Nonmelanoma skin cancer in survivors of childhood and adolescent cancer: a report from the childhood cancer survivor study. J Clin Oncol 2005;23:3733–41.

40. Watt TC, Inskip PD, Stratton K, et al. Radiation-related risk of basal cell carcinoma: a report from the Childhood Cancer Survivor Study. J Natl Cancer Inst 2012;104:1240–50.

41. Boukheris H, Stovall M, Gilbert ES, et al. Risk of salivary gland cancer after childhood cancer: a report from the Childhood Cancer Survivor Study. Int J Radiat Oncol Biol Phys 2013;85:776–83.

42. Allard A, Haddy N, Le Deley MC, et al. Role of radiation dose in the risk of secondary leukemia after a solid tumor in childhood treated between 1980 and 1999. Int J Radiat Oncol Biol Phys 2010;78:1474–82.

43. Allodji RS, Schwartz B, Veres C, et al. Risk of subsequent leukemia after a solid tumor in childhood: impact of bone marrow radiation therapy and chemotherapy. Int J Radiat Oncol Biol Phys 2015;93:658–67.

44. Haddy N, Le Deley MC, Samand A, et al. Role of radiotherapy and chemotherapy in the risk of secondary leukaemia after a solid tumour in childhood. Eur J Cancer 2006;42:2757–64.

45. Le Deley MC, Leblanc T, Shamsaldin A, et al. Risk of secondary leukemia after a solid tumor in childhood according to the dose of epipodophyllotoxins and anthracyclines: a case-control study by the Societe Francaise d'Oncologie Pediatrique. J Clin Oncol 2003;21:1074–81.

46. Tucker MA, Meadows AT, Boice JD Jr, et al. Leukemia after therapy with alkylating agents for childhood cancer. J Natl Cancer Inst 1987;78:459–64.

47. Advani PG, Schonfeld SJ, Curtis RE, et al. Risk of therapy-related myelodysplastic syndrome/acute myeloid leukemia after childhood cancer: a population-based study. Leukemia 2019;33:2947–78.

48. Cotter SE, McBride SM, Yock TI. Proton radiotherapy for solid tumors of childhood. Technol Cancer Res Treat 2012;11:267–78.

49. Veldeman L, Madani I, Hulstaert F, et al. Evidence behind use of intensity-modulated radiotherapy: a systematic review of comparative clinical studies. Lancet Oncol 2008;9:367–75.

50. Casey DL, Friedman DN, Moskowitz CS, et al. Second cancer risk in childhood cancer survivors treated with intensity-modulated radiation therapy (IMRT). Pediatr Blood Cancer 2015;62:311–6.

51. Schneider U, Lomax A, Pemler P, et al. The impact of IMRT and proton radiotherapy on secondary cancer incidence. Strahlenther Onkol 2006;182:647–52.

52. Miralbell R, Lomax A, Cella L, et al. Potential reduction of the incidence of radiation-induced second cancers by using proton beams in the treatment of pediatric tumors. Int J Radiat Oncol Biol Phys 2002;54:824–9.

53. Eaton BR, MacDonald SM, Yock TI, et al. Secondary malignancy risk following proton radiation therapy. Front Oncol 2015;5:261.

54. Hall EJ. Intensity-modulated radiation therapy, protons, and the risk of second cancers. Int J Radiat Oncol Biol Phys 2006;65:1–7.

55. Turcotte LM, Liu Q, Yasui Y, et al. Chemotherapy and risk of subsequent malignant neoplasms in the childhood cancer survivor study cohort. J Clin Oncol 2019;37(34):3310–9.

56. Pui CH, Ribeiro RC, Hancock ML, et al. Acute myeloid leukemia in children treated with epipodophyllotoxins for acute lymphoblastic leukemia. N Engl J Med 1991;325(24):1682–7.

57. Pendleton M, Lindsey RH, Felix CA, et al. Topoisomerase II and leukemia. Ann N Y Acad Sci 2014;1310:98–110.

58. Morton LM, Dores GM, Curtis RE, et al. Stomach cancer risk after treatment for Hodgkin Lymphoma. J Clin Oncol 2013;31(27):3369–77.

59. Schaapveld M, Aleman BM, van Eggermond AM, et al. Second cancer risk up to 40 years after treatment for Hodgkin's lymphoma. N Engl J Med 2015;373(26):2499–511.

60. Henderson TO, Moskowitz CS, Chou JF, et al. Breast cancer risk in childhood cancer survivors without a history of chest radiotherapy: a report from the childhood cancer survivor study. J Clin Oncol 2016;34(9):910–8.

61. Veiga LHS, Bhatti P, Ronckers CM, et al. Chemotherapy and thyroid cancer risk: a report from the childhood cancer survivor study. Cancer Epidemiol Biomarkers Prev 2012;21(1):92–101.

62. Travis LB, Gospodarowicz M, Curtis RE, et al. Lung cancer following chemotherapy and radiotherapy for Hodgkin's disease. J Natl Cancer Inst 2002;94(3):182–92.

63. Ehrhardt MJ, Howell CR, Hale K, et al. Subsequent Breast Cancer in Female Childhood Cancer Survivors in the St Jude Lifetime Cohort Study (SJLIFE). J Clin Oncol 2019;37(19):1647–56.

64. Swerdlow AJ, Cooke R, Bates A, et al. Breast cancer risk after supradiaphragmatic radiotherapy for Hodgkin's Lymphoma in England and Wales: A National Cohort Study. J Clin Oncol 2012;30(22):2745–52.

65. De Bruin ML, Sparidans J, van't Veer MB, et al. Breast cancer risk in female survivors of Hodgkin's lymphoma: lower risk after smaller radiation volumes. J Clin Oncol 2009;27(26):4239–46.

66. Cooke R, Jones ME, Cunningham D, et al. Breast cancer risk following Hodgkin lymphoma radiotherapy in relation to menstrual and reproductive factors. Br J Cance 2013;108(11):2399–406.

67. Krul IM, Opstal-van Winden AWJ, Aleman BMP, et al. Breast cancer risk after radiation therapy for hodgkin lymphoma: influence of gonadal hormone exposure. Int J Radiat Oncol Biol Phys 2017;99(4):843–53.

68. Morton LM, Savage SA, Bhatia S, et al. Schottenfeld & Fraumeni: cancer epidemiology & prevention. 4th edition. New York: Oxford University Press; 2017. p. 1155–92.

69. Mai PL, Best AF, Peters JA, et al. Risks of first and subsequent cancers among TP53 mutation carriers in the National Cancer Institute Li-Fraumeni syndrome cohort. Cancer 2016;122(23):3673–81.

70. Dommering CJ, Marees T, van der Hout AH, et al. RB1 mutations and second primary malignancies after hereditary retinoblastoma. Fam Cancer 2012;11:225–33.

71. Kleinerman RA, Yu CL, Little MP, et al. Variation of second cancer risk by family history of retinoblastoma among long-term survivors. J Clin Oncol 2012;30:950–7.

72. Marees T, Moll AC, Imhof SM, et al. Risk of second malignancies in survivors of retinoblastoma: more than 40 years of follow-up. J Natl Cancer Inst 2008;100:1771–9.

73. Marees T, van Leeuwen FE, Schaapveld M, et al. Risk of third malignancies and death after a second malignancy in retinoblastoma survivors. Eur J Cancer 2010;46:2052–8.

74. Michailidou K, Lindstrom S, Dennis J, et al. Association analysis identifies 65 new breast cancer risk loci. Nature 2017;551:92–4.

75. Maas P, Barrdahl M, Joshi AD, et al. Breast cancer risk from modifiable and nonmodifiable risk factors among white women in the United States. JAMA Oncol 2016;2:1295–302.

76. Cline MS, Liao RG, Parsons MT, et al. BRCA challenge: BRCA Exchange as a global resource for variants in BRCA1 and BRCA2. PLoS Genet 2018;14:e1007752.

77. Bhatia S. Genetic variation as a modifier of association between therapeutic exposure and subsequent malignant neoplasms in cancer survivors. Cancer 2015;121:648–63.

78. Gramatges MM, Bhatia S. Evidence for genetic risk contributing to long-term adverse treatment effects in childhood cancer survivors. Annu Rev Med 2018;69:247–62.

79. Sapkota Y, Turcotte LM, Ehrhardt MJ, et al. Genome-wide association study in irradiated childhood cancer survivors identifies HTR2A for subsequent basal cell carcinoma. J Invest Dermatol 2019;139:2042–5.e8.

80. Morton LM, Sampson JN, Armstrong GT, et al. Genome-wide association study to identify susceptibility loci that modify radiation-related risk for breast cancer after childhood cancer. J Natl Cancer Inst 2017;109(11):djx058.

81. Opstal-van Winden AWJ, de Haan HG, Hauptmann M, et al. Genetic susceptibility to radiation-induced breast cancer after Hodgkin lymphoma. Blood 2019;133:1130–9.

82. Knight JA, Skol AD, Shinde A, et al. Genome-wide association study to identify novel loci associated with therapy-related myeloid leukemia susceptibility. Blood 2009;113:5575–82.

83. Best T, Li D, Skol AD, et al. Variants at 6q21 implicate PRDM1 in the etiology of therapy-induced second malignancies after Hodgkin's lymphoma. Nat Med 2011;17:941–3.

84. Wang Z, Wilson CL, Easton J, et al. Genetic risk for subsequent neoplasms among long-term survivors of childhood cancer. J Clin Oncol 2018;36:2078–87.

85. Villani A, Shore A, Wasserman JD, et al. Biochemical and imaging surveillance in germline TP53 mutation carriers with Li-Fraumeni syndrome: 11 year follow-up of a prospective observational study. Lancet Oncol 2016;17(9):1295–305.

86. Koskenvuo L, Pitkaniemi J, Rantanen M, et al. Impact of Screening on Survival in Familial Adenomatous Polyposis. J Clin Gastroenterol 2016;50(1):40–4.

87. Gareth ED, Nisha K, Yit L, et al. MRI breast screening in high-risk women: Cancer detection and survival analysis. Breast Cancer Res Treat 2014;145:663–72.

88. Hodgson DC, Cotton C, Crystal P, et al. Impact of Early Breast Cancer Screening on Mortality Among Young Survivors of Childhood Hodgkin's Lymphoma. J Natl Cancer Inst 2016;108(7):djw010.

89. Landier W, Bhatia S, Eshelman DA, et al. Development of risk based guidelines for pediatric cancer survivors: the Children's Oncology Group Long Term Follow Up Guidelines from the Children's Oncology Group Late Effects Committee and Nursing Discipline. J Clin Oncol 2016;22:4979–90.

90. Barratt A, Irwin L, Glasziou P, et al. How to use guidelines and recommendations about screening. JAMA 1999;281(2):2029–34.

91. Fidler MM, Frobisher C, Hawkins MM, et al. Challenges and opportunities in the care of survivors of adolescent and young adult cancers. Pediatr Blood Cancer 2019;66:e27668.

92. Long-Term Follow-Up Guidelines for Survivors of Childhood, Adolescent and Young Adult Cancers, version 4.0. Available at: http://www.survivorshipguidelines.org. Accessed November 9, 2019.

93. National Comprehensive Cancer Network Clinical Practice Guidelines in Oncology; Adolescent and Young Adult Oncology Version 1.2020. Available at: https://www.nccn.org/professionals/physician_gls/pdf/aya.pdf. Accessed November 9, 2019.

94. Kremer LC, Mulder RL, Oeffinger KC, et al. A worldwide collaboration to harmonize guidelines for the long-term follow-up of childhood and young adult cancer survivors: A report from the International Late Effects of Childhood Cancer Guideline Harmonization Group. Pediatr Blood Cancer 2013;60:543–9.

95. Mulder RL, Kremer LCM, Hudsom MM, et al. Recommendations for breast cancer surveillance for female survivors of childhood, adolescent, and young adult cancer given chest radiation: a report from the International Late Effects of Childhood Cancer Guideline Harmonization Group. Lancet Oncol 2013;14:e621–9.

96. Clement SC, Kremer LCM, Verburg FA, et al. Balancing the benefits and harms of thyroid cancer surveillance in survivors of Childhood, adolescent and young adult cancer: Recommendations from the international Late Effects of Childhood Cancer Guideline Harmonization Group in collaboration with the PanCare-SurFup Consortium. Cancer Treat Rev 2018;63:28–39.

97. Hudson MM, Leisenring W, Stratton KK, et al. Increasing cardiomyopathy screening in at-risk adult survivors of pediatric malignancies: a randomized controlled trial. J Clin Oncol 2014;32(35):3974–81.

98. Oeffinger KC, Ford J, Moskowitz CS, et al. The EMPOWER study: promoting breast cancer screening—a randomized controlled trial (RCT) in the childhood cancer survivor study (CCSS). J Clin Oncol 2016;34(15_suppl):10506.

99. Berg CJ, Stratton E, Esiashvili N, et al. Young adult cancer survivors' experience with cancer treatment and follow-up care and perceptions of barriers to engaging in recommended care. J Cancer Educ 2016;31(3):430–42.

100. Casillas J, Oeffinger KC, Hudson MM, et al. Identifying predictors of longitudinal decline in the level of medical care received by adult survivors of childhood cancer: a report from the childhood cancer survivor study. Health Serv Res 2015; 50(4):1021–42.

101. Nathan PC, Agha M, Pole JD, et al. Predictors of attendance at specialized survivor clinics in a population-based cohort of adult survivors of childhood cancer. J Cancer Surviv 2016;10(4):611–8.

102. Suh E, Daugherty CK, Wroblewski K, et al. General internists' preferences and knowledge about the care of adult survivors of childhood cancer: a cross-sectional survey. Ann Intern Med 2014;160(1):11–7.

103. Nathan PC, Daugherty CK, Wroblewski KE, et al. Family physician preferences and knowledge gaps regarding the care of adolescent and young adult survivors of childhood cancer. J Cancer Surviv 2013;7(3):275–82.

104. Cox CL, Oeffinger KC, Montgomery M, et al. Determinants of mammography screening participation in adult childhood cancer survivors: results from the Childhood Cancer Survivor Study. Oncol Nurs Forum 2009;36(3):335–44.

105. Daniel CL, Kohler CL, Stratton KL, et al. Predictors of colorectal cancer surveillance among survivors of childhood cancer treated with radiation: a report from the Childhood Cancer Survivor Study. Cancer 2015;121(11):1856–63.

106. Baxstrom K, Peterson BA, Lee C, et al. A pilot investigation on impact of participation in a long-term follow-up clinic (LTFU) on breast cancer and cardiovascular screening among women who received chest radiation for Hodgkin lymphoma. Support Care Cancer 2018;26(7):2361–8.

107. Oeffinger KC, Ford JS, Moskowitz CS, et al. Breast cancer surveillance practices among women previously treated with chest radiation for a childhood cancer. JAMA 2009;301(4):404–14.

108. Nathan PC, Ness KK, Mahoney MC, et al. Screening and surveillance for second malignant neoplasms in adult survivors of childhood cancer: a report from the childhood cancer survivor study. J Cancer Surviv 2019;13:713–29.

109. Institute of Medicine and National Research Council. From cancer patient to cancer survivor: lost in transition. Washington, DC: The National Academies Press; 2006. https://doi.org/10.17226/11488.

110. Haupt R, Essiaf S, Dellacasa C, et al. PanCareSurFup, ENCCA Working Group; ExPo-r-Net Working Group. The 'Survivorship Passport' for childhood cancer survivors. Eur J Cancer 2018;102:69–81.

111. Michel G, Mulder RL, van der Pal HJH, et al. Evidence based recommendations for the organization of long-term follow-up care for childhood and adolescent cancer survivors: a report from the PanCareSurFup Guidelines Working Group. J Cancer Surviv 2019;13(5):759–72.

112. Jacobsen PB, DeRosa AP, Henderson TO, et al. Systematic review of the impact of cancer survivorship care plans on health outcomes and health care delivery. J Clin Oncol 2018;36(20):2088–100.

113. Zabih V, Kahane A, O'Neill NE, et al. Interventions to improve adherence to surveillance guidelines in survivors of childhood cancer: a systematic review. J Cancer Surviv 2019;13:713–29.

114. Steele JR, Wall M, Salkowski N, et al. Predictors of risk-based medical follow-up: a report from the childhood cancer survivor study. J Cancer Surviv 2013;7(3): 379–91.

115. Kadan-Lottick NS, Ross WL, Mitchell H-R, et al. Randomized trial of the impact of empowering childhood cancer survivors with survivorship care plans. J Natl Cancer Inst 2018;110:1352–9.

116. Oeffinger KC, Hudson MM, Mertens AC, et al. Increasing rates of breast cancer and cardiac surveillance among high-risk survivors of childhood Hodgkin lymphoma following a mailed, one-page survivorship care plan. Pediatr Blood Cancer 2011;56(5):818–24.
117. Zhang J, Walsh MF, Wu G, et al. Germline mutations in predisposition genes in pediatric cancer. N Engl J Med 2015;373:2336–46.
118. Kratz CP, Achatz MI, Brugieres L, et al. Cancer screening recommendations for individuals with Li-Fraumeni syndrome. Clin Cancer Res 2017;23(11):e38–45.
119. Kalish JM, Doros L, Lee J, et al. Surveillance recommendations for children with overgrowth syndromes and predisposition to Wilms tumors and hepatoblastoma. Clin Cancer Res 2017;23(11):e115–22.
120. Brodeur GM, Nichols KE, Plon SE, et al. Pediatric cancer predisposition and surveillance: an overview, and a tribute to Alfred G. Knudson JR. Clin Cancer Res 2017;23(11):e1–5.
121. Majzner RG, Heitzeneder S, Mackall CL. Harnessing the Immunotherapy Revolution for the Treatment of Childhood Cancers. Cancer Cell 2017;31:476–85.
122. Mackall CL, Merchant MS, Fry TJ. Immune-based therapies for childhood cancer. Nat Rev Clin Oncol 2014;11:693–703.
123. Bhatti P, Veiga LH, Ronckers CM, et al. Risk of second primary thyroid cancer after radiotherapy for a childhood cancer in a large cohort study: an update from the childhood cancer survivor study. Radiat Res 2010;174:741–52.
124. Lorigan P, Radford J, Howell A, et al. Lung cancer after treatment for Hodgkin's lymphoma: a systematic review. Lancet Oncol 2005;6:773–9.
125. van Leeuwen FE, Klokman WJ, Stovall M, et al. Roles of radiotherapy and smoking in lung cancer following Hodgkin's disease. J Natl Cancer Inst 1995;87:1530–7.
126. Friedman DL, Whitton J, Leisenring W, et al. Subsequent neoplasms in 5-year survivors of childhood cancer: the Childhood Cancer Survivor Study. J Natl Cancer Inst 2010;102:1083–95.
127. Limacher JM, Frebourg T, Natarajan-Ame S, et al. Two metachronous tumors in the radiotherapy fields of a patient with Li-Fraumeni syndrome. Int J Cancer 2001;96:238–42.
128. Birch JM, Alston RD, McNally RJ, et al. Relative frequency and morphology of cancers in carriers of germline TP53 mutations. Oncogene 2001;20:4621–8.
129. Talwalkar SS, Yin CC, Naeem RC, et al. Myelodysplastic syndromes arising in patients with germline TP53 mutation and Li-Fraumeni syndrome. Arch Pathol Lab Med 2010;134:1010–5.
130. Kleinerman RA, Tucker MA, Tarone RE, et al. Risk of new cancers after radiotherapy in long-term survivors of retinoblastoma: an extended follow-up. J Clin Oncol 2005;23:2272–9.
131. Draper GJ, Sanders BM, Kingston JE. Second primary neoplasms in patients with retinoblastoma. Br J Cancer 1986;53:661–71.
132. Sharif S, Ferner R, Birch JM, et al. Second primary tumors in neurofibromatosis 1 patients treated for optic glioma: substantial risks after radiotherapy. J Clin Oncol 2006;24:2570–5.
133. Bhatia S, Chen Y, Wong FL, et al. Subsequent Neoplasms After a Primary Tumor in Individuals With Neurofibromatosis Type 1. J Clin Oncol 2019;37:3050–8.
134. Swift M, Morrell D, Massey RB, et al. Incidence of cancer in 161 families affected by ataxia-telangiectasia. N Engl J Med 1991;325:1831–6.

135. Bernstein JL, Haile RW, Stovall M, et al. Radiation exposure, the ATM Gene, and contralateral breast cancer in the women's environmental cancer and radiation epidemiology study. J Natl Cancer Inst 2010;102:475–83.

136. Brooks JD, Teraoka SN, Reiner AS, et al. Variants in activators and downstream targets of ATM, radiation exposure, and contralateral breast cancer risk in the WECARE study. Hum Mutat 2012;33:158–64.

137. Travis LB, Demark Wahnefried W, Allan JM, et al. Aetiology, genetics and prevention of secondary neoplasms in adult cancer survivors. Nat Rev Clin Oncol 2013;10:289–301.

138. Olsen JH, Hahnemann JM, Borresen-Dale AL, et al. Breast and other cancers in 1445 blood relatives of 75 Nordic patients with ataxia telangiectasia. Br J Cancer 2005;93:260–5.

139. Allan JM. Genetic susceptibility to radiogenic cancer in humans. Health Phys 2008;95:677–86.

140. Kalow W, Ozdemir V, Tang BK, et al. The science of pharmacological variability: an essay. Clin Pharmacol Ther 1999;66:445–7.

141. Evans WE, McLeod HL. Pharmacogenomics–drug disposition, drug targets, and side effects. N Engl J Med 2003;348:538–49.

142. Wang X, Sun CL, Hageman L, et al. Clinical and genetic risk prediction of subsequent cns tumors in survivors of childhood cancer: a report from the COG AL-TE03N1 Study. J Clin Oncol 2017;35:3688–96.

143. Furzer J, Tessier L, Hodgson D, et al. Cost-utility of early breast cancer surveillance in survivors of thoracic radiation-treated adolescent Hodgkin lymphoma. J Natl Cancer Inst 2020;112(1):63–70.

144. Bhatia S, Palomares M, Hageman L, et al. Low-Dose Tamoxifen (LDTam) As a Breast Cancer (BC) Risk-Reduction Strategy in Lymphoma Survivors Exposed to Chest Radiation Therapy (RT) during adolescence/young adulthood – a randomized, placebo- controlled double blinded phase IIb trial. Blood 2019; 134(Issue supplement_1):2843.

Cardiovascular and Pulmonary Challenges After Treatment of Childhood Cancer

Henk Visscher, MD, PhD[a,b,*], Maria Otth, MD[c,d],
E.A.M. (Lieke) Feijen, PhD[b], Paul C. Nathan, MD, MSc[e],
Claudia E. Kuehni, MD[c,f]

KEYWORDS

- Late effects • Childhood cancer survivor • Cardiovascular • Pulmonary

KEY POINTS

- Cardiovascular disease and pulmonary disease are the second leading nonrecurrence causes of death in childhood cancer survivors.
- Anthracyclines and radiotherapy to heart, head, and neck cause substantial cardiovascular disease, in particular, congestive heart failure, ischemic and valvular heart disease, and stroke.
- Bleomycin, busulfan, nitrosoureas, chest radiation, and lung surgery are the main contributors to pulmonary disease.
- Prevention and regular screening according to established are crucial because treatment options are limited once disease becomes clinically manifest.
- Childhood cancer survivors should be encouraged to adopt healthy lifestyles (exercise, healthy diet, and no smoking) and modifiable risk factors should be addressed.

INTRODUCTION

Both cardiovascular disease and pulmonary disease occur with increased frequency in childhood cancer survivors (CCSs), although both might not become apparent until many years after treatment.[1] These late effects of cancer therapy can vary from subclinical to life threatening and can substantially increase mortality and morbidity. After

[a] Division of Haematology/Oncology, Hospital for Sick Children, 555 University Avenue, Toronto, Ontario M5G 1X8, Canada; [b] Princess Máxima Center for Pediatric Oncology, Heidelberglaan 25, Utrecht 3584 CS, The Netherlands; [c] Childhood Cancer Research Platform, Institute of Social and Preventive Medicine, University of Bern, Mittelstrasse 43, Bern 3012, Switzerland; [d] Division of Hematology-Oncology, Department of Pediatrics, Kantonsspital Aarau, Switzerland; [e] AfterCare Program, Division of Haematology/Oncology, Hospital for Sick Children, 555 University Avenue, Toronto, Ontario M5G 1X8, Canada; [f] Department of Pediatrics, Inselspital, Bern University Hospital, University of Bern, Mittelstrasse 43, Bern 3012, Switzerland
* Corresponding author. Princess Maxima Center for Pediatric Oncology, Heidelberglaan 25, Utrecht 3584 CS, The Netherlands.
E-mail address: h.visscher-6@prinsesmaximacentrum.nl

Pediatr Clin N Am 67 (2020) 1155–1170
https://doi.org/10.1016/j.pcl.2020.07.007
0031-3955/20/© 2020 Elsevier Inc. All rights reserved.

subsequent malignancies, cardiovascular disease and pulmonary disease are the leading nonrecurrence causes of death in CCSs.[2–4]

In particular, there is a 5-fold to 10-fold increase in mortality due to cardiovascular disease (CVD),[2–4] which is in large part due to the 5-fold to 15-fold increased risk of congestive heart failure (CHF)[5] and more than 10-fold increased risk of ischemic heart disease and stroke.[6] Similarly, the risk of death from a pulmonary event is 7-times to 14-times higher in CCSs compared with the general population,[2,7,8] and hospitalization due to respiratory conditions is 2-times to 5-times higher in survivors.[9–11]

The purpose of this review is to describe the current knowledge of cardiac and pulmonary late effects, including risk factors, early detection, possible treatments, and opportunities for prevention.

CARDIOVASCULAR DISEASE

CVD after childhood cancer usually manifests as left ventricular (LV) systolic dysfunction/heart failure, ischemic (coronary artery) heart disease, or stroke.[1,12–15] Patients, however, also can develop pericardial disease, arrhythmias, or valvular and peripheral vascular dysfunction.[13,16] Both chemotherapy and radiotherapy can contribute to these conditions either alone or in combination. For example, in a study of 5845 CCSs, those who received both cardiotoxic chemotherapy and radiotherapy involving the heart (7%) had a cumulative incidence of heart failure 40 years after diagnosis of 28%, whereas patients who received only cardiotoxic chemotherapy or only radiotherapy involving the heart had cumulative incidence of 11% and 3%, respectively.[17]

Risk Factors and Pathophysiology

The increased risk of CVD in CCSs is due mainly to exposure to anthracyclines and radiotherapy involving the heart.[4–6,13,18] Other conventional chemotherapeutic drugs, radiotherapy to head and neck, and a growing list of newer targeted agents that increasingly are used in children, however, all can affect this risk **(Table 1)**.[4,6,13,15,16,18–21] In addition, standard risk factors for CVD, such as hypertension, dyslipidemia, diabetes mellitus, and obesity, many of which are more prevalent in CCSs, contribute to the increased CVD risk.[22–24]

Conventional chemotherapy

Anthracyclines (eg, doxorubicin, daunorubicin, idarubicin, and epirubicin), including the anthraquinone, mitoxantrone, commonly are used to treat a variety of childhood cancers and have been known for several decades to cause dose-dependent cardiotoxicity that can range from subclinical, with only mildly reduced shortening fraction,[25,26] to severe overt clinical heart failure.[13,17,27]

Anthracycline cardiotoxicity (ACT) historically has been described based on the time of onset, which can be acute, early (within the first year of treatment), or late (after the first year). Although early-onset ACT can resolve without intervention, some patients continue to have LV systolic dysfunction, which might be progressive, whereas others develop late-onset ACT after a latency period free of symptoms, suggesting this might be a continuum rather than clearly different entities and that additional myocardial injury or stress might contribute to developing later symptoms.[28–30]

The effects of anthracyclines are dose dependent and increase over time with CCSs who received a cumulative doxorubicin-equivalent dose greater than or equal to 250 mg/m^2, having a 30-year follow-up cumulative incidence of CHF of 8% to 13%.[17,27] Not all anthracyclines are equally cardiotoxic, with mitoxantrone carrying the highest risk for CHF and hence the conversion into doxorubicin equivalents.[31]

Table 1
List of treatments for childhood cancer associated with cardiovascular disease

Treatment Modality	Late Effect/Disease	References
Chemotherapy		
Anthracyclines (eg, doxorubicin, daunorubicin, idarubicin, and mitoxantrone)	LV systolic dysfunction/heart failure, pericardial disease, and arrhythmia	5,13,17,25–28
Alkylators (eg, cyclophosphamide, carmustine, lomustine, and ifosfamide)	Stroke, LV systolic dysfunction/heart failure, pericardial disease, and arrhythmias	6,15–17,19,27,35–37
Antimetabolites (eg, cytarabine and 5-Fluorouracil)	Pericardial disease, arrhythmias, ischemic heart disease, and heart failure	16,35
Platinums (eg, cisplatin)	Stroke, arrhythmias, vascular disease, and ischemic heart disease	6,16,35
Vinca alkaloids (eg, vincristine and vinblastine)	Ischemic heart disease	4,38
Radiotherapy		
Chest (heart)	Ischemic heart disease, valvular disease, pericardial disease, arrhythmia, and heart failure	5,6,13,17,27
Head/neck	Stroke	6,15,19,37
New targeted agents		
BCR-ABL TKIs (eg, imatinib, dasatinib, and ponatinib)	LV systolic dysfunction/heart failure, arrhythmias, ischemic heart disease, stroke, and vascular disease	39
Immune checkpoint inhibitors (eg, nivolumab, ipilimumab, and pembrolizumab)	Myocarditis and heart failure	21,40
Proteasome inhibitors (eg, bortezomib)	Heart failure, ischemic heart disease, and arrythmias	20
VEGF inhibitors or TKIs with anti-VEGF activity (eg, bevacizumab and sorafenib)	Vascular disease, ischemic heart disease, stroke, and cardiomyopathy/heart failure	20,41

Patients who were younger during the exposure and, although not consistently, female, also seem to be at higher risk.[5,17,27]

Despite being studied extensively, the exact mechanism of anthracycline toxicity has not been fully unraveled. Many preclinical studies have focused on redox cycling of anthracyclines and generation of reactive oxygen species (ROS), with cardiomyocytes particularly susceptible to ROS,[32] whereas others have found mitochondrial iron accumulation to be involved.[33] Another important mediator of ACT is topoisomerase IIb (Top2b): cardiomyocyte-specific deletion of this gene, which is one of the forms of topoisomerase 2, the presumed cellular target of doxorubicin, protects mice from doxorubicin cardiotoxicity.[34] Several of genetic risk factors for ACT that have been found (discussed later) are in genes related to ROS and iron metabolism or that interact with Top2b.

Alkylators are another large group of drugs commonly used in childhood cancer or hematopoietic stem cell transplantation (HSCT), some of which have been associated with different types of CVD. Most of these toxicities initially were reported in adults but can occur in children.[16,35] In particular, cyclophosphamide at higher doses, such as in myeloablative HSCT conditioning, can cause acute myocarditis with subsequent LV systolic dysfunction and acute CHF, although most patients recover.[16,35] Similarly, ifosfamide can cause CHF as well as arrhythmias. More recently, cyclophosphamide, but not ifosfamide, was found to be associated with CHF in long-term CCSs.[17] Another study linked cyclophosphamide to pericardial disease, but not CHF.[27] Alkylators also were associated with a higher risk of stroke,[6,19,36] although this might be limited to certain subgroups, such as patients with brain tumors.[15,19,37]

Case reports in adults have noted pericarditis, arrhythmias, and CHF after high doses of the antimetabolite cytarabine.[35] While cytarabine frequently is used in children, it is unclear how often, if at all, cardiotoxicities occur and what the long-term outcomes are. Similarly, the antimetabolite 5-fluorouracil, although used only occasionally in children, has been linked to ischemic heart disease, arrhythmias, and heart failure, including in some pediatric case reports.[16]

Platinums, specifically cisplatin, have been found to cause arrhythmias, possibly through electrolyte disturbances.[35] In addition, vascular dysfunction, either through vasospasm or endothelial damage and platelet aggregation, can lead to myocardial infarction and stroke.[6,16,35]

Vinca alkaloids, such as vincristine and vinblastine, seem to increase risk for ischemic heart disease in adults.[38] Results in CCSs are more conflicting; one study found an increased risk of cardiovascular death after vinca alkaloid exposure,[4] whereas others failed to find such an association[13,17] or found even lower risk of myocardial infarction.[27] Possibly, the increased CVD death could be due to the often concomitant exposure to alkylators.[4]

Radiotherapy

Radiation involving the heart has been known for decades to cause ischemic heart disease and pericardial and valvular disease, and radiotherapy also can increase the risk of anthracycline-induced heart failure.[5,6,13,17,27] Arrhythmias also are common but might occur only after longer follow-up. These effects also are dose dependent, with patients treated with higher doses, in particular those greater than or equal to 35 Gy, at highest risk.[5,6,27]

Radiation to head and neck both has been consistently associated with stroke in CCSs, including transient ischemic attacks, cerebral infarction, and intracranial hemorrhage.[6,15,19,37] Again, this effect is dose-dependent, with patients receiving greater than or equal to 30 Gy to the brain at highest risk, in particular patients treated for brain tumors.[6,19] The risk of stroke increases over time and can be as high as 20% in high risk patients by age 50.[6,15,19] The toxic effect of radiotherapy is presumed to be through the cerebral vasculature, with radiation causing an inflammatory response in the vessel wall, leading to luminal narrowing and weakening of the wall that can over time result in occlusion or hemorrhage.[14]

New targeted agents

Better understanding of the biology and molecular pathways involved in cancers has led to the discovery and use of many new targeted agents, which have revolutionized the treatment of some cancers. Although these agents were developed against cancer-specific molecules or aberrant pathways, many have specific toxicities both on-target/off-tumor (target also expressed elsewhere) as well as off-target (drug not specific for the target), including the cardiovascular system.[20] Because some of these agents increasingly are used in children, the long-term impact of these toxicities in

CCSs needs to be considered, especially because these agents are given in addition to conventional treatments.[21]

BCR-ABL–directed tyrosine kinase inhibitors (TKIs), such as imatinib, but also the newer dasatinib and ponatinib, commonly are used in pediatric Philadelphia (Ph)-positive acute lymphoblastic leukemia (ALL) and chronic myelogenous leukemia (CML) and block the BCR-ABL fusion gene kinase. Newer TKIs, especially, have been associated with a variety of CVD toxicities, including LV dysfunction/cardiomyopathy, ischemic heart disease, stroke, and vascular disease.[39] Although they were developed primarily for targeting BCR-ABL, they are multikinase inhibitors that also affect kinases in the cardiovascular system, in particular vascular endothelial growth factor (VEGF) (discussed later), which might explain this toxicity.[39] Because some patients require long-term treatment with TKIs (eg, CML and Ph + ALL), these toxicities are becoming more important.

Immune checkpoint inhibitors restore antitumor immunity by blocking inhibitory signals or receptors on tumors or immune cells, such as PD-1, PD-L1 or CTLA-4.[40] Commonly used drugs in adults, such as nivolumab, ipilimumab, and pembrolizumab, are studied and used in children.[21] Blocking the inhibitory pathways, however, can shift the balance toward autoimmunity, including myocarditis with associated heart failure, which carries a high fatality rate.[40]

Proteasome inhibitors have been found to cause heart failure, ischemic heart disease, and arrythmias, although this risk might be lower for bortezomib, which is used for pediatric relapsed or refractory ALL.[20]

VEGF inhibitors or TKIs with anti-VEGF activity can have various cardiovascular toxic effects similar to BCR-ABL–directed TKIs. VEGF inhibitors, such as bevacizumab, used in certain central nervous system tumors (eg, gliomas), inhibit tumor angiogenesis by directly blocking VEGF, whereas the anti-VEGF effect of TKIs, including FLT3 inhibitors, such as sorafenib, used in certain high-risk acute myelogenous leukemia patients, is off-target.[41] Cardiovascular toxicity include thromboembolic events leading to ischemic heart disease, stroke, and cardiomyopathy with heart failure, which is mediated partly through an increased risk of hypertension.[20,41] These toxicities are important in CCSs, especially for acute myelogenous leukemia patients, who often receive anthracyclines and FLT3 inhibitors.

Genetic risk factors

In addition to exposure to specific therapies, certain germline genetic variations also have been found to modify CVD risk, in particular for ACT. Studies that focused specifically on ACT in CCSs have found variants in genes related to anthracycline transport and metabolism ($SLC28A3$,[42,43] $UGT1A6$,[42,43] $CBR3$,[44,45] $SLC22A7$,[46] $SLC22A17$,[46] and $ABCC5$[47]), iron metabolism (HFE[48]), oxidative stress (CAT,[49] $GSTP1$,[50] $NOS3$,[47] and $HAS3$[51]), hypertension ($PLCE1$[52] and $ATP2B1$[52]), cardiac physiology or structure ($HAS3$,[51] $CELF4$,[53] $GPR35$,[54] and TTN[55]), and DNA damage ($RARG$[56]). Some variants have been replicated in multiple cohorts, whereas others have not, and the functional consequences of these variants have been explored only partly.[57]

Diagnosis, Surveillance, Treatment, and Prevention

Echocardiography remains the mainstay for screening and diagnosis of cardiac disease in CCSs, in particular for LV dysfunction after anthracyclines and chest radiotherapy, measuring shortening or ejection fraction.[58] Echocardiography also can diagnose valvular abnormalities, diastolic dysfunction, and pericardial disease. When more sensitive parameters, such as global longitudinal strain, are used, echocardiography can detect more subclinical systolic dysfunction than by measuring ejection fraction alone.[59] Cardiac magnetic resonance imaging is even more sensitive but also more costly and not readily available in every center.[58] Imaging to detect vascular or cerebrovascular disease are not used routinely to screen asymptomatic CCSs.

Currently, international harmonized guidelines provide recommendations for screening for cardiomyopathy in CCSs using echocardiography.[58] Further refinement of risk for CVD using clinical risk factors[5,6] or incorporating genetic variants[60] might aid to decide which CCSs to screen and how often, thereby likely improving screening cost effectiveness.[58,61,62]

Electrocardiography at baseline is recommended by most CCS long-term follow-up guidelines,[61,62] but its role to detect conduction abnormalities in asymptomatic CCSs is unclear.[63]

Cardiac biomarkers, such as troponins or the N-terminal prohormone of brain natri-uretic peptide, have been studied extensively in CCSs, but although elevations of these markers during treatment might predict long-term LV dysfunction, their role for screening asymptomatic survivors is limited due to their low sensitivity.[58,64] These markers may be used to monitor or screen symptomatic patients similar to the general population.[58]

Prevention

To prevent cardiovascular toxicities from occurring, treatment protocols have evolved over time, reducing, omitting, or replacing certain chemotherapeutic agents and radio-therapy without affecting cancer treatment outcome. For example, maximum cumula-tive doses for anthracyclines are recommended in many protocols, and radiotherapy has been successfully reduced in the treatment of Hodgkin disease.[16] Risk prediction models might identify patients who will benefit most from these preventative mea-sures.[5,6,57,60] Newer radiation techniques, including intensity-modulated radiation therapy or proton therapy, might further reduce the harmful effects to cardiovascular structures.[16] Cardioprotective agents, specifically dexrazoxane, have been studied extensively, and dexrazoxane seems to reduce ACT without affecting antitumor effi-cacy or increasing secondary malignancies.[65]

Secondary prevention, aimed at preventing CVD after treatment exposures, relies in part on screening and early detection of subclinical disease to initiate pharmaco-logic treatment, as discussed previously for heart failure. In adult cancer survivors, the combination of angiotensin-converting enzyme (ACE) inhibitors and β-blockers was shown to help recover cardiac function after early detection of LV dysfunction, even in asymptomatic survivors.[30] Although the role of pre-emptive heart failure treatment in asymptomatic CCSs is less clear, it still is employed often.[16,66] Other strategies focus on targeting modifiable risk factors, such as hypertension, dyslipi-demia, diabetes mellitus, obesity, and adopting a healthy lifestyle (ie, regular exer-cise, healthy diet, and no smoking),[16,24] which have been incorporated in survivor guidelines.[61,62]

Treatment

Treatment of CVD in CCSs depends on the type of disease and usually is managed similar to the general population.[16] Childhood Cancer Survivors patients with heart failure commonly are treated with ACE inhibition often in combination with β-blockers, although the evidence in children is scarce.[16,67,68] Once symptoms occur, heart func-tion can rapidly decline and become refractory to treatment necessitating mechanical support or heart transplant.[16]

PULMONARY DISEASE

Pulmonary disease is another important long-term complication in CCSs with high morbidity and mortality. It is due to a range of pulmonary conditions, such as fibrosis, emphysema, recurrent pneumonia, or chronic cough, that affects survivors throughout their life and increases in frequency with longer time elapsed from cancer treatment.[1,69,70]

Risk Factors and Pathophysiology

Several important treatment modalities, such as bleomycin, busulfan, lomustine (CCNU) or carmustine (BCNU), radiation of the thorax, and surgery to the lung or chest wall, impart a risk of pulmonary damage. Patients after HSCT are at particular risk because their treatment often incorporates more than one treatment-related risk factor. Unlike in CVD, no studies have systematically investigated genetic risk factors for pulmonary toxicity.

Chemotherapy

For most categories of chemotherapeutic agents and their combinations, reports of chemotherapy-induced lung injuries have been published, although often only as case reports or case series. Consistent and robust evidence for pulmonary toxicity is available for bleomycin, busulfan, and nitrosoureas (BCNU and CCNU).[71–73]

Bleomycin is used to treat Hodgkin lymphoma and germ cell tumors. The lung is vulnerable to this agent because it lacks the bleomycin-inactivating enzyme bleomycin hydrolase. This leads to free radical formation and oxidative damage to lung tissues. Subsequent inflammatory processes eventually cause alveolar damage, hypersensitivity reaction, pneumonitis, and pulmonary fibrosis (**Table 2**). Reported prevalence of bleomycin-induced pneumonitis (BIP) ranges from 0% to 46%. BIP usually develops during treatment, resulting in cough, dyspnea, and fever.[74] Data on long-term prognosis after BIP are inconsistent. One review concluded that radiographic changes and lung function abnormalities usually resolve completely.[74] However, 2 studies that assessed lung function by spirometry, body plethysmography, and measurement of diffusion capacity for carbon monoxide (DLCO) in children, 2 years and 4 years after exposure to bleomycin, found that 41% and 52% of children, respectively, had pathologic test results at these time points.[75,76] The toxicity is dose dependent and more common with doses greater than 400 U/m^2, which seldom are used in pediatrics. Simultaneous or subsequent radiotherapy to the lung, exposure to elevated oxygen concentrations, renal dysfunction, smoking, and higher age at treatment may exacerbate bleomycin toxicity.[72,74,77]

Busulfan is an alkylating agent used mainly to condition children before autologous or allogeneic HSCT. The exact mechanism of lung injury is unknown, and the dose-response relationship is unclear. It seems, however, that cumulative doses less than 500 mg do not cause pulmonary injury in adults.[72,73,78] As with bleomycin, concomitant irradiation may magnify the toxic effect of busulfan.[72]

Nitrosoureas, including CCNU and BCNU, mainly are used to treat brain tumors and to condition patients for autologous HSCT. Nitrosoureas are risk factors for pneumonitis and pulmonary fibrosis (see **Table 2**). Pulmonary fibrosis usually develops slowly over years or decades with asymptomatic periods of various length.[79] In nitrosourea-induced pulmonary fibrosis, inflammatory reactions followed by depletion of type I pneumocytes and hyperplasia of type II pneumocytes lead to increased collagen deposition.[80] Higher cumulative doses are associated with increasing risk of lung injury. Patients exposed to thoracic irradiation may develop lung injury at lower doses of nitrosoureas than those not exposed.[72,73,81] A case series followed 17 long-term

Table 2
List of treatments for childhood cancer associated with pulmonary disease

Treatment Modality	Late Effect/Disease	References
Chemotherapy		
Bleomycin	Acute respiratory distress syndrome Interstitial or hypersensitivity pneumonitis Bronchiolitis obliterans organizing pneumonia Pulmonary veno-occlusive disease Pulmonary fibrosis	72–76
Busulfan	Acute respiratory distress syndrome Alveolar proteinosis Pulmonary fibrosis	72,73,78
Nitrosoureas (carmustine, and lomustine)	Hypersensitivity pneumonitis Alveolitis Pulmonary veno-occlusive disease Pulmonary fibrosis	72,73,79,81,82
Radiotherapy to the chest	Bronchiolitis obliterans organizing pneumonia Interstitial pneumonitis Impaired chest wall growth Pulmonary fibrosis	71–73,83,84
Surgery		
(eg, pulmonary lobectomy, pulmonary wedge resection, pulmonary metastasectomy, and chest wall resection)	Restrictive lung function impairment Scoliosis Chest wall deformity	72,85
Stem cell transplantation		
Lung toxic agents used for conditioning	See Busulfan and Nitrosoureas	
Transplant-specific noninfectious pulmonary complications	IPS BOS Bronchiolitis obliterans organizing pneumonia DAH	72,86,87

brain tumor survivors treated with high-dose BCNU and spinal irradiation (n = 12) for up to 25 years. Half (53%) of the survivors died of pulmonary fibrosis, whereas all 7 patients who were still alive after 25 years of follow-up showed radiologic and physiologic (ie, lung function) evidence of pulmonary fibrosis.[79,82]

Radiotherapy

Direct irradiation of the lung, but also scattered radiation after radiotherapy to the chest wall, abdomen, or spine, increases the risk for pulmonary damage. Radiation can lead to DNA strand breaks and trigger lung injury by starting a cascade of inflammatory reactions, with capillary leaks and alveolar and interstitial exudate, which later organizes into collagen. Acute radiation pneumonitis usually develops within 6 weeks to 3 months after radiotherapy (see **Table 2**). The most frequent symptoms are dyspnea and cough. Although early stages of radiation pneumonitis can be self-limited and resolve completely, most patients develop progressive fibrosis.[80] Toxicity due to radiation depends on the irradiated lung volume; total dose; method of irradiation, such as dose fraction; and application of radiosensitizer. At least 10% of the lung volume has to be irradiated to produce significant toxicity. Radiation pneumonitis rarely develops in cases of fractionated radiotherapy with a total dose less than 20 Gy, but is common if the cumulative dose exceeds 40 Gy to 60 Gy.[71,73,83,84]

Surgery
Extensive pulmonary and chest wall surgery can alter pulmonary function.[85] Lobectomy or resection of multiple metastases leads to reduced lung volumes. Removal of ribs or part of the chest wall can cause restrictive ventilation impairment due to a reduction in expansibility of the chest wall.

Hematopoietic stem cell transplantation
Children treated with HSCT face transplant-specific pulmonary complications and late effects, in addition to those discussed previously. Approximately 37% of patients after HSCT develop pulmonary complications.[86] Pulmonary complications are divided in infectious and noninfectious, depending on the underlying cause. The noninfectious complications generally are transplant-specific, such as bronchiolitis obliterans syndrome (BOS), diffuse alveolar hemorrhage (DAH), and idiopathic pneumonia syndrome (IPS) (see **Table 2**). DAH and IPS typically present with an acute onset of respiratory failure within the first 30 days and 120 days after HSCT, respectively.[86] Both diseases have a high mortality, but no data on long-term outcomes exist.[86] BOS typically is diagnosed greater than 100 days after transplantation.[86,87] The main symptoms of BOS are dry cough and dyspnea. BOS has a variable clinical course, but most patients have slowly progressive airflow obstruction. Stabilization or improvement of lung function is rare.[87]

Diagnosis, Surveillance, Treatment and Prevention

Lung function tests
Lung function impairment in CCSs is assessed by pulmonary function tests. Pulmonary symptoms, such as chronic cough or dyspnea at exertion, are late signs of pulmonary dysfunction. One study found that only 24% of those with restrictive disease diagnosed by lung function tests reported symptoms using the Medical Research Council dyspnea questionnaire.[88]

Lung function usually is assessed by spirometry, body plethysmography, and measurement of the diffusing capacity for carbon monoxide (DLCO), with restrictive, obstructive, mixed restrictive-obstructive patterns, and decreased diffusion capacity having been reported. Decreased diffusion capacity is the most frequent abnormality (35%–45%), followed by restrictive (13%–32%) and obstructive disease (1%–4%).[75,76,88–91] Few studies have assessed lung function longitudinally, so that knowledge on long-term prognosis is scarce. Repeated lung function tests in survivors after HSCT found 3 phases in lung function trajectories: (1) an initial decrease in lung function after completion of treatment, lasting for 3 months to 6 months; (2) a subsequent recovery until 1 year to 2 years after completion, usually not reaching baseline values; and (3) stable values or slow deterioration in the long-term follow-up.[92–94]

Multiple breath washout tests (MBWs) might be more sensitive to identify early changes. They measure ventilation inhomogeneity in the lung, which is increased in case of central and peripheral airway obstruction. One study assessed pulmonary function in adults (n = 225) with BOS after HSCT with MBW and found the test highly sensitive for detecting abnormal lung function in their cohort (95% abnormal MBW test compared with 56% abnormal forced expiratory volume in the first second of expiration/forced vital capacity [FEV1/FVC]).[95] Whether this test will be valuable in the early detection of lung function impairment in CCSs still must be evaluated. Additional examinations, such as imaging or lung biopsy, are used in case of suspected pulmonary disease but not in regular follow-up care.

Surveillance

National and international follow-up guidelines concerning pulmonary late effects specify that the use of the chemotherapeutic agents (discussed previously), radiotherapy to the chest, and thoracic surgery are indications for pulmonary follow-up using lung function tests.[61,62,96] The available evidence is scarce, however, and the effect of other chemotherapies unclear, so more dedicated research is needed.

Treatment and prevention

Treatment options for pulmonary diseases and functional impairment in CCSs depend on the underlying disease. In general, treatment options are limited but the field is evolving quickly. This article focuses on treatment options for noninfectious pulmonary diseases beyond the acute-phase. BOS can be treated with systemic steroids, but these can increase the risk of pulmonary infection.[97,98] Inhaled bronchodilators do not improve pulmonary function in these patients.[98] One case series reported that patients with BOS who received inhaled fluticasone, azithromycin, and montelukast (FAM) could reduce their doses of systemic steroids compared with those not treated with FAM, thereby sparing them from the serious toxicities associated with long-term steroid use.[98] The subsequent phase II study confirmed that the FAM-regimen with reduced doses of systemic steroids was well tolerated and resulted in a reduction in pulmonary function decline in most patients.[99] Systemic steroid therapy improves radiation pneumonitis, but most experts agree that corticosteroid therapy is ineffective for the treatment of pulmonary fibrosis.[71,73] A few newer drugs, such as the TKI nintedanib, are available for adults with idiopathic pulmonary fibrosis. Data for the use in children are lacking. Nintedanib slows lung function decline and acute exacerbations in patients with idiopathic pulmonary fibrosis.[100,101]

Because treatment options are limited, prevention of pulmonary damage has high priority. Bleomycin no longer is a first-line therapy for lymphoma, although it remains a core component of germ cell tumor therapy, and radiotherapy has been reduced in many protocols, but avoidance of pulmonary toxic chemotherapy or radiation not always is possible. Therefore, any additional damage to the lung should be avoided throughout a survivor's life. Survivors must be counseled to not smoke and to avoid secondhand smoke exposure. Pneumococcal and influenza vaccinations should be considered in survivors with established pulmonary disease. Survivors should be advised to inform anesthetists about previous bleomycin treatment in cases of general anesthesia, because high fraction of inspired oxygen (>30%) concentration may further affect preexisting pulmonary damage.[102] Also survivors who desire to scuba dive should have a pulmonary consultation prior to undertaking the activity.[61,62,96]

SUMMARY

Cardiovascular disease and pulmonary disease after childhood cancer treatment impose great challenges for survivors. The cardiovascular system and lungs can be severely affected by cancer treatment in many ways, resulting in increased morbidity and mortality. Treatment options once disease becomes clinically manifest are focused on decreasing symptoms but do not cure cardiovascular or pulmonary disease. Therefore, prevention and regular screening according to established follow-up guidelines are crucial, even in the absence of symptoms, which generally occur rather late. Survivors should be encouraged to adopt a healthy lifestyle, and modifiable risk factors should be addressed. Close collaboration and early referral to experienced specialists (eg, cardiologist and pulmonologist) are essential for optimal diagnosis and management.

ACKNOWLEDGMENTS

This study was supported by the Swiss Cancer Research (grant no: 04157-02-2017) to C.E. Kuehni.

DISCLOSURE

Authors have nothing to disclose.

REFERENCES

1. Armstrong GT, Kawashima T, Leisenring W, et al. Aging and risk of severe, disabling, life-threatening, and fatal events in the childhood cancer survivor study. J Clin Oncol 2014;32(12):1218–27.
2. Armstrong GT, Liu Q, Yasui Y, et al. Late mortality among 5-year survivors of childhood cancer: a summary from the Childhood Cancer Survivor Study. J Clin Oncol 2009;27(14):2328–38.
3. Fidler MM, Reulen RC, Henson K, et al. Population-based long-term cardiac-specific mortality among 34 489 five-year survivors of childhood cancer in great Britain. Circulation 2017;135(10):951–63.
4. Tukenova M, Guibout C, Oberlin O, et al. Role of cancer treatment in long-term overall and cardiovascular mortality after childhood cancer. J Clin Oncol 2010; 28(8):1308–15.
5. Chow EJ, Chen Y, Kremer LC, et al. Individual prediction of heart failure among childhood cancer survivors. J Clin Oncol 2015;33(5):394–402.
6. Chow EJ, Chen Y, Hudson MM, et al. Prediction of ischemic heart disease and stroke in survivors of childhood cancer. J Clin Oncol 2018;36(1):44–52.
7. Schindler M, Belle FN, Grotzer MA, et al. Childhood cancer survival in Switzerland (1976-2013): Time-trends and predictors. Int J Cancer 2017; 140(1):62–74.
8. Fidler MM, Reulen RC, Bright CJ, et al. Respiratory mortality of childhood, adolescent and young adult cancer survivors. Thorax 2018;73(10):959–68.
9. Smith L, Glaser AW, Peckham D, et al. Respiratory morbidity in young people surviving cancer: Population-based study of hospital admissions, treatment-related risk factors and subsequent mortality. Int J Cancer 2019;145(1):20–8.
10. Kirchhoff AC, Fluchel MN, Wright J, et al. Risk of hospitalization for survivors of childhood and adolescent cancer. Cancer Epidemiol Biomarkers Prev 2014; 23(7):1280–9.
11. Brewster DH, Clark D, Hopkins L, et al. Subsequent hospitalisation experience of 5-year survivors of childhood, adolescent, and young adult cancer in Scotland: a population based, retrospective cohort study. Br J Cancer 2014; 110(5):1342–50.
12. Lipshultz SE, Landy DC, Lopez-Mitnik G, et al. Cardiovascular status of childhood cancer survivors exposed and unexposed to cardiotoxic therapy. J Clin Oncol 2012;30(10):1050–7.
13. van der Pal HJ, van Dalen EC, van Delden E, et al. High risk of symptomatic cardiac events in childhood cancer survivors. J Clin Oncol 2012;30(13):1429–37.
14. Morris B, Partap S, Yeom K, et al. Cerebrovascular disease in childhood cancer survivors: a children's oncology group report. Neurology 2009;73(22):1906–13.
15. van Dijk IW, van der Pal HJ, van Os RM, et al. Risk of symptomatic stroke after radiation therapy for childhood cancer: a long-term follow-up cohort analysis. Int J Radiat Oncol Biol Phys 2016;96(3):597–605.

16. Lipshultz SE, Adams MJ, Colan SD, et al. Long-term cardiovascular toxicity in children, adolescents, and young adults who receive cancer therapy: pathophysiology, course, monitoring, management, prevention, and research directions: a scientific statement from the American Heart Association. Circulation 2013;128(17):1927–95.

17. Feijen E, Font-Gonzalez A, Van der Pal HJH, et al. Risk and temporal changes of heart failure among 5-year childhood cancer survivors: a DCOG-LATER study. J Am Heart Assoc 2019;8(1):e009122.

18. Haddy N, Diallo S, El-Fayech C, et al. Cardiac diseases following childhood cancer treatment: cohort study. Circulation 2016;133(1):31–8.

19. Bowers DC, Liu Y, Leisenring W, et al. Late-occurring stroke among long-term survivors of childhood leukemia and brain tumors: a report from the Childhood Cancer Survivor Study. J Clin Oncol 2006;24(33):5277–82.

20. Moslehi JJ. Cardiovascular toxic effects of targeted cancer therapies. N Engl J Med 2016;375(15):1457–67.

21. Chow EJ, Antal Z, Constine LS, et al. New agents, emerging late effects, and the development of precision survivorship. J Clin Oncol 2018;36(21):2231–40.

22. van Waas M, Neggers SJ, Pieters R, et al. Components of the metabolic syndrome in 500 adult long-term survivors of childhood cancer. Ann Oncol 2010; 21(5):1121–6.

23. Meacham LR, Sklar CA, Li S, et al. Diabetes mellitus in long-term survivors of childhood cancer. Increased risk associated with radiation therapy: a report for the childhood cancer survivor study. Arch Intern Med 2009;169(15):1381–8.

24. Armstrong GT, Oeffinger KC, Chen Y, et al. Modifiable risk factors and major cardiac events among adult survivors of childhood cancer. J Clin Oncol 2013; 31(29):3673–80.

25. Lipshultz SE, Lipsitz SR, Sallan SE, et al. Chronic progressive cardiac dysfunction years after doxorubicin therapy for childhood acute lymphoblastic leukemia. J Clin Oncol 2005;23(12):2629–36.

26. van der Pal HJ, van Dalen EC, Hauptmann M, et al. Cardiac Function in 5-Year Survivors of Childhood Cancer: A Long-term Follow-up Study. Arch Intern Med 2010;170(14):1247–55.

27. Mulrooney DA, Yeazel MW, Kawashima T, et al. Cardiac outcomes in a cohort of adult survivors of childhood and adolescent cancer: retrospective analysis of the Childhood Cancer Survivor Study cohort. BMJ 2009;339:b4606.

28. Steinherz LJ, Steinherz PG, Tan CT, et al. Cardiac toxicity 4 to 20 years after completing anthracycline therapy. JAMA 1991;266(12):1672–7.

29. Lipshultz SE, Cochran TR, Franco VI, et al. Treatment-related cardiotoxicity in survivors of childhood cancer. Nat Rev Clin Oncol 2013;10(12):697–710.

30. Cardinale D, Colombo A, Bacchiani G, et al. Early detection of anthracycline cardiotoxicity and improvement with heart failure therapy. Circulation 2015; 131(22):1981–8.

31. Feijen EAM, Leisenring WM, Stratton KL, et al. Derivation of anthracycline and anthraquinone equivalence ratios to doxorubicin for late-onset cardiotoxicity. JAMA Oncol 2019;5(6):864–71.

32. Simunek T, Sterba M, Popelova O, et al. Anthracycline-induced cardiotoxicity: overview of studies examining the roles of oxidative stress and free cellular iron. Pharmacol Rep 2009;61(1):154–71.

33. Ichikawa Y, Ghanefar M, Bayeva M, et al. Cardiotoxicity of doxorubicin is mediated through mitochondrial iron accumulation. J Clin Invest 2014;124(2):617–30.

34. Zhang S, Liu X, Bawa-Khalfe T, et al. Identification of the molecular basis of doxorubicin-induced cardiotoxicity. Nat Med 2012;18(11):1639–42.
35. Fulbright JM. Review of cardiotoxicity in pediatric cancer patients: during and after therapy. Cardiol Res Pract 2011;2011:942090.
36. Campen CJ, Kranick SM, Kasner SE, et al. Cranial irradiation increases risk of stroke in pediatric brain tumor survivors. Stroke 2012;43(11):3035–40.
37. Bowers DC, McNeil DE, Liu Y, et al. Stroke as a late treatment effect of Hodgkin's Disease: a report from the Childhood Cancer Survivor Study. J Clin Oncol 2005; 23(27):6508–15.
38. Floyd JD, Nguyen DT, Lobins RL, et al. Cardiotoxicity of cancer therapy. J Clin Oncol 2005;23(30):7685–96.
39. Moslehi JJ, Deininger M. Tyrosine kinase inhibitor-associated cardiovascular toxicity in chronic myeloid leukemia. J Clin Oncol 2015;33(35):4210–8.
40. Martins F, Sofiya L, Sykiotis GP, et al. Adverse effects of immune-checkpoint inhibitors: epidemiology, management and surveillance. Nat Rev Clin Oncol 2019; 16(9):563–80.
41. Touyz RM, Herrmann SMS, Herrmann J. Vascular toxicities with VEGF inhibitor therapies-focus on hypertension and arterial thrombotic events. J Am Soc Hypertens 2018;12(6):409–25.
42. Visscher H, Ross CJ, Rassekh SR, et al. Pharmacogenomic prediction of anthracycline-induced cardiotoxicity in children. J Clin Oncol 2012;30(13): 1422–8.
43. Visscher H, Ross CJ, Rassekh SR, et al. Validation of variants in SLC28A3 and UGT1A6 as genetic markers predictive of anthracycline-induced cardiotoxicity in children. Pediatr Blood Cancer 2013;60(8):1375–81.
44. Blanco JG, Leisenring WM, Gonzalez-Covarrubias VM, et al. Genetic polymorphisms in the carbonyl reductase 3 gene CBR3 and the NAD(P)H:quinone oxidoreductase 1 gene NQO1 in patients who developed anthracycline-related congestive heart failure after childhood cancer. Cancer 2008;112(12): 2789–95.
45. Blanco JG, Sun CL, Landier W, et al. Anthracycline-related cardiomyopathy after childhood cancer: role of polymorphisms in carbonyl reductase genes–a report from the Children's Oncology Group. J Clin Oncol 2012;30(13):1415–21.
46. Visscher H, Rassekh SR, Sandor GS, et al. Genetic variants in SLC22A17 and SLC22A7 are associated with anthracycline-induced cardiotoxicity in children. Pharmacogenomics 2015;16(10):1065–76.
47. Krajinovic M, Elbared J, Drouin S, et al. Polymorphisms of ABCC5 and NOS3 genes influence doxorubicin cardiotoxicity in survivors of childhood acute lymphoblastic leukemia. Pharmacogenomics J 2016;16(6):530–5.
48. Lipshultz SE, Lipsitz SR, Kutok JL, et al. Impact of hemochromatosis gene mutations on cardiac status in doxorubicin-treated survivors of childhood high-risk leukemia. Cancer 2013;119(19):3555–62.
49. Rajic V, Aplenc R, Debeljak M, et al. Influence of the polymorphism in candidate genes on late cardiac damage in patients treated due to acute leukemia in childhood. Leuk Lymphoma 2009;50(10):1693–8.
50. Windsor RE, Strauss SJ, Kallis C, et al. Germline genetic polymorphisms may influence chemotherapy response and disease outcome in osteosarcoma: a pilot study. Cancer 2012;118(7):1856–67.
51. Wang X, Liu W, Sun CL, et al. Hyaluronan synthase 3 variant and anthracycline-related cardiomyopathy: a report from the children's oncology group. J Clin Oncol 2014;32(7):647–53.

52. Hildebrandt MAT, Reyes M, Wu X, et al. Hypertension susceptibility loci are associated with anthracycline-related cardiotoxicity in long-term childhood cancer survivors. Sci Rep 2017;7(1):9698.

53. Wang X, Sun CL, Quinones-Lombrana A, et al. CELF4 variant and anthracycline-related cardiomyopathy: a children's oncology group genome-wide association study. J Clin Oncol 2016;34(8):863–70.

54. Ruiz-Pinto S, Pita G, Patino-Garcia A, et al. Exome array analysis identifies GPR35 as a novel susceptibility gene for anthracycline-induced cardiotoxicity in childhood cancer. Pharmacogenet Genomics 2017;27(12):445–53.

55. Garcia-Pavia P, Kim Y, Restrepo-Cordoba MA, et al. Genetic variants associated with cancer therapy-induced cardiomyopathy. Circulation 2019;140(1):31–41.

56. Aminkeng F, Bhavsar AP, Visscher H, et al. A coding variant in RARG confers susceptibility to anthracycline-induced cardiotoxicity in childhood cancer. Nat Genet 2015;47(9):1079–84.

57. Tripaydonis A, Conyers R, Elliott DA. Pediatric anthracycline-induced cardiotoxicity: mechanisms, pharmacogenomics, and pluripotent stem-cell modeling. Clin Pharmacol Ther 2019;105(3):614–24.

58. Armenian SH, Hudson MM, Mulder RL, et al. Recommendations for cardiomyopathy surveillance for survivors of childhood cancer: a report from the International Late Effects of Childhood Cancer Guideline Harmonization Group. Lancet Oncol 2015;16(3):e123–36.

59. Armstrong GT, Joshi VM, Ness KK, et al. Comprehensive echocardiographic detection of treatment-related cardiac dysfunction in adult survivors of childhood cancer: results from the St. Jude Lifetime Cohort Study. J Am Coll Cardiol 2015;65(23):2511–22.

60. Aminkeng F, Ross CJD, Rassekh SR, et al. Pharmacogenomic screening for anthracycline-induced cardiotoxicity in childhood cancer. Br J Clin Pharmacol 2017;83(5):1143–5.

61. Children's Oncology Group. Long term follow-up guidelines for survivors of childhood, adolescent and young adult cancers, version 5.0. 2018. Available at: http://www.survivorshipguidelines.org/pdf/2018/COG_LTFU_Guidelines_v5.pdf. Accessed November 13, 2019.

62. Dutch Childhood Oncology Group. Guidelines for follow-up in survivors of childhood cancer 5 years after diagnosis. Available at: https://www.skion.nl/voor-patienten-en-ouders/late-effecten/533/richtlijn-follow-up-na-kinderkanker/. Accessed November 13, 2019.

63. Pourier MS, Mavinkurve-Groothuis AM, Loonen J, et al. Is screening for abnormal ECG patterns justified in long-term follow-up of childhood cancer survivors treated with anthracyclines? Pediatr Blood Cancer 2017;64(3). https://doi.org/10.1002/pbc.26243.

64. Leerink JM, Verkleij SJ, Feijen EAM, et al. Biomarkers to diagnose ventricular dysfunction in childhood cancer survivors: a systematic review. Heart 2019;105(3):210–6.

65. Reichardt P, Tabone MD, Mora J, et al. Risk-benefit of dexrazoxane for preventing anthracycline-related cardiotoxicity: re-evaluating the European labeling. Future Oncol 2018;14(25):2663–76.

66. Silber JH, Cnaan A, Clark BJ, et al. Enalapril to prevent cardiac function decline in long-term survivors of pediatric cancer exposed to anthracyclines. J Clin Oncol 2004;22(5):820–8.

67. Kirk R, Dipchand AI, Rosenthal DN, et al. The International Society for Heart and Lung Transplantation Guidelines for the management of pediatric heart failure: Executive summary. [Corrected]. J Heart Lung Transplant 2014;33(9):888–909.

68. Cheuk DK, Sieswerda E, van Dalen EC, et al. Medical interventions for treating anthracycline-induced symptomatic and asymptomatic cardiotoxicity during and after treatment for childhood cancer. Cochrane Database Syst Rev 2016;(8):CD008011.

69. Mertens AC, Yasui Y, Liu Y, et al. Pulmonary complications in survivors of childhood and adolescent cancer. A report from the Childhood Cancer Survivor Study. Cancer 2002;95(11):2431–41.

70. Kasteler R, Weiss A, Schindler M, et al. Long-term pulmonary disease among Swiss childhood cancer survivors. Pediatr Blood Cancer 2018;65(1). https://doi.org/10.1002/pbc.26749.

71. Skinner R, Kaplan R, Nathan PC. Renal and pulmonary late effects of cancer therapy. Semin Oncol 2013;40(6):757–73.

72. Huang TT, Hudson MM, Stokes DC, et al. Pulmonary outcomes in survivors of childhood cancer: a systematic review. Chest 2011;140(4):881–901.

73. Abid SH, Malhotra V, Perry MC. Radiation-induced and chemotherapy-induced pulmonary injury. Curr Opin Oncol 2001;13(4):242–8.

74. Sleijfer S. Bleomycin-induced pneumonitis. Chest 2001;120(2):617–24.

75. De A, Guryev I, LaRiviere A, et al. Pulmonary function abnormalities in childhood cancer survivors treated with bleomycin. Pediatr Blood Cancer 2014;61(9):1679–84.

76. Zorzi AP, Yang CL, Dell S, et al. Bleomycin-associated Lung Toxicity in Childhood Cancer Survivors. J Pediatr Hematol Oncol 2015;37(8):e447–52.

77. Liles A, Blatt J, Morris D, et al. Monitoring pulmonary complications in long-term childhood cancer survivors: guidelines for the primary care physician. Cleve Clin J Med 2008;75(7):531–9.

78. Jenney ME. Malignant disease and the lung. Paediatr Respir Rev 2000;1(3):279–86.

79. Lohani S, O'Driscoll BR, Woodcock AA. 25-year study of lung fibrosis following carmustine therapy for brain tumor in childhood. Chest 2004;126(3):1007.

80. Hinkle AS, Proukou C, Chen Y. Pulmonary Effects of Antineoplastic Therapy. In: Schwartz CL, Hobbie WL, Constine LS, et al, editors. Survivors of Childhood and Adolescent Cancer. A Multidisciplinary Approach. 2nd Edition. Berlin Heidelberg: Springer-Verlag; 2005.

81. Aronin PA, Mahaley MS Jr, Rudnick SA, et al. Prediction of BCNU pulmonary toxicity in patients with malignant gliomas: an assessment of risk factors. N Engl J Med 1980;303(4):183–8.

82. O'Driscoll BR, Hasleton PS, Taylor PM, et al. Active lung fibrosis up to 17 years after chemotherapy with carmustine (BCNU) in childhood. N Engl J Med 1990;323(6):378–82.

83. Bolling T, Konemann S, Ernst I, et al. Late effects of thoracic irradiation in children. Strahlenther Onkol 2008;184(6):289–95.

84. Venkatramani R, Kamath S, Wong K, et al. Correlation of clinical and dosimetric factors with adverse pulmonary outcomes in children after lung irradiation. Int J Radiat Oncol Biol Phys 2013;86(5):942–8.

85. Denbo JW, Zhu L, Srivastava D, et al. Long-term pulmonary function after metastasectomy for childhood osteosarcoma: a report from the St Jude lifetime cohort study. J Am Coll Surg 2014;219(2):265–71.

86. Diab M, ZazaDitYafawi J, Soubani AO. Major pulmonary complications after hematopoietic stem cell transplant. Exp Clin Transplant 2016;14(3):259–70.

87. Soubani AO, Pandya CM. The spectrum of noninfectious pulmonary complications following hematopoietic stem cell transplantation. Hematol Oncol Stem Cell Ther 2010;3(3):143–57.

88. Armenian SH, Landier W, Francisco L, et al. Long-term pulmonary function in survivors of childhood cancer. J Clin Oncol 2015;33(14):1592–600.

89. Green DM, Zhu L, Wang M, et al. Pulmonary function after treatment for childhood cancer. A report from the St. Jude Lifetime Cohort Study (SJLIFE). Ann Am Thorac Soc 2016;13(9):1575–85.

90. Mulder RL, Thonissen NM, van der Pal HJ, et al. Pulmonary function impairment measured by pulmonary function tests in long-term survivors of childhood cancer. Thorax 2011;66(12):1065–71.

91. Record E, Williamson R, Wasilewski-Masker K, et al. Analysis of risk factors for abnormal pulmonary function in pediatric cancer survivors. Pediatr Blood Cancer 2016;63(7):1264–71.

92. Green DM, Merchant TE, Billuyps CA, et al. Pulmonary function after treatment for embryonal brain tumors on SJMB03 that included craniospinal irradiation. Int J Radiat Oncol Biol Phys 2015;93(1):47–53.

93. Wieringa J, van Kralingen KW, Sont JK, et al. Pulmonary function impairment in children following hematopoietic stem cell transplantation. Pediatr Blood Cancer 2005;45(3):318–23.

94. Inaba H, Yang J, Pan J, et al. Pulmonary dysfunction in survivors of childhood hematologic malignancies after allogeneic hematopoietic stem cell transplantation. Cancer 2010;116(8):2020–30.

95. Nyilas S, Baumeler L, Tamm M, et al. Inert Gas Washout in Bronchiolitis Obliterans Following Hematopoietic Cell Transplantation. Chest 2018;154(1):157–68.

96. Skinner R, Wallace WHB, Levitt GA. Practice Statement: Therapy Based Long Term Follow-up. United Kingdom Children's Cancer Study Group Late Effects Group. 2nd Edition; 2005.

97. Uhlving HH, Buchvald F, Heilmann CJ, et al. Bronchiolitis obliterans after alloSCT: clinical criteria and treatment options. Bone Marrow Transplant 2012; 47(8):1020–9.

98. Norman BC, Jacobsohn DA, Williams KM, et al. Fluticasone, azithromycin and montelukast therapy in reducing corticosteroid exposure in bronchiolitis obliterans syndrome after allogeneic hematopoietic SCT: a case series of eight patients. Bone Marrow Transplant 2011;46(10):1369–73.

99. Williams KM, Cheng GS, Pusic I, et al. Fluticasone, azithromycin, and montelukast treatment for new-onset bronchiolitis obliterans syndrome after hematopoietic cell transplantation. Biol Blood Marrow Transplant 2016;22(4):710–6.

100. Richeldi L, du Bois RM, Raghu G, et al. Efficacy and safety of nintedanib in idiopathic pulmonary fibrosis. N Engl J Med 2014;370(22):2071–82.

101. Raghu G, Rochwerg B, Zhang Y, et al. An Official ATS/ERS/JRS/ALAT clinical practice guideline: treatment of idiopathic pulmonary fibrosis. an update of the 2011 clinical practice guideline. Am J Respir Crit Care Med 2015;192(2): e3–19.

102. Mathes DD. Bleomycin and hyperoxia exposure in the operating room. Anesth Analg 1995;81(3):624–9.

Endocrine Health in Childhood Cancer Survivors

Hanneke M. van Santen, MD, PhD[a,b,]*, Wassim Chemaitilly, MD, PhD[c],
Lillian R. Meacham, MD, PhD[d], Emily S. Tonorezos, MD, MPH[e],
Sogol Mostoufi-Moab, MD, PhD, MSCE[f,g]

KEYWORDS

- Growth hormone deficiency • Metabolic syndrome • Hypothyroidism • Bone health
- Late effects • Childhood cancer survivor • Radiation effects
- Secondary thyroid cancer

KEY POINTS

- Endocrine late effects, including reproductive disorders, have been reported in up to 50% of childhood cancer survivors (CCS).
- Radiation-induced hypothalamic-pituitary dysfunction may present several months or many years after treatment, with multiple disorders appearing over time, growth hormone deficiency being the most common deficiency.
- CCS who have been exposed to external radiation or meta-iodobenzylguanidine are at risk for primary hypothyroidism, radiation thyroiditis, hyperthyroidism as well as benign nodules and differentiated thyroid cancer.
- CCS with a history of total body irradiation, abdominal radiotherapy, cranial radiotherapy, surgery to the hypothalamus, or corticosteroids are at increased risk for the development of metabolic syndrome or its components.
- Skeletal abnormalities owing to bone toxicity is common in CCS. The spectrum ranges from mild bone pain to debilitating osteonecrosis.

[a] Department of Pediatric Endocrinology, Wilhelmina Children's Hospital, UMCU, PO Box 85090, Utrecht 3505 AB, the Netherlands; [b] Princess Máxima Center for Pediatric Oncology, Utrecht, the Netherlands; [c] Division of Endocrinology, St. Jude Children's Research Hospital, Memphis, TN, USA; [d] Division of Hematology/Oncology/BMT, Department of Pediatrics, Emory University, Atlanta, GA, USA; [e] Department of Medicine, Memorial Sloan Kettering and Weill Cornell Medical College, Memorial Sloan Kettering Cancer Center, 485 Lexington Avenue, 2nd Floor, New York, NY 10017, USA; [f] Division of Endocrinology, Department of Pediatrics, The Children's Hospital of Philadelphia, Roberts Pediatric Clinical Research Building, 2716 South Street, Philadelphia, PA 19146, USA; [g] Division of Oncology, Department of Pediatrics, The Children's Hospital of Philadelphia, Roberts Pediatric Clinical Research Building, 2716 South Street, Philadelphia, PA 19146, USA
* Corresponding author. Department of Pediatric Endocrinology, Wilhelmina Children's Hospital, UMCU, PO Box 85090, Utrecht 3505 AB, the Netherlands.
E-mail address: h.m.vansanten@umcutrecht.nl

Pediatr Clin N Am 67 (2020) 1171–1186
https://doi.org/10.1016/j.pcl.2020.08.002
0031-3955/20/© 2020 The Author(s). Published by Elsevier Inc. This is an open access article under the CC BY license (http://creativecommons.org/licenses/by/4.0/).

INTRODUCTION

Endocrine late effects have been reported in up to 50% of childhood cancer survivors (CCS) >5 years after treatment.[1–4] Most endocrine disorders are amenable to treatment; awareness of symptoms is therefore of great importance. Timely treatment of endocrine disorders improves quality of life in CCS and may prevent possible consequences, such as short stature, bone and cardiovascular disorders, and depression. However, recognition of these symptoms may be delayed because many are nonspecific. At-risk CCS must therefore be regularly monitored and systematically screened. This article provides a summary of the most commonly reported endocrine late effects in CCS, with the exception of late effects affecting the reproductive system, which are described in a separate article.

HYPOTHALAMIC-PITUITARY DYSFUNCTION

CCS with tumors arising near the hypothalamic-pituitary (HP) region and those treated with surgery or radiotherapy involving this region are at risk for HP dysfunction (**Table 1**). HP dysfunction includes growth hormone (GH) deficiency, luteinizing hormone (LH)/follicle stimulating hormone (FSH) deficiency, thyroid stimulating hormone (TSH) deficiency, adrenocorticotrophic hormone (ACTH) deficiency, central precocious puberty (CPP), hyperprolactinemia, and central diabetes insipidus (CDI).

Tumor and surgery involving the HP region are major risk factors for HP dysfunction.[5] In this setting, multiple HP disorders, including CDI, may occur in the immediate postoperative setting. By contrast, radiation-induced HP dysfunction frequently presents several months or years after treatment, with multiple disorders appearing over time.

The reported prevalence of HP dysfunction depends on follow-up time, age, and kind of CCS included in the studied cohort. In a large cohort of 3141 CCS with a median follow-up time of 24.1 years, prevalence of GH deficiency, TSH deficiency, LH/FSH deficiency, ACTH deficiency, and CPP was 22.2%, 5.5%, 5.1%, 4.1%, and 1.1%, respectively, in all and 40.2%, 11.1%, 10.6%, 3.2%, and 0.9%, respectively, among those treated with HP radiotherapy.[2] As the cumulative incidence of radiation-induced HP disorders increases with length of time in follow-up, at-risk CCS require lifelong monitoring.[3] CDI, which is reported in 2.6% of pediatric central nervous system (CNS) tumors patients at time of diagnosis or after neurosurgery, does not occur as a late effect.[6]

Growth Hormone Deficiency

GH is the most common HP deficiency following cranial radiation (CRT)[7–9] (**Fig. 1**). The likelihood of developing GH deficiency and a shortened time to onset is directly related to radiation dose whereas inversely related to the number of fractions used to deliver the radiation.[10,11] GH deficiency has been reported after a single fraction of 10 Gy, has been reported after fractioned doses of 12 Gy given as total body irradiation (TBI), and is common after conformal radiotherapy used to treat CNS tumors.[12] Likewise, GH deficiency is seen after doses of 18 to 24 Gy used to treat acute leukemia.[13] Treatment before puberty, and especially at a younger age, may increase the risk for compromised final adult height.[13–16] Data on rates of GH deficiency after proton beam irradiation are limited at this time.

GH deficiency after traditional chemotherapy is unlikely; however, newer agents, such as immune checkpoint inhibitors and tyrosine kinase inhibitors (TKI), appear to interfere with normal growth.[17–19] The checkpoint inhibitors have been associated with autoimmune hypophysitis.[17,20] TKI may interfere with GH/insulin-like growth factor 1 (IGF-1)

Table 1
Radiotherapy-associated endocrine late effects

Radiotherapy Field	Treated Conditions	Possible Late Effects
Cranial, includes • Whole brain • Infratemporal • Nasopharyngeal • Orbital • Waldeyer ring	CNS tumors ALL with CNS disease Nonbrain solid tumors: • Rhabdomyosarcoma • Nasopharyngeal carcinoma • Retinoblastoma	Anterior pituitary disorders[a] Obesity Metabolic syndrome
Craniospinal	Medulloblastoma PNET	Anterior pituitary disorders[a] Obesity Short stature Primary hypothyroidism Hyperthyroidism Thyroid nodules Differentiated thyroid cancer Premature ovarian insufficiency
Total body irradiation	Conditioning for HSCT	Growth hormone deficiency Obesity Short stature Primary hypothyroidism Hyperthyroidism Thyroid nodules Differentiated thyroid cancer Premature ovarian insufficiency Male germ cell failure Decreased bone mineral density Abnormal glucose metabolism Metabolic syndrome
Neck, thorax, mediastinum • Neck • Chest • Lung • Mantle • Nasopharyngeal • Oropharyngeal • Supraclavicular	Hodgkin lymphoma Solid tumor located within field: • Rhabdomyosarcoma • Neuroblastoma • Ewing sarcoma • Nasopharyngeal carcinoma	Primary hypothyroidism Hyperthyroidism Thyroid nodules Differentiated thyroid cancer
Abdominal, pelvic, genitourinary, includes • Flank or hemiabdomen • Whole abdomen • Inverted Y • Bladder • Vaginal • Prostate, testes • Iliac • Inguinal, femoral	Hodgkin lymphoma Solid tumor located within field: • Rhabdomyosarcoma • Neuroblastoma ALL	Premature ovarian insufficiency Male germ cell failure Leydig cell failure Abnormal glucose metabolism
^{131}I-MIBG	Neuroblastoma	Primary hypothyroidism Thyroid nodules Differentiated thyroid cancer Premature ovarian insufficiency

Abbreviation: PNET, primitive neuroectodermal tumors.
[a] Includes GH, LH/FSH, TSH, and ACTH deficiency, CPP, and hyperprolactinemia.
Adapted from Chemaitilly W, Sklar CA. Childhood Cancer Treatments and Associated Endocrine Late Effects: A Concise Guide for the Pediatric Endocrinologist. *Horm Res Paediatr.* 2019;91(2):74-82. https://doi.org/10.1159/000493943; with permission.

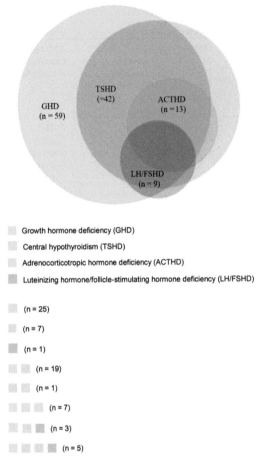

Growth hormone deficiency (GHD)

Central hypothyroidism (TSHD)

Adrenocorticotropic hormone deficiency (ACTHD)

Luteinizing hormone/follicle-stimulating hormone deficiency (LH/FSHD)

(n = 25)

(n = 7)

(n = 1)

(n = 19)

(n = 1)

(n = 7)

(n = 3)

(n = 5)

Fig. 1. Relative proportions and overlap among anterior pituitary deficiencies following cranial radiotherapy for childhood cancer. ACTHD, adrenocorticotropic hormone deficiency; GHD, growth hormone deficiency; TSHD, thyroid-stimulating hormone deficiency.[3] (*From* Chemaitilly W, Li Z, Huang S, et al. Anterior hypopituitarism in adult survivors of childhood cancers treated with cranial radiotherapy: a report from the St Jude Lifetime Cohort study. *J Clin Oncol.* 2015;33(5):492-500. https://doi.org/10.1200/JCO.2014.56.7933, p. 496.; with permission.)

signaling pathways or affect the growth plates.[18,19,21] There is conflicting evidence regarding catch-up growth in patients following treatment with TKIs.[18,22,23]

There are many causes of poor growth in CCS that are not associated with GH deficiency. Poor nutrition, suboptimal body mass index (BMI), and long-term treatment with glucocorticoids can cause transient decreases in growth velocity.[24] Treatment with cis-Retinoic acid is associated with short stature secondary to premature closure of the growth plates and therefore is not amenable to GH treatment.[25] Spinal radiation, especially at young age, may result in disproportionate growth with deficits in the upper segment resulting in arm span being greater than standing height.[14,26] Last, the timing and velocity of puberty can complicate the interpretation of growth. GH deficiency can be masked in children with early-onset puberty and seemingly normal growth rate, often resulting in delayed diagnosis of GH deficiency.

Screening for GH deficiency is done by measuring height, sitting height, weight, BMI percentiles, and height velocity every 6 months and should be interpreted in light of past height percentiles, mid–parental height, and Tanner stage. It is not recommended to rely solely on serum IGF-1 levels in CCS exposed to HP axis radiotherapy to make the diagnosis of GH deficiency.[27] When GH deficiency is suspected, GH stimulation tests must be done to confirm the diagnosis.

The risks and benefits of replacement therapy with human recombinant GH (hGH) should be discussed with the family. It should be mentioned that hGH may exacerbate scoliosis and increase the risk for slipped capital femoral epiphysis. There is currently no definitive evidence that the administration of hGH treatment increases the risk of cancer recurrence or secondary neoplasms.[28] Although the Childhood Cancer Survivor Study reported a 2- to 3-fold increase in risk for subsequent neoplasms, other reports suggest no significant increased risk for second cancers.[28–34]

GH replacement is typically delayed at least until 1 year after completion of cancer therapy,[27] although in children with low-grade neoplasms, such as craniopharyngioma, there may be arguments to commence earlier. GH treatment regimens used in the general population appear to also be appropriate for CCS.[27] In CCS treated with GH, height velocity will improve, but other factors, including end-organ resistance owing to radiation damage, timing, and velocity of puberty and other concurrent endocrinopathies, may limit final height.[35] Increased weight-to-height ratio, decreased lean muscle mass, muscle weakness, poor exercise tolerance, and frailty have been described in adult GH-deficient CCS,[36] but the presence of these conditions is less well documented in pediatric-aged CCS with GH deficiency. While treating with hGH, it is prudent to maintain IGF-1 levels in the normal range for age, sex, and pubertal status.[27] The risks and benefits of long-term GH replacement in adult CCS are not well established and represent areas of active research.[3]

Luteinizing hormone/follicle stimulating hormone deficiency

Depending on the attained stage of puberty at the time of onset of LH/FSH deficiency, survivors may present differently. Prepubertal children may present with pubertal delay; peripubertal children may present with arrested puberty, and postpubertal survivors may present with signs of hypogonadism, such as secondary amenorrhea in women and symptoms of androgen deficit (decreased libido and erectile dysfunction) in men. Untreated, LH/FSH deficiency may have repercussions on bone health, cardiovascular morbidity, and quality of life.[37] Low or declining serum estradiol (women) or morning testosterone (men) without elevation in LH levels is suggestive of the diagnosis. The treatment relies on sex-hormone replacement therapy.[27]

Thyroid stimulating hormone deficiency

Decreased or progressively declining serum free thyroxine (FT4) levels with low or inappropriately normal TSH levels are suggestive of the diagnosis TSH deficiency.[38] Untreated individuals may experience increased cardiovascular risk.[38] Treatment relies on replacement with levothyroxine.[27]

Adrenocorticotrophic hormone deficiency

Patients with ACTH deficiency may present with symptoms of adrenal insufficiency, including fatigue and vulnerability to medical stressors. Untreated, ACTH deficiency exposes survivors to the risk of adrenal crisis, which if not expeditiously managed could lead to shock, hypoglycemia, seizures, and death.[27] The diagnosis relies on the measurement of a low cortisol level after stimulation with low-dose or high-dose ACTH.[39] Treatment requires replacement with hydrocortisone at maintenance doses and stress dosing during illness.[27]

Central precocious puberty

Increased intracranial pressure or neoplasms in the HP region are risk factors for developing CPP. Children with CPP present with pubertal development and growth acceleration before the age of 8 years in girls (breast development) and 9 years in boys (testicular enlargement). Testicular volume enlargement may not be a reliable sign in boys treated with gonadotoxic therapies, such as alkylating agents or testicular radiotherapy,[40] and growth acceleration may be lacking because of the presence of GH deficiency. Untreated, CPP may lead to short stature and psychosocial adjustment issues.[41] The treatment relies on pubertal suppression using gonadotropic-releasing hormone agonists.[27]

Hyperprolactinemia

Radiation-induced hyperprolactinemia is rarely symptomatic, and treatment of hyperprolactinemia for its suppressive effects on gonadotropins is almost never necessary.[42]

Central diabetes insipidus

CDI is not considered a late effect of CCS but is most frequently present from the outset or immediately after neurosurgery in patients with neoplasms near the HP region (craniopharyngioma, germinoma, Langerhans cell histiocytosis). Patients with CDI present with polyuria and polydipsia owing to antidiuretic hormone deficiency.[43] A small subset, with extensive hypothalamic injury, experiences loss of thirst sensation. Management relies on treatment with desmopressin and monitoring fluid intake and output.[43,44]

THYROID DISORDERS

CCS, mainly those who have been exposed to radiation to a field including the thyroid gland, are at increased risk for primary hypothyroidism, subclinical (compensated) hypothyroidism, radiation thyroiditis, Graves hyperthyroidism followed by hypothyroidism as well as benign nodules and differentiated thyroid cancer (DTC).[45–48]

Thyroid Dysfunction

Radiation to a field including the thyroid gland and treatment with ^{131}I-meta-iodobenzylguanidine (MIBG) are the main risk factors for thyroid function disorders in CCS.[49] Survivors of neuroblastoma and Hodgkin lymphoma have the highest rate of hypothyroidism, with a prevalence up to 50% and 32%, respectively.[14,50] The risk for hypothyroidism increases with radiation dose, with 50% of CCS exposed to doses $\geq$45 Gy developing hypothyroidism by 20 years of follow-up.[51] Additional risk factors include younger age at radiotherapy and female gender.

Some evidence suggests that chemotherapy may affect thyroid function[52] (**Table 2**). In a study of the Late Effects Surveillance System in Germany, thyroid disorders were reported in survivors of sarcoma treated with chemotherapy alone.[53] Thyroid disorders have also been reported in up to 30% of survivors of hematopoietic stem cell transplantation (HSCT) conditioned with chemotherapy alone.[54] No difference was found in risk to develop hypothyroidism between a TBI or busulphan-based regimen. The BEAM (carmustine, etoposide, cytarabin and melphalan) combination used for conditioning was associated with a higher prevalence of thyroid disorders when compared with busulfan and fludarabine-based regimens.[55]

Immunotherapy, such as treatment with cytokines and check-point inhibitors, may cause thyroiditis resulting in an increased or decreased thyroid function.[56] Treatment with TKIs may result in thyroid dysfunction probably because of thyroiditis, although

Table 2
Chemotherapeutic agents associated with endocrine late effects

Category	Drug	Possible Late Effects
Alkylating agents	Busulfan Carmustine Chlorambucil Cyclophosphamide Dacarbazine Ifosfamide Lomustine Mechlorethamine Melphalan Procarbazine Temozolomide Thiotepa	Premature ovarian insufficiency Male germ cell failure Leydig cell dysfunction (subclinical mostly) Primary hypothyroidism (busulfan)
Heavy metals	Carboplatin Cisplatin	Premature ovarian insufficiency Male germ cell failure
Glucocorticoids	Dexamethasone Prednisone	Obesity Decreased bone mineral density Metabolic syndrome
Tyrosine kinase inhibitors	Imatinib Sorafenib Sunitinib	Impaired linear growth Primary hypothyroidism
Immunomodulator	Interferon	Autoimmune thyroiditis
Immune checkpoint inhibitor–anti-CTLA4 monoclonal antibody	Ipilimumab	Immune hypophysitis with anterior pituitary disorders[a] Autoimmune thyroiditis
Other	Retinoic acid Hedgehog pathway inhibitor	Skeletal dysplasia–short stature

[a] Includes GH, LH/FSH, TSH, and ACTH deficiency.
Adapted from Chemaitilly W, Sklar CA. Childhood Cancer Treatments and Associated Endocrine Late Effects: A Concise Guide for the Pediatric Endocrinologist. *Horm Res Paediatr.* 2019;91(2):74-82. https://doi.org/10.1159/000493943; with permission.

other mechanisms have been proposed.[57] A transient period of thyrotoxicosis may precede definitive hypothyroidism in individuals with thyroiditis. Effects of immunotherapy and TKIs are mainly seen in the first months after treatment.

Monitoring of thyroid function is recommended with yearly determination of TSH and FT4 in all CCS whose thyroid was potentially exposed to radiotherapy or therapeutic ^{131}I-MIBG.[27] Persistently high concentrations of TSH may increase the risk for thyroid nodules, but evidence is lacking in regards to an association with thyroid cancer.[58] In the case of hypothyroidism, it is recommended to replace thyroid hormone using regimens similar to those used in noncancer populations. It is currently not advised to screen thyroid function in CCS after treatment with chemotherapy alone.[58]

Thyroid Neoplasia

CCS treated with radiation therapy that includes the thyroid gland or with ^{131}I-MIBG are at an increased risk of developing benign thyroid nodules and DTC.[58–60] Neuroblastoma survivors who were treated with external beam irradiation to a field including the thyroid gland have been shown to have an increased risk for DTC when compared with Hodgkin survivors.[58,61] The risk for DTC is linear up to approximately 10 Gy, plateaus between 10 and 30 Gy, and declines at higher radiation doses (**Fig. 2**).[62] Because of the fact that DTC has been reported after thyroid radiation doses of less than 1 Gy and in individuals who received doses exceeding 40 Gy, all CCS with thyroid radiation exposure should be considered as having increased risk for DTC. Female CCS seem to be at increased risk when compared with male CCS[63]; however, other studies have reported no association with gender.[58]

Chemotherapy may increase the risk to develop thyroid cancer, although this has not been consistently reported. In a pooled analysis of 4 studies, the relative risk for DTC following treatment with anthracyclines was 4.5 (95% confidence interval [CI], 1.4–17.8) in nonirradiated patients.[63] This finding has been confirmed in an updated pooled analysis of 12 studies, in which exposure to chemotherapy was significantly associated with thyroid cancer (see **Fig. 2**).[62]

DTC has an excellent prognosis. There is no evidence that DTC in CCS has a different behavior or prognosis than sporadic DTC, although it may be argued that it is favorable to diagnose DTC in CCS at an early stage.[64,65] The workup for a thyroid nodule possibly indicating DTC and treatment of DTC should be the same as in non-CCS. An expert panel of the International Guideline Harmonization Group evaluated evidence for the benefits and harms related to surveillance for DTC in CCS with thyroid ultrasound versus neck palpation. It was recommended that survivors be advised of the disadvantages (false negatives and subsequent unnecessary evaluations) versus the advantages (early detection of DTC) of both surveillance modalities and to decide by shared decision making between the health care provider and the survivor if thyroid ultrasounds would be obtained.[58]

METABOLIC SYNDROME

Adults diagnosed with the metabolic syndrome have at least three of the following criteria: elevated blood pressure, elevated fasting triglycerides, elevated fasting glucose, low high-density lipoprotein cholesterol level, and increased waist circumference and are at increased risk for cardiovascular morbidity. CCS with a history of TBI, abdominal radiotherapy, CRT, surgery to the hypothalamus, or corticosteroids use are

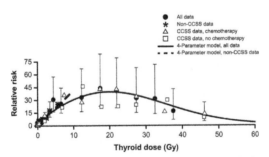

Fig. 2. Relative risk to develop thyroid cancer after radiation and chemotherapy in CCS. Category-specific relative risks for thyroid radiation dose for all data (*solid circle*) with selected 95% CIs, for non-CCSS data (*star*) and CCSS data for those who were (*open triangle*) or were not (*open square*) treated with chemotherapy, and the 4-parameter fitted dose-response model to all data (*solid line*) and to non-CCSS data only (*dash line*). Display includes full range of doses.[62] CCSS, childhood cancer survivor studies. (*From* Veiga LHS, Holmberg E, Anderson H, et al. Thyroid Cancer after Childhood Exposure to External Radiation: An Updated Pooled Analysis of 12 Studies. Radiat. Res. 2016; 185: 473-484; with permission © 2020 Radiation Research Society.)

at increased risk for the development of metabolic syndrome or its components. In light of the risk for cardiovascular morbidity and early mortality among CCS,[66–68] attention to the metabolic syndrome in this population is essential to high-quality care.

Evidence suggests that the prevalence of the metabolic syndrome is increased among CCS, compared with the general population.[69] In the St. Jude Lifetime Cohort Study, 508 of 1598 (31.8%) CCS (median age 32.7 years) met criteria for metabolic syndrome.[70] The highest risk was among acute lymphoblastic leukemia (ALL) survivors with a history of CRT. Among ALL survivors, individual metabolic late effects, including obesity, insulin resistance, dyslipidemia, hypertension, and cardiovascular events, have been reported.[70,71] In an analysis of the Childhood Cancer Survivor Study, CCS were more likely to take medications for hypertension (odds ratio [OR], 1.9; 95% CI, 1.6–2.2), dyslipidemia (OR, 1.6; 95% CI, 1.3–2.0), or diabetes (OR, 1.7; 95% CI, 1.2–2.3) than their siblings; however, they were not more likely to be obese or to have the cardiovascular risk factor cluster. CCS at highest risk were those who had a history of TBI or radiation to the chest or abdomen and also those who were physically inactive or were older at the time of follow-up.[72]

Causes for the Metabolic Syndrome in Childhood Cancer Survivors

HP deficiencies and obesity caused by (neurosurgical) damage to the HP region increase the risk for metabolic syndrome.[73] Survivors of craniopharyngioma are especially at risk for hypothalamic obesity, because of destruction of the ventromedial hypothalamus,[74] which may induce severe hyperphagia. In addition, insulin resistance may result from excess insulin secretion from the β cell of the pancreas because of overactive vagal neural transmission.

Corticosteroids have been repeatedly implicated in the observed metabolic risk for CCS. Acutely, corticosteroid administration may disturb glucose levels while causing weight gain and height loss.[75] Corticosteroids are also known to increase circulating free fatty acids, resulting in dyslipidemia and inhibition of myocellular glucose transport, increased gluconeogenesis and fatty acid synthesis, with decreased adiponectin levels.[76] Furthermore, corticosteroids can alter appetite regulation and have been reported to result in decreased physical activity, both contributing to metabolic risk. The metabolic impact of corticosteroids does not appear to end with discontinuation. A recent retrospective analysis of 184 children with ALL found that weight gain and height loss that occurred during the corticosteroid-containing reinduction phase persisted throughout intensification, maintenance, and survivorship.[77]

Multiple chemotherapy agents, most notably heavy metals and alkylating agents, have been associated with metabolic syndrome components.[76]

CCS with a history of TBI, radiation to the chest or abdomen, and CRT are at increased risk for the metabolic syndrome.[72] As noted above, GH deficiency following CRT may be implicated in the observed metabolic risk in this setting. However, metabolic syndrome and its components have also been described in survivors with a history of CRT without GH deficiency.[78] Survivors with a history of exposure to abdominal radiation were at 3.4-fold increased risk for diabetes when compared with siblings, after adjusting for BMI.[79]

TBI may cause the metabolic syndrome without obesity.[80] In a large single-institution study of 1885 one-year HSCT survivors (52% with a history of TBI), the prevalence of cardiovascular risk factors was significantly higher among transplant recipients, compared with community controls. Transplant recipients with a history of TBI were at highest risk for cardiovascular risk factors.

Similar to the general population, physical inactivity and poor-quality diet are significant contributors to metabolic and cardiovascular risk among CCS.[81] Subsequent studies have suggested that higher levels of physical activity and adherence to a Mediterranean diet are associated with better cardiometabolic risk factor profiles in CCS.[82,83]

BONE TOXICITY IN CHILDHOOD CANCER SURVIVORS

Skeletal abnormalities owing to bone toxicity are common in CCS. The spectrum ranges from mild bone pain to debilitating osteonecrosis (ON) and fractures.[84] The growing skeleton is particularly vulnerable to the effects of childhood cancer therapies and complications that interfere with skeletal metabolism and result in muscle deficits or poor muscle function. Musculoskeletal abnormalities can be recognized at the time of cancer diagnosis and during treatment and/or persist as long-term sequelae after treatment. Osteotoxic chemotherapy, prolonged treatment with glucocorticoids, poor nutrition, vitamin D insufficiency, and poor muscle mass are recognized risk factors that contribute to bone pathologic condition during and after cancer therapy, resulting in negative skeletal outcomes.[85]

ALL is associated with significant skeletal morbidity, including vertebral compression fractures, severe bone mineral density (BMD) deficit (BMD Z score ≤ -2), and ON.[86] The prevalence of severe vertebral compression fractures in children with newly diagnosed ALL is as high as 16% and associated with substantial risk for subsequent vertebral as well as nonvertebral fractures during and after completion of ALL treatment.[87] Prolonged therapy with glucocorticoids can also result in ON that further contributes to bone morbidity and altered quality of life. Although skeletal recovery in ALL survivors is noted after completion of therapy, BMD deficits may still persist over years depending on other chronic health conditions and lifestyle factors.[88]

The cause for BMD deficits in HSCT recipients may be due to the direct effect of leukemia on bone structure or as a consequence of treatments including glucocorticoids and transplant-related complications. Additional risk factors are TBI or CRT, young age at treatment, graft-versus-host disease, GH deficiency, and LH/FSH deficiency.[89] CCS treated with retinoids are at marked risk for reduced longitudinal bone growth, abnormal osteoblast differentiation, and premature epiphyseal closure.[25] Changes in bone remodeling and hyperparathyroidism have recently been described in pediatric patients treated with prolonged TKI.[21]

Recommendation for early detection of an abnormal BMD are inconsistent. An international guideline harmonization working group is developing an international guideline on this topic (www.ighg.org). If a diagnostic test is needed for bone health assessment after childhood cancer therapy, dual-energy x-ray absorptiometry is recommended.[90] Treatments for low BMD in CCS include treatment of hormonal deficiencies, repletion of vitamin D deficiency, supplementation of poor calcium intake, and consultation about the benefits of regular physical activity and deleterious effects of smoking and alcohol consumption.[91]

Current treatment options for ON include analgesia, limited weight bearing, physical therapy, and surgical procedures, including core decompression and/or joint replacement.[92] Alternative treatments have not shown clear benefits. Although treatment with bisphosphonates contributes to pain improvement with a reduced requirement in oral analgesia, their use has failed to demonstrate the prevention, destruction, and subsequent collapse in most affected weight-bearing joints, such as the hip joint.[93]

SUMMARY

Endocrine, metabolic, and bone disorders are frequent in CCS. Because recognition of the symptoms of HP deficiency may be masked, the (pediatric) endocrinologist should be part of the late-effects team for early recognition and treatment. CCS should be counseled on risk factors for bone and metabolic problems, and regular physical activity and healthy diet should be encouraged. Active counseling regarding BMI and timely treatment of HP disorders may improve quality of life of the survivors.

DISCLOSURE

H.M. van Santen has received speakers fees from Pfizer BV and Ferring BV. The remaining authors have nothing to disclose.

REFERENCES

1. Chemaitilly W, Sklar CA. Childhood cancer treatments and associated endocrine late effects: a concise guide for the pediatric endocrinologist. Horm Res Paediatr 2019;91:74–82.
2. van Iersel L, Li Z, Srivastava DK, et al. Hypothalamic-pituitary disorders in childhood cancer survivors: prevalence, risk factors and long-term health outcomes. J Clin Endocrinol Metab 2019;104(12):6101–15.
3. Chemaitilly W, Li Z, Huang S, et al. Anterior hypopituitarism in adult survivors of childhood cancers treated with cranial radiotherapy: a report from the St Jude Lifetime Cohort Study. J Clin Oncol 2015;33:492–500.
4. Barnes N, Chemaitilly W. Endocrinopathies in survivors of childhood neoplasia. Front Pediatr 2014;2:1–12.
5. Gan HW, Phipps K, Aquilina K, et al. Neuroendocrine morbidity after pediatric optic gliomas: a longitudinal analysis of 166 children over 30 years. J Clin Endocrinol Metab 2015;100:3787–99.
6. Clement SC, Schouten-van Meeteren AY, Boot AM, et al. Prevalence and risk factors of early endocrine disorders in childhood brain tumor survivors: a nationwide, multicenter study. J Clin Oncol 2016;34:4362–70.
7. Schmiegelow M, Lassen S, Poulsen HS, et al. Cranial radiotherapy of childhood brain tumours: growth hormone deficiency and its relation to the biological effective dose of irradiation in a large population based study. Clin Endocrinol (Oxf) 2000;53:191–7.
8. Shalet SM, Beardwell CG, Pearson CG, et al. The effect of varying doses of cerebral irradiation on growth hormone production in childhood. Clin Endocrinol (Oxf) 1976;5:287–90.
9. Shalet SM, Beardwell CG, Aarons BM, et al. Growth hormone deficiency in children with brain tumors. Cancer 1976;37:1144–8.
10. Merchant TE, Goloubeva O, Pritchard DL, et al. Radiation dose-volume effects on growth hormone secretion. Int J Radiat Oncol Biol Phys 2002;52:1264–70.
11. Darzy KH, Shalet SM. Hypopituitarism as a consequence of brain tumours and radiotherapy. Pituitary 2005;8:203–11.
12. Brennan BMD, Shalet SM. Endocrine late effects after bone marrow transplant. Br J Haematol 2002;118:58–66.
13. Viana MB, Vilela MIOP. Height deficit during and many years after treatment for acute lymphoblastic leukemia in children: a review. Pediatr Blood Cancer 2008;50:509–16.
14. Chow EJ, Friedman DL, Yasui Y, et al. Decreased adult height in survivors of childhood acute lymphoblastic leukemia: a report from the Childhood Cancer Survivor Study. J Pediatr 2007;150:370–5.
15. Dalton VK, Rue M, Silverman LB, et al. Height and weight in children treated for acute lymphoblastic leukemia: relationship to CNS treatment. J Clin Oncol 2003;21:2953–60.

16. Gurney JG, Ness KK, Stovall M, et al. Final height and body mass index among adult survivors of childhood brain cancer: Childhood Cancer Survivor Study. J Clin Endocrinol Metab 2003;88:4731–9.

17. Corsello SM, Barnabei A, Marchetti P, et al. Endocrine side effects induced by immune checkpoint inhibitors. J Clin Endocrinol Metab 2013;98:1361–75.

18. Narayanan KR, Bansal D, Walia R, et al. Growth failure in children with chronic myeloid leukemia receiving imatinib is due to disruption of GH/IGF-1 axis. Pediatr Blood Cancer 2013;60:1148–53.

19. Tauer JT, Hofbauer LC, Jung R, et al. Impact of long-term exposure to the tyrosine kinase inhibitor imatinib on the skeleton of growing rats. PLoS One 2015;10: e0131192.

20. Joshi MN, Whitelaw BC, Palomar MTP, et al. Immune checkpoint inhibitor-related hypophysitis and endocrine dysfunction: clinical review. Clin Endocrinol 2016;85: 331–9.

21. Lodish MB, Stratakis CA. Endocrine side effects of broad-acting kinase inhibitors. Endocr Relat Cancer 2010;17:R233–44.

22. Shima H, Tokuyama M, Tanizawa A, et al. Distinct impact of imatinib on growth at prepubertal and pubertal ages of children with chronic myeloid leukemia. J Pediatr 2011;159:676–81.

23. Rastogi MV, Stork L, Druker B, et al. Imatinib mesylate causes growth deceleration in pediatric patients with chronic myelogenous leukemia. Pediatr Blood Cancer 2012;59:840–5.

24. Meacham LR, Mason PW, Sullivan KM. Auxologic and biochemical characterization of the three phases of growth failure in pediatric patients with brain tumors. J Pediatr Endocrinol Metab 2004;17:711–7.

25. Mostoufi-Moab S. Skeletal impact of retinoid therapy in childhood cancer survivors. Pediatr Blood Cancer 2016;63:1884–5.

26. Clayton PE, Shalet SM. The evolution of spinal growth after irradiation. Clin Oncol 1991;3:220–2.

27. Sklar CA, Antal Z, Chemaitilly W, et al. Hypothalamic–pituitary and growth disorders in survivors of childhood cancer: an Endocrine Society Clinical Practice Guideline. J Clin Endocrinol Metab 2018;103:2761–84.

28. Sklar CA, Mertens AC, Mitby P, et al. Risk of disease recurrence and second neoplasms in survivors of childhood cancer treated with growth hormone: a report from the Childhood Cancer Survivor Study. J Clin Endocrinol Metab 2002;87: 3136–41.

29. Ergun-Longmire B, Mertens AC, Mitby P, et al. Growth hormone treatment and risk of second neoplasms in the childhood cancer survivor. J Clin Endocrinol Metab 2006;91:3494–8.

30. Woodmansee WW, Zimmermann AG, Child CJ, et al. Incidence of second neoplasm in childhood cancer survivors treated with GH: an analysis of GeNeSIS and HypoCCS. Eur J Endocrinol 2013;168:565–73.

31. Raman S, Grimberg A, Waguespack SG, et al. Risk of neoplasia in pediatric patients receiving growth hormone therapy - a report from the pediatric Endocrine Society Drug and Therapeutics Committee. J Clin Endocrinol Metab 2015;100: 2192–203.

32. Mackenzie S, Craven T, Gattamaneni HR, et al. Long-term safety of growth hormone replacement after CNS irradiation. J Clin Endocrinol Metab 2011;96: 2756–61.

33. Brignardello E, Felicetti F, Castiglione A, et al. GH replacement therapy and second neoplasms in adult survivors of childhood cancer: a retrospective study from a single institution. J Endocrinol Invest 2015;38:171–6.

34. Allen DB, Backeljauw P, Bidlingmaier M, et al. GH safety workshop position paper: a critical appraisal of recombinant human GH therapy in children and adults. Eur J Endocrinol 2016;174:P1–9.

35. Brownstein CM, Mertens AC, Mitby PA, et al. Factors that affect final height and change in height standard deviation scores in survivors of childhood cancer treated with growth hormone: a report from the Childhood Cancer Survivor Study. J Clin Endocrinol Metab 2004;89:4422–7.

36. Ness KK, Krull KR, Jones KE, et al. Physiologic frailty as a sign of accelerated aging among adult survivors of childhood cancer: a report from the St Jude Lifetime Cohort Study. J Clin Oncol 2013;31:4496–503.

37. Fleseriu M, Hashim IA, Karavitaki N, et al. Hormonal replacement in hypopituitarism in adults: an Endocrine Society Clinical Practice Guideline. J Clin Endocrinol Metab 2016;101:3888–921.

38. van Iersel L, Xu J, Potter BS, et al. Clinical importance of free thyroxine concentration decline after radiotherapy for pediatric and adolescent brain tumors. J Clin Endocrinol Metab 2019;104:4998–5007.

39. Patterson BC, Truxillo L, Wasilewski-Masker K, et al. Adrenal function testing in pediatric cancer survivors. Pediatr Blood Cancer 2009;53:1302–7.

40. Sklar CA, Robison LL, Nesbit ME, et al. Effects of radiation on testicular function in long-term survivors of childhood acute lymphoblastic leukemia: a report from the Children Cancer Study Group. J Clin Oncol 1990;8:1981–7.

41. Chemaitilly W, Merchant TE, Li Z, et al. Central precocious puberty following the diagnosis and treatment of paediatric cancer and central nervous system tumours: presentation and long-term outcomes. Clin Endocrinol (Oxf) 2016;84: 361–71.

42. Constine LS, Woolf PD, Constine CD, et al. Hypothalamic-pituitary dysfunction after radiation for brain tumors. N Engl J Med 1993;328:87–94.

43. Di Iorgi N, Napoli F, Allegri AE, et al. Diabetes insipidus - diagnosis and management. Horm Res Paediatrics 2012;77:69–84.

44. Mishra G, Chandrashekhar SR. Management of diabetes insipidus in children. Indian J Endocrinol Metab 2011;15(Suppl 3):S180–7.

45. Waguespack SG. Thyroid sequelae of pediatric cancer therapy. Horm Res Paediatrics 2019;91:104–17.

46. Hancock SL, McDougall IR, Constine LS. Thyroid abnormalities after therapeutic external radiation. Int J Radiat Oncol Biol Phys 1995;31:1165–70.

47. Hancock SL, Cox RS, Mcdougall IR. Thyroid diseases after treatment of Hodgkin's disease. N Engl J Med 1991;325:599–605.

48. Inskip PD, Veiga LHS, Brenner AV, et al. Hyperthyroidism after radiation therapy for childhood cancer: a report from the Childhood Cancer Survivor Study. Int J Radiat Oncol Biol Phys 2019;104:415–24.

49. Jereczek-Fossa BA, Alterio D, Jassem J, et al. Radiotherapy-induced thyroid disorders. Cancer Treat Rev 2004;30:369–84.

50. Clement SC, van Rijn RR, van Eck-Smit BL, et al. Long-term efficacy of current thyroid prophylaxis and future perspectives on thyroid protection during 131I-metaiodobenzylguanidine treatment in children with neuroblastoma. Eur J Nucl Med Mol Imaging 2015;42:706–15.

51. Sklar C, Whitton J, Mertens A, et al. Abnormalities of the thyroid in survivors of Hodgkin's disease: data from the childhood cancer survivor study. J Clin Endocrinol Metab 2000;85:3227–32.

52. Berger C, Le-Gallo B, Donadieu J, et al. Late thyroid toxicity in 153 long-term survivors of allogeneic bone marrow transplantation for acute lymphoblastic leukaemia. Bone Marrow Transplant 2005;35:991–5.

53. Paulides M, Dörr HG, Stöhr W, et al. Thyroid function in paediatric and young adult patients after sarcoma therapy: a report from the Late Effects Surveillance System. Clin Endocrinol (Oxf) 2007;66:727–31.

54. Sanders JE, Hoffmeister PA, Woolfrey AE, et al. Thyroid function following hematopoietic cell transplantation in children: 30 years' experience. Blood 2009; 113:306–8.

55. Veiga LH, Bhatti P, Ronckers CM, et al. Chemotherapy and thyroid cancer risk: a report from the Childhood Cancer Survivor Study. Cancer Epidemiol Biomarkers Prev 2012;21:92–101.

56. Cima LN, Martin SC, Lambrescu IM, et al. Long-term thyroid disorders in pediatric survivors of hematopoietic stem cell transplantation after chemotherapy-only conditioning. J Pediatr Endocrinol Metab 2018;31:869–78.

57. Torino F, Corsello SM, Longo R, et al. Hypothyroidism related to tyrosine kinase inhibitors: an emerging toxic effect of targeted therapy. Nat Rev Clin Oncol 2009;6:219–28.

58. Clement SC, Kremer LCM, Verburg FA, et al. Balancing the benefits and harms of thyroid cancer surveillance in survivors of childhood, adolescent and young adult cancer: recommendations from the international Late Effects of Childhood Cancer Guideline Harmonization Group in collaboration with the PanCareSurFup Consortium. Cancer Treat Rev 2018;63:28–39.

59. Bhatti P, Veiga LH, Ronckers CM, et al. Risk of second primary thyroid cancer after radiotherapy for a childhood cancer in a large cohort study: an update from the Childhood Cancer Survivor Study. Radiat Res 2010;174:741–52.

60. van Santen HM, Tytgat GA, van de Wetering MD, et al. Differentiated thyroid carcinoma after 131I-MIBG treatment for neuroblastoma during childhood: description of the first two cases. Thyroid 2012;22:643–6.

61. de Vathaire F, François P, Schlumberger M, et al. Epidemiological evidence for a common mechanism for neuroblastoma and differentiated thyroid tumour. Br J Cancer 1992;65:425–8.

62. Veiga LHS, Holmberg E, Anderson H, et al. Thyroid cancer after childhood exposure to external radiation: an updated pooled analysis of 12 studies. Radiat Res 2016;185:473–84.

63. Veiga LHS, Lubin JH, Anderson H, et al. A pooled analysis of thyroid cancer incidence following radiotherapy for childhood cancer. Radiat Res 2012;178:365–76.

64. Acharya S, Sarafoglou K, LaQuaglia M, et al. Thyroid neoplasms after therapeutic radiation for malignancies during childhood or adolescence. Cancer 2003;97: 2397–403.

65. Clement SC, Kremer LC, Links TP, et al. Is outcome of differentiated thyroid carcinoma influenced by tumor stage at diagnosis? Cancer Treat Rev 2015;41:9–16.

66. Chen Y, Chow EJ, Oeffinger KC, et al. Traditional cardiovascular risk factors and individual prediction of cardiovascular events in childhood cancer survivors. J Natl Cancer Inst 2019. https://doi.org/10.1093/jnci/djz108.

67. Armstrong GT, Oeffinger KC, Chen Y, et al. Modifiable risk factors and major cardiac events among adult survivors of childhood cancer. J Clin Oncol 2013;31: 3673–80.

68. Van Nimwegen FA, Schaapveld M, Janus CPM, et al. Cardiovascular disease after Hodgkin lymphoma treatment: 40-year disease risk. JAMA Intern Med 2015; 175:1007–17.

69. Talvensaari KK, Lanning M, Tapanainen P, et al. Long-term survivors of childhood cancer have an increased risk of manifesting the metabolic syndrome. J Clin Endocrinol Metab 1996;81:3051–5.

70. Smith WA, Li C, Nottage KA, et al. Lifestyle and metabolic syndrome in adult survivors of childhood cancer: a report from the St. Jude Lifetime Cohort Study. Cancer 2014;120:2742–50.

71. Malhotra J, Tonorezos ES, Rozenberg M, et al. Atherogenic low density lipoprotein phenotype in long-term survivors of childhood acute lymphoblastic leukemia. J Lipid Res 2012;53:2747–54.

72. Meacham LR, Chow EJ, Ness KK, et al. Cardiovascular risk factors in adult survivors of pediatric cancer-a report from the childhood cancer survivor study. Cancer Epidemiol Biomarkers Prev 2010;19:170–81.

73. Nandagopal R, Laverdière C, Mulrooney D, et al. Endocrine late effects of childhood cancer therapy: a report from the children's oncology group. Horm Res 2008;69:65–74.

74. Schwartz MW, Woods SC, Porte D, et al. Central nervous system control of food intake. Nature 2000;404:661–71.

75. Arguelles B, Barrios V, Buno M, et al. Anthropometric parameters and their relationship to serum growth hormone-binding protein and leptin levels in children with acute lymphoblastic leukemia: a prospective study. Eur J Endocrinol 2000; 143:243–50.

76. Rosen GP, Nguyen HT, Shaibi GQ. Metabolic syndrome in pediatric cancer survivors: a mechanistic review. Pediatr Blood Cancer 2013;60:1922–8.

77. Touyz LM, Cohen J, Neville KA, et al. Changes in body mass index in long-term survivors of childhood acute lymphoblastic leukemia treated without cranial radiation and with reduced glucocorticoid therapy. Pediatr Blood Cancer 2017;64(4): e26344.

78. Gurney JG, Ness KK, Sibley SD, et al. Metabolic syndrome and growth hormone deficiency in adult survivors of childhood acute lymphoblastic leukemia. Cancer 2006;107:1303–12.

79. Meacham LR, Sklar CA, Li S, et al. Diabetes mellitus in long-term survivors of childhood cancer - increased risk associated with radiation therapy: a report for the childhood cancer survivor study. Arch Intern Med 2009;169:1381–8.

80. Adachi M, Oto Y, Muroya K, et al. Partial lipodystrophy in patients who have undergone hematopoietic stem cell transplantation during childhood: an institutional cross-sectional survey. Clin Pediatr Endocrinol 2017;26:99–108.

81. Florin TA, Fryer GE, Miyoshi T, et al. Physical inactivity in adult survivors of childhood acute lymphoblastic leukemia: a report from the childhood cancer survivor study. Cancer Epidemiol Biomarkers Prev 2007;16:1356–63.

82. Järvelä LS, Kemppainen J, Niinikoski H, et al. Effects of a home-based exercise program on metabolic risk factors and fitness in long-term survivors of childhood acute lymphoblastic leukemia. Pediatr Blood Cancer 2012;59:155–60.

83. Tonorezos ES, Robien K, Eshelman-Kent D, et al. Contribution of diet and physical activity to metabolic parameters among survivors of childhood leukemia. Cancer Causes Control 2013;24:313–21.

84. Mostoufi-Moab S, Ward LM. Skeletal morbidity in children and adolescents during and following cancer therapy. Horm Res Paediatrics 2019;91:137–51.

85. Chemaitilly W, Cohen L, Mostoufi-Moab S, et al. Endocrine late effects in childhood cancer survivors. J Clin Oncol 2018;36:2153–9.

86. Mostoufi-Moab S, Halton J. Bone morbidity in childhood leukemia: epidemiology, mechanisms, diagnosis, and treatment. Curr Osteoporos Rep 2014;12:300–12.

87. Cummings EA, Ma J, Fernandez CV, et al. Incident vertebral fractures in children with leukemia during the four years following diagnosis. J Clin Endocrinol Metab 2015;100:3408–17.

88. Gurney JG, Kaste SC, Liu W, et al. Bone mineral density among long-term survivors of childhood acute lymphoblastic leukemia: results from the St. Jude Lifetime Cohort Study. Pediatr Blood Cancer 2014;61:1270–6.

89. Mostoufi-Moab S, Ginsberg JP, Bunin N, et al. Bone density and structure in long-term survivors of pediatric allogeneic hematopoietic stem cell transplantation. J Bone Miner Res 2012;27:760–9.

90. Crabtree NJ, Arabi A, Bachrach LK, et al. Dual-energy x-ray absorptiometry interpretation and reporting in children and adolescents: the revised 2013 ISCD pediatric official positions. J Clin Densitom 2014;17:225–42.

91. Hudson MM, Ness KK, Gurney JG, et al. Clinical ascertainment of health outcomes among adults treated for childhood cancer. JAMA 2013;309:2371–81.

92. Barr RD, Sala A. Osteonecrosis in children and adolescents with cancer. Pediatr Blood Cancer 2008;50:483–5.

93. Padhye B, Dalla-Pozza L, Little DG, et al. Use of zoledronic acid for treatment of chemotherapy related osteonecrosis in children and adolescents: a retrospective analysis. Pediatr Blood Cancer 2013;60:1539–45.

Reproductive Complications in Childhood Cancer Survivors

Hanneke M. van Santen, MD, PhD[a,b,*],
Marianne D. van de Wetering, MD, PhD[b],
Annelies M.E. Bos, MD, PhD[c],
Marry M. vd Heuvel-Eibrink, MD, PhD[b],
Helena J. van der Pal, MD, PhD[b], William Hamish Wallace, MD, PHD[d]

KEYWORDS

- Infertility • Gonadal failure • Late effects • Childhood cancer survivor
- Premature ovarian failure • Radiation effects • Fertility preservation

KEY POINTS

- Male and female childhood cancer survivors (CCSs) may be at risk for gonadal insufficiency, resulting in pubertal delay or pubertal arrest, reduced bone mass, sexual impairment, and infertility.
- Best practice for CCSs should include consultation on the risk for gonadotoxicity, infertility, future obstetric risk, and sexuality, because this greatly influences their quality of survival.
- CCSs at risk for gonadal dysfunction should be screened according to the recent recommendations and be referred upon indication to a (pediatric) endocrinologist, andrologist, gynecologist, or fertility specialist with experience in CCSs.

INTRODUCTION

Gonadal dysfunction and infertility after cancer treatment is of major concern to childhood cancer survivors (CCSs) and their parents.[1] Uncertainty about fertility or being diagnosed with infertility has a negative impact on quality of survival.[2] This article reviews determinants of gonadal damage and their impact on fertility and pregnancies. It

[a] Department of Pediatric Endocrinology, Wilhelmina Children's Hospital, UMCU, PO Box 85090, Utrecht 3505 AB, The Netherlands; [b] Princess Máxima Center for Pediatric Oncology, Heidelberglaan 25, Utrecht 3584 CS, The Netherlands; [c] Department of Reproductive Medicine and Gynecology, University Medical Centre, Utrecht, Postbus 85500, Utrecht 3508 GA, the Netherlands; [d] Department of Pediatric Haematology and Oncology, Royal Hospital for Sick Children, Edinburgh, Scotland
* Corresponding author. Department of Pediatric Endocrinology, Wilhelmina Children's Hospital, UMCU, PO Box 85090, Utrecht, 3505 AB, The Netherlands.
E-mail address: h.m.vansanten@umcutrecht.nl

Pediatr Clin N Am 67 (2020) 1187–1202
https://doi.org/10.1016/j.pcl.2020.08.003 **pediatric.theclinics.com**
0031-3955/20/© 2020 The Author(s). Published by Elsevier Inc. This is an open access article under the CC BY license (http://creativecommons.org/licenses/by/4.0/).

also provides specific recommendations for screening and treatment of gonadal function to enable timely treatment of gonadal insufficiency and its effects, such as stunted linear growth, delayed pubertal development, effects on bone health, and sexual functioning. Options for fertility preservation are discussed.

FEMALE GONADAL TOXICITY, FERTILITY, AND REPRODUCTIVE COMPLICATIONS
Definition

Premature ovarian insufficiency (POI) is a clinical condition that develops under the age of 40 years and is characterized by the absence of menstrual cycles for greater than or equal to 4 months and 2 sequential elevated follicle-stimulating hormone (FSH) levels in the postmenopausal range.[3]

Risk Factors

Overall, female CCSs have an estimated nonsurgical cumulative risk of developing POI of approximately 8%.[4] A large nationwide retrospective cohort study demonstrated that a majority of CCSs did not show signs of reduced ovarian reserve; however, specific subgroups of CCSs are at high risk.[5] CCSs at high risk for POI are those who have been treated with alkylating agents or radiotherapy to a field, including the ovaries (**Box 1, Fig. 1**).

The human ovary is sensitive to cytotoxic agents.[6] Commonly used alkylating and similar DNA interstrand cross-linking agents in pediatric oncology are the alkylating agents (busulfan, chlorambucil, cyclophosphamide, ifosfamide, mechlorethamine [nitrogen mustard], melphalan, and thiotepa), the triazenes (procarbazine, dacarbazine, and temozolomide), the nitrosoureas (carmustine [BCNU] and lomustine [CCNU]), and platinum agents (carboplatin and cisplatin). A dose-dependent relation for developing POI has been shown for alkylating agents. For use of a single drug, a high level of evidence has been found for busulfan and melphalan; however, for other single agents, the level of evidence is much lower,[6] which is due mainly to the fact that in most studies patients are treated with combination therapy, making it difficult to determine the independent absolute risk of a single alkylating agent. To combine and compare cumulative dosages of different alkylating agents for survivor outcomes, such as POI, the cyclophosphamide equivalent dose (CED) has been shown useful.[7] International consensus is that a high risk for infertility is likely when the CED is greater than or equal to 6000 mg/m^2 to 8000 mg/m^2, and a lower risk after CED is 6000 mg/m^2 to 8000 mg/m^2.

Radiation exposure is another acknowledged risk factor for damaging the ovarian tissue and the uterus.[6] The magnitude of the radiation effect is related to dose, fractionation, and age at time of radiation exposure. A mathematical model has been developed in which threshold doses for POI are calculated for infants (20.3 Gy), children up to 10 years of age (18.4 Gy), and adolescents up to 20 years of age (16.5 Gy), illustrating that the older the patient, the lower the dose needed to deplete the nongrowing follicle pool and thus cause POI.[4] POI has been described after treatment with ^{131}I-meta-iodobenzylguanidine MIBG and surgery for neuroblastoma.[8] In CCSs who were treated with ^{131}I for differentiated thyroid carcinoma, transient effects on female gonadal function have been reported.[9] The effect of ^{131}I and ^{131}I-MIBG on the human ovary should be investigated further. Interindividual variability in susceptibility to therapy-related gonadal impairment suggests a role for genetic variation. This issue is being addressed in the PanCareLIFE study, Europe's largest clinical cohort to study the impact of treatment regimens on the quality of life of CCSs.[10]

Box 1
Harmonized recommendations for premature ovarian insufficiency surveillance in survivors of childhood, adolescent, and young adult cancer

General recommendation
  Survivors treated with 1 or more potentially gonadotoxic treatments,[a] and their providers, should be aware of the risk of POI and its implications for future fertility (level A and level C evidence).

Who needs surveillance?
  Counselling regarding the risk of POI and its implications for future fertility is recommended for survivors treated with
  • Alkylating agents in general (level A evidence)
  • Cyclophosphamide and procarbazine (level C evidence)
  • Radiotherapy, potentially exposing the ovaries (level A evidence)

Which surveillance modality should be used for prepubertal and peripubertal survivors?
  Monitoring of growth (height) and pubertal development and progression (Tanner stage) is recommended for pre-pubertal survivors treated with potentially gonadotoxic chemotherapy and/or radiotherapy, potentially exposing the ovaries (expert opinion/no literature search).[a,b]
  FSH and estradiol are recommended for evaluation of POI in prepubertal survivors treated with potentially gonadotoxic chemotherapy and/or radiotherapy, potentially exposing the ovaries,[a] who fail to initiate or progress through puberty (expert opinion/no literature search).[c,d]

Which surveillance modality should be used for postpubertal survivors?
  A detailed history and physical examination with specific attention for POI symptoms (eg, amenorrhea and irregular cycles) are recommended for postpubertal survivors treated with potentially gonadotoxic chemotherapy and/or radiotherapy, potentially exposing the ovaries (expert opinion/no literature search).[a]
  FSH and estradiol are recommended for evaluation of POI in postpubertal survivors treated with potentially gonadotoxic chemotherapy and/or radiotherapy, potentially exposing the ovaries,[a] who present with menstrual cycle dysfunction suggesting POI or who desire assessment about potential for future fertility. Hormone replacement therapy should be discontinued prior to laboratory evaluation when applicable (expert opinion/no studies).[d,e]

AMH is not recommended as the primary surveillance modality for evaluation of POI in survivors treated with potentially gonadotoxic chemotherapy and/or radiotherapy, potentially exposing the ovaries,[a] who desire assessment about potential future fertility (expert opinion/ no studies).

AMH may be reasonable in conjunction with FSH and estradiol for identification of POI in survivors treated with potentially gonadotoxic chemotherapy and/or radiotherapy, potentially exposing the ovaries,[a] aged >25 years who present with menstrual cycle dysfunction suggesting POI or who desire assessment about potential for future fertility (expert opinion/no studies).

When should prepubertal and peripubertal survivors be referred?
  Referral to pediatric endocrinology/gynecology is recommended for any survivor who has
  • No signs of puberty by 13 years of age
  • Primary amenorrhea by 16 years of age
  • Failure of pubertal progression[f] (expert opinion/no literature search)

When should postpubertal survivors be referred?
  Referral to gynecology/reproductive medicine/endocrinology (according to local referral pathways) is recommended for postpubertal survivors treated with potentially gonadotoxic chemotherapy and/or radiotherapy potentially exposing the ovaries[a] who present with menstrual cycle dysfunction suggesting POI (expert opinion/no literature search).

What should be done when abnormalities are identified in prepubertal, peripubertal, and postpubertal survivors?

◀ Consideration of sex steroid replacement therapy is recommended for prepubertal, peripubertal, and postpubertal survivors diagnosed with POI by referral to gynecology/endocrinology (expert opinion/no literature search).

What should be done when potential for future fertility is questioned?
Referral to gynecology/reproductive medicine/endocrinology according to local referral pathways) is recommended for postpubertal female CCSs treated with potentially gonadotoxic chemotherapy and/or ovarian irradiation[a] without signs and symptoms of POI who desire assessment about potential for future fertility (expert opinion/no literature search).

Abbreviations: level A, high level of evidence; level B, moderate/low level of evidence; level C, very low level of evidence. [a] Treatments with evidence of causing POI include alkylating agents in general (level A evidence), cyclophosphamide, procarbazine (level C evidence), and radiotherapy to a field that includes the ovaries (level A evidence). [b] At least annually, with increasing frequency as clinically indicated based on growth and pubertal progression. [c] At least for girls of 11 years of age and older, and for girls with primary amenorrhea (age 16). [d] If amenorrhea, measure FSH and estradiol randomly; if oligomenorrhea, measure during early follicular phase (day 2–5). [e] This assessment should be performed after ending oral contraceptive pill/sex steroid replacement therapy use, ideally after 2 months without oral contraceptive pills. [f] The absence of initiation of puberty (Tanner stage 2 breast development) in girls 13 years or older or failure to progress in pubertal stage for $\geq$12 months.

From van Dorp W, Mulder RL, Kremer LC et al. Recommendations for premature ovarian insufficiency surveillance for female survivors of childhood, adolescent, and young adult cancer: A report from the International Late Effects of Childhood Cancer Guideline Harmonization Group in collaboration with the PanCareSurFup Consortium. Journal of Clinical Oncology 2016; 34:3440–3450; with permission.

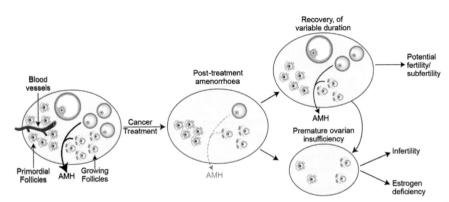

Fig. 1. Representation of the effects of gonadotoxic treatment on the ovary. Illustration of the key effects of cancer treatment on the ovary, highlighting the variable recovery after treatment such that some patients have permanent POI with infertility and estrogen deficiency, but others show recovery allowing fertility, although their reproductive life span may be shortened. (*From* Jayasinghe YL, Wallace WHB, Anderson RA. Ovarian function, fertility and reproductive lifespan in cancer patients. Expert Review of Endocrinology and Metabolism 2018; 13:125–136; with permission.)

Consequences of ovarian damage may be decreased production of estrogen (and to a lesser extent androgen), resulting in pubertal delay or failure, primary or secondary amenorrhea, osteoporosis, cardiovascular disorders, psychosocial problems, infertility, and sexual health issues. Radiation to the uterus has been associated with miscarriage, premature delivery, placental abnormalities and stillbirth.[4,11]

Screening for Premature Ovarian Insufficiency

In young prepubertal and peripubertal CCSs, clinical assessment for POI is advised by measurement of height, plotted in a growth chart in relation to target height, and calculating height velocity, in conjunction with clinical examination of pubertal stage. Determination of the FSH concentration is the recommended screening tool in girls at risk for POI age 12 or up[6] (see **Box 1**). The serum antimüllerian hormone (AMH) concentration is an endocrine marker for age-dependent decline in ovarian reserve.[12] A validated normative model for AMH from birth to senescence has been made, describing a transition period in early adulthood, after which AMH reflects the progressive loss of the nongrowing follicle pool.[13] For women and girls under 24 years of age, the interpretation of AMH as indirect marker of ovarian reserve remains speculative, which makes the value of AMH in predicting early menopause in CCSs uncertain.[14] Also, a very low AMH in young adolescent CCSs does not exclude spontaneous pregnancy. Furthermore, AMH concentrations seem to be influenced not only by treatment but also by the general disease state.[15] For all these reasons, AMH currently has not been recommended as screening tool for POI in CCSs[3] (see **Box 1**). Measuring AMH concentrations may be considered, however, after finding an increased FSH concentration, because the combination of an increased FSH with undetectable AMH has been related to ovarian insufficiency.

It is strongly advised to refer CCSs with signs of gonadal failure after treatment of childhood cancer to a pediatric endocrinologist for estrogen and progestogen treatment and, upon request, also to a fertility specialist for fertility counseling (see **Box 1**). A pediatric endocrinologist induces puberty with gradual administration of sex steroids, aiming to mimic the timing and key milestones of normal puberty. The need for puberty induction should be anticipated in girls who have been exposed to high-risk therapy.[4,6] For adult CCSs, an endocrinologist or gynecologist considers hormone replacement for optimization of bone mineralization or relieve of symptoms, such as hot flushes, joint pain, and tiredness. Hormone replacement generally is recommended until the age of natural menopause.[4]

Fertility Preservation in Female Childhood Cancer Survivors

CCSs who have been exposed to cytotoxic drugs, radiation therapy including the ovaries in the radiation field or to surgery near the ovaries radiotherapy, or surgery, including the ovaries, deserve counseling regarding the available fertility preservation methods that may apply to them.[6,16,17] It is important that the attending physician actively counsels and informs the survivor whether there are questions about fertility, pregnancy, or sexuality during the long-term follow-up visits. In a questionnaire among 484 survivors, fewer than half of the women reported to have received information about their treatment's impact on fertility, and only 14% reported that they received information about fertility preservation.[18]

Counseling CCSs at risk for POI includes first providing information on established and experimental options for preservation of gonadal function after cancer treatment.[19]

Autotransplantation of previously cryopreserved ovarian cortex tissue in CCSs can be done for fertility restoration or endocrine replacement. After reimplantation of ovarian tissue, ovarian activity is restored in more than 95% of cases. The mean duration of ovarian function after reimplantation is 4 years to 5 years, but the function can persist for up to 7 years, depending on the follicular density at the time of ovarian-tissue cryopreservation.[20] The first successful pregnancy after replacement of cryopreserved ovarian tissue was reported in 2004.[21] At present, more than 130 live births have been described, with a pregnancy rate of 29% to 41% and a live birth rate of 23% to 36%.[17,20]

Also, successful puberty induction has been described in two 13-year-old girls with hypergonadotropic hypogonadism.[22,23] Although these reports are of scientific and clinical importance because they prove that follicular growth may be activated in pre-pubertally cryopreserved ovarian tissue, they also open the discussion upon the subject if this procedure is beneficial for an adolescent or not.[24] Tissue replacement for puberty induction has many disadvantages, such as escalation of estrogen dose, early exposure to progesterone, the fact that it has only temporary effect (loss of valuable tissue), and the potential risk of malignant contamination.[17,24] For all these reasons, endocrine substitution therapy is recommended by exogenous hormonal replacement therapy over tissue replacement.

For postpubertal CCSs at risk for developing POI who did not receive prior fertility preservation methods, oocyte cryopreservation is a feasible fertility preservation technique. This may be offered to selected female CCSs at risk for POI, if hormonal treatment intervention is allowed from an oncological perspective.[25]

For CCSs with full-blown POI and no egg cell reserve, currently, no techniques are possible to restore fertility. For these survivors, however, it is important to stress that replacement of estrogen may influence growth of the uterus, enabling possible future pregnancy by donor oocytes.[26,27] The latter may not hold for CCSs who have been treated with radiotherapy to a field, including the uterus, such as in survivors with ovarian failure secondary to total body irradiation of 20 Gy to 30 Gy in which hormone replacement therapy did not seem to increase uterine size, blood flow, or endometrial thickness.[28]

Female fertility outcomes and reproductive complications

The overall reduction in the likelihood of pregnancy in female CCSs aged under 40 compared with the general population has been reported to be 38%.[29] In a large Swedish cohort of CCSs, the hazard ratio (HR) for having a first live birth in CCSs was significantly lower than in healthy controls,[30] although it was lower only for CCSs with malignancy of the eye, central nervous system (CNS) tumors, or leukemia. Women surviving childhood cancer have a lower HR for having a first live birth compared with women diagnosed with cancer in adolescence (HR 0.47 vs 0.89, respectively).[30] CCSs who have received abdominal or cranial radiotherapy take significantly longer to become pregnant than their siblings.[31]

Uterine radiotherapy with doses greater than 5 Gy (relative risk 2.48; 95% CI, 1.54–4.01) significantly increases the risk of infertility.[31] As a consequence of radiation exposure to the uterus or lack of sex steroids, female CCSs may be at increased risk for miscarriage, fetal growth restrictions, perinatal deaths, preterm births, delivery of small-for-gestational-age infants, preeclampsia, and abnormal placentation.[3,28]

The fact that survivors of CNS tumors have the lowest HRs for the chance to become pregnant (HR 0.53 and HR 0.62 for male CCSs and female CCSs, respectively[30]) not only may be the consequence of pituitary damage resulting in hypogonadism or a toxic effect of chemotherapy on the gonads but also may be a reflection of the fact that achieving pregnancy requires an adequate neurocognitive development. Impaired cognitive impairment is in turn associated with lower educational level, higher unemployment, less independent living, and a higher risk of never getting married. All these factors may influence the chance for pregnancy.[32]

There seems to be no increased risk for congenital abnormalities in the offspring of CCSs.[33]

Referral and Treatment of Female Childhood Cancer Survivors with Gonadal Dysfunction

CCSs with gonadal insufficiency should be referred for treatment to the appropriate health care provider like a dedicated (onco-) endocrine and/or fertility expert.

Sex steroid hormone replacement therapy is indicated in all girls and women age less than 40 with hypogonadism to restore pubertal development and remediate or prevent the consequences of premature estrogen deficiency, such as loss of bone mass, loss of self-esteem, and decrease in sexual activity.[34] In postpubertal girls and women, replacement of estrogens has a positive influence on bone health and cardiovascular status.[35] There is insufficient evidence that androgen replacement therapy in women with POI has beneficial effect on sexual function, bone mineral density, or quality of life.[36]

For prepubertal female CCSs, timing and dosing of estrogen substitution are essential to enable a normal pubertal and bone development as well as a normal social development during the teenage years. CCSs less than 18 years of age should be referred to an experienced pediatric endocrinologist. Estrogen supplementation is given, with monitoring of Tanner stage in relation to age, growth velocity, and skeletal maturation at regular basis. This may be challenging in girls who have been exposed to gonadotoxic agents in combination with cranial radiation or a tumor in the sellar region resulting in hypopituitarism. In this case, simultaneous growth hormone (GH) deficiency, luteinizing hormone (LH)/FSH deficiency, and primary gonadal failure may be present, influencing growth velocity and bone maturation. It also makes interpretation of laboratory values, such as insulinlike growth factor 1, LH, and FSH, challenging.

The association between sex steroid replacement therapy and risk of developing breast cancer was evaluated by the Childhood Cancer Survivor Study, in which a lower of developing breast cancer was found for CCSs with POI and treatment with estrogen replacement than CCSs without POI.[37]

The timing, dosage, and route of estrogen replacement is the same as those recommended for non-CCSs.[38–40] There is some evidence that transdermal versus oral replacement therapy in female CCSs may be of advantage[35,41]; however, this evidence was considered insufficiently strong.[6,35] Treatment with estrogen needs to be combined with progestin for endometrial cycling.

In cases of simultaneous GH deficiency, it may be chosen to start GH replacement therapy first before estrogen replacement therapy, to ensure an adequate pubertal growth velocity. These choices should be made individually by the pediatric endocrinologist and should be discussed with the teen survivor, balancing the advantages of estrogen replacement and pubertal development versus delaying this and optimizing final height.

MALE GONADAL TOXICITY, FERTILITY, AND REPRODUCTIVE COMPLICATIONS

In male CCSs, primary gonadal failure due to Leydig cell failure is defined as having decreased androgen concentrations in combination with elevated LH and FSH levels or failure to develop signs of puberty by age 14 or no change in pubertal stage for at least 6 months at the age at which progression would be expected in combination with elevated levels of LH and FSH.[42] Impaired spermatogenesis is the consequence of Sertoli cell failure and is defined as having azoospermia or oligozoospermia. Male gonadal function may be hampered by damage to the testes or due to hypothalamic-pituitary (HP) damage resulting in central hypogonadism (**Table 1**).

In the testes, 2 distinct cell types are present: the Sertoli cells, which are important for spermatogenesis, and the Leydig cells, which are responsible for steroidogenesis (testosterone production). Spermatogenesis can be impaired without manifest damage to steroidogenesis. Although survival of the germ cells is most crucial for future fertility, the Sertoli cells (somatic stem cells) play an important role for fertility, because they create the environment that is needed to support development and survival of the germ cells. If these germ cells are lost, no restoration of spermatogenesis occurs.[43] In addition, decreased testosterone production may lead to sexual dysfunction or impaired spermatogenesis leading to subsequent impaired fertility. Leydig cell failure and Leydig cell dysfunction recently have been associated with impaired glucose tolerance, insulin resistance, increased abdominal/body fat, and decreased quality of life.[44]

Risk Factors for Male Gonadal Failure

The function of the Leydig cells, Sertoli cells, or testicular germ cells may be distorted as a consequence of surgery, chemotherapy, or radiation to a field involving the testes.[42] Damage to the testicular vessels, changes in pituitary hormone concentrations, growth factors, or the structure of the seminiferous tubule structure also may cause dysfunction of the Sertoli cells or Leydig cells. This also holds for interstitial effects on the Leydig cells, leading to alterations in hormones or growth factors that may have an impact on germ cells directly or indirectly (eg, testosterone deficiency) through effects on other somatic cell populations. Gonadal function also already may be hampered before the start of treatment.[45]

In a large CCSs study, the prevalence rates of Leydig cell failure and Leydig cell dysfunction were reported to be 6.9% and 14.7%, respectively, after a mean follow-up time of 22 years after cancer diagnosis.[44] Independent risk factors for Leydig cell failure included an age of 26 years or older at assessment, testicular radiotherapy at any dose, and alkylating agents at CED greater than or equal to 4000 mg/m^2.[44]

In male CCSs treated for leukemia with alkylating agents, long-term depletion of the spermatogonial pool was seen whereas survivors without alkylating agents remained within normative reference values for prepubertal boys.[46] Spermatogenesis in male CCSs was described to be impaired after treatment with busulfan, cyclophosphamide, mechlorethamine (nitrogen mustard), ifosfamide, fludarabine/melphalan, and procarbazine.[42] Treatment with cyclophosphamide with a CED greater than or equal to 5 g/m^2 has been reported to induce impaired spermatogenesis.[47]

Although possible recovery of gonadal function in male CCSs has been reported even long after discontinuation of cancer treatment,[48] recent data demonstrated an increasing risk for Leydig cell failure, with increasing age at follow-up indicating that there may be an association with longer follow-up time and Leydig cell function.[44] Recovery or further decline of male gonadal function in time should be studied further in prospective cohorts.

Radiotherapy, including total body irradiation to a field, including the testes, has been associated with an increased risk for androgen deficiency.[42] The threshold for Leydig cell damage has been shown to be 12 Gy; however, spermatogenesis can already be impaired even after exposure to a radiation dose greater than 2 Gy.[32]

Table 1
Cancer treatments and risk factors associated with male adverse reproductive outcomes

Treatment	Reproductive Outcome		
	Impaired Spermatogenesis	Testosterone Deficiency	Sexual Dysfunction
Chemotherapy			
Alkylating agents	CED[a] >5 g/m^2	Possible, CED >20 g/m^2 or combinations	Possible, secondary to testosterone deficiency
Radiation			
Testicular	Low risk <12 Gy [c] High risk >12 Gy	Moderate risk >12 Gy High risk >20 Gy	Possible, secondary to testosterone deficiency
Pelvis, spine, lower extremities	Scatter or incidental dose to testes ≥2–3 Gy	Unlikely	Spinal field T11 and below, radiation field that includes genitourinary organs
Hypothalamus, pituitary, optic pathway	≥30 Gy	≥30 Gy	Possible, secondary to testosterone deficiency
Surgery			
Orchiectomy-unilateral[b]	Testicular cancer—possible reduced spermatogenesis	Testicular cancer—possible premature hormonal aging	Unlikely
Pelvic	Unlikely	Unlikely	Retroperitoneal lymph node dissection, Prostatectomy, Rectal surgery
Spinal	Unlikely	Unlikely	T11 and below
HP, optic pathway	Possible, tumor invasion of hypothalamus	Possible, tumor invasion of hypothalamus	Possible, secondary to testosterone deficiency

[a] An established unit for quantifying therapeutic exposure to different alkylating agents based on hematologic toxicity; for specific calculations, see Green and colleagues.[7]

[b] Data derived from studies with survivors of testicular cancer.

[c] Some evidence suggests that spermatogenesis may be impaired after radiation to the testes of 5 Gy. The risk for impaired spermatogenesis increases with increasing radiation dose.

Adapted from Kenney LB, Antal Z, Ginsberg JP, et al. Improving Male Reproductive Health After Childhood, Adolescent, and Young Adult Cancer: Progress and Future Directions for Survivorship Research. J Clin Oncol. 2018;36(21):2160-2168. https://doi.org/10.1200/JCO.2017.76.3839; with permission.

Impaired spermatogenesis may be reversible or permanent, depending on the combinations of treatment and on the cumulative dose of chemotherapy given. When counseling CCSs with impaired gonadal function, the survivor must be informed that infertility in male CCSs may be the result of a combination of factors, such as impaired spermatogenesis, androgen insufficiency, HP function, and sexual dysfunction. Each of these factors, in turn, can be a result of direct toxic effects of the given therapy or can be a consequence of psychosocial effects of having had cancer as a child.

Screening for Male Gonadal Failure

Different recommendations for screening of male gonadal failure exist. Due to discrepancies within the existing recommendations, the International Guideline Harmonization Group (IGHG) has formed a collaborative for recommendations on whom and how to screen for testicular insufficiency after treatment of childhood cancer.[42,49] Consensus was found to recommend that all CCSs treated with 1 or more potentially gonadotoxic agents should be advised and counseled about the risk of impaired spermatogenesis and its implications for future fertility.[42]

The assessment of gonadal failure in male CCSs should consist at least of a detailed history of the survivor, including physical examination, monitoring of height, body mass index, Tanner stage, and testicular volume in prepubertal and peripubertal boys. In older boys and adolescents, attention should be paid to the sexual history (onset of puberty, libido, presence of erections, and sexual activity).

For prepubertal boys at risk for gonadal insufficiency, it has been recommended to monitor height and pubertal development and progression (Tanner stage, including testicular volume); in postpubertal men, early morning serum testosterone and LH/FSH concentrations can be measured to monitor for gonadal insufficiency.[42] Semen analysis generally is considered the gold standard to evaluate male fertility and it should be offered to all postpubertal male CCSs when information on fertility is requested.

Inhibin B is secreted by the Sertoli cells. Therefore, it has been evaluated for use in screening for gonadal damage in male CCSs. In male CCSs treated for childhood Hodgkin lymphoma with combination chemotherapy (Adriamycin/epirubicin, bleomycin, vinblastine, and dacarbazine) with or without mechlorethamine, vincristine, prednisone, and procarbazine (MOPP), inhibin B concentrations were correlated independently with sperm concentration.[50] In prepubertal boys, it was found to be a potential marker, when used in combination with FSH, for semen quality. Even in this study, however, semen analysis still was suggested as the gold standard.[50] Two other studies that investigated the diagnostic value of inhibin B and FSH concentrations for detecting azoospermia and oligospermia showed that measurements of FSH, inhibin B concentrations, and using the inhibin-FSH ratio all show fairly diagnostic value for detecting azoospermia.[51,52] With these studies in mind, it has been concluded that inhibin B measurements may be useful but are not as reliable as the gold standard, and, therefore, should not be recommended as the standard screening tool.

The accuracy of FSH as a predictor of azoospermia in adult CCSs remains controversial, with conflicting results. Strong supporting evidence was found for the use of serum FSH as a surrogate biomarker for azoospermia in adult CCSs, with an optimal FSH threshold of 10.4 IU/L to detect azoospermia (specificity of 81% and sensitivity of 83%).[53] The IGHG recommended that if survivors require assessment of fertility, semen analysis is preferred to determination of FSH or inhibin B serum concentrations.[42]

Treatment of Male Gonadal Failure

Consequences of androgen (testosterone) deficiency in male CCSs can be pubertal delay or pubertal arrest, gynecomastia, reduced bone mass, lethargy, fatigue, diminished muscle mass, abdominal obesity, and sexual impairment. A recent study associated Leydig cell failure in CCSs with diabetes mellitus and all-cause mortality.[44] Timely diagnosis of androgen deficiency is important because most of the consequences of androgen deficiency may be overcome with testosterone replacement therapy.

Also, considering that sexual health has been shown to be important for overall health and quality of life, awareness and screening for sexual impairment in CCSs deserve attention. Sexual impairment may be present not only in CCSs with gonadal failure but also after surgery or radiation involving the lower spinal cord, prostate, distal colon, or rectum, due to disruption of the innervation required for erection and ejaculation.[32] These CCSs may be referred to an (andro-) urology department for specific techniques to improve sexual function.

Fertility Preservation in Boys Treated for Childhood Cancer

There are several experimental and established techniques for preservation of male fertility.[42] For pubertal and postpubertal male CCSs at potential risk of infertility due to treatment with alkylating agents, radiotherapy to volumes exposing the testes, hematopoietic stem cell transplantation, cisplatin, or orchiectomy or cranial radiotherapy, it has been recommended by the IGHG to offer semen cryopreservation before start of gonadotoxic therapy. Also, in male CCSs with high risk of recurrent disease and subsequent high risk of impairing further testicular function, sperm banking may be offered. In postpubertal male CCSs, sperm may be banked by cryopreservation after masturbation, or, if masturbation is not possible and there is a high risk of infertility, alternative techniques, such as vibration, electroejaculation, and microsurgical epididymal sperm aspiration or testicular sperm cell extraction, have been described.[54,55] In prepubertal boys, no proved fertility preservation option is available. The IGHG moderately recommends offering testicular tissue harvesting for cryopreservation in a research setting to prepubertal childhood, adolescent, and young adult (CAYA) cancer patients with high risk for infertility. In theory, this can be autotransplanted at the time the CCS is ready for it, after screening for residual malignant cells. Research is done by different groups to expand the spermatogonial stem cells in vitro.[32] Although the research in this field is active, there currently is no treatment possible for male CCSs with azoospermia after cancer treatment, except for pregnancy using donor sperm.

Male Fertility Outcomes

Male CCSs have been shown to have a reduced chance of siring a pregnancy than siblings (HR 0.56; 95% CI, −0.49–0.63), with increased risk for males after exposure to more than 7.5-Gy radiotherapy to both testes and higher cumulative doses of alkylating chemotherapy (CED >4000 mg/m^2).[56]

Referral and Treatment of Male Childhood Cancer Survivors with Gonadal Dysfunction

The most optimal timing to start testosterone supplementation in CCS boys depends on the decline in serum testosterone concentration, the growth height velocity, and bone age in combination with the development of and wish for secondary sexual characteristics. Testosterone may be administered orally, intramuscularly, or topically. The goal of sex steroid replacement in male CCSs is to obtain adequate pubertal develop-ment in combination with optimization of final height, accrual of bone and muscle mass, and satisfaction upon secondary sexual characteristics and sexual functioning. In CCSs with central hypogonadism and no previous exposure to gonadotoxic drugs, stimulation of the testes for pubertal induction may be done using HCG. In this situa-tion, during the virilization phase, the testes enlarge, which may give the developing teenager more self-confidence and improve body satisfaction. Disadvantages of HCG versus testosterone replacement therapy are the manner of administration and the cost effectiveness; HCG is more expensive and should be administered twice weekly subcutaneously. These advantages and disadvantages should be discussed with the teen survivor by an experienced pediatric endocrinologist. There seems to be no difference in effect of treatment with HCG versus testosterone replacement therapy on virilization (in case of sufficient testes) or fertility outcome.

CENTRAL HYPOGONADISM (FEMALE AND MALE)

Central hypogonadism results from inadequate or failing pulsatile release of gonadotropin-releasing hormone from the hypothalamus and/or inadequate FSH/LH secretion from the anterior pituitary. The most common causes for this condition are either a tumor in the sellar or suprasellar hypothalamic region or radiation exposure to a field that includes the HP region.[57] In rare cases, combined primary gonadal insuf-ficiency and central hypogonadism exist due to the combination of treatment with gonadotoxic chemotherapy and damage to the HP region.

Central hypogonadism, or hypogonadotropic hypogonadism, leads to pubertal delay or arrest in peripubertal and postpubertal CCSs as well to signs and symptoms of sex steroid deficiency in adolescents, including all the possible consequences, as discussed previously. When there has been no exposure to gonadotoxic treatments, fertility may not be impaired because the gonads can be stimulated by FSH, human chorionic gonadotropin (HCG), or a combination treatment.[58] This should be coun-seled with the survivor, because the survivor may not be aware of the differences be-tween hyperpogonadotropic (primary) and hypogonadotropic (central) hypogonadism with regard to fertility outcome.

Central hypogonadism may be diagnosed after cranial radiation, including the HP region, with greater than 22 Gy to 30 Gy, in survivors with tumors in the sellar or supra-sellar region, such as craniopharyngeoma or germinoma, or after neurosurgery in the HP region, such as in patients with low-grade glioma.[59] The overall incidence of hypo-gonadotropic hypogonadism in CCSs was reported to be 6.3%.[60] In a Dutch cohort of 481 childhood brain tumor survivors age 12 years or older, 4.2% were found to have hypogonadotropic hypogonadism after a median onset of 4.5 years.[61] In 748 children followed for a median period of 27.3 years after cranial irradiation, the prevalence of LH/FSH deficiency was found to be 10.8% and was associated significantly with male sex and obesity.[59] Strikingly, hypogonadism was not treated in 78.5% of individ-uals, and presence of hypogonadism could be associated with hypertension, dyslipi-demia, low bone mineral density, slow walking, abdominal obesity, low energy expenditure, and muscle weakness. These results emphasize the need for adequate screening and timely treatment of androgen deficiency.

PSYCHOLOGICAL CONSEQUENCES

Worries and uncertainty about gonadal or sexual dysfunction and fertility may have a great impact on CCSs. Dealing with infertility, even if it has been anticipated, needs time and professional guidance. For this reason, psychological support must be present and offered to the survivor and is part of the expert oncofertility team and/or late effects clinic team.[1]

SUMMARY

Male and female CCSs may be at risk for gonadal insufficiency, resulting in pubertal delay or pubertal arrest, reduced bone mass, lethargy, fatigue, and sexual impairment. In addition, male CCSs may present with gynecomastia, diminished muscle mass, and abdominal obesity and female CCSs with hot flushes and sweating. Best practice is that all CCSs should be informed about their risk for gonadal toxicity, infertility, future obstetric risk, and reduced sexuality, because this greatly influences their quality of survival. Consultation about fertility preservation options and alternative family planning should be done for CCSs at high risk before transition toward adult survivorship clinics and repeated at appropriate time intervals based on international established guidelines for fertility preservation.

CCSs at risk should be screened according to recent recommendations and be referred on indication to a pediatric endocrinologist, andrologist, gynecologist, or fertility specialist with experience in CCSs. Before and during pregnancy, risk factors for premature delivery should be considered and discussed with obstetric medicine care experts.

DISCLOSURE

H.M. van Santen has received speakers fee from Pfizer BV and Ferring BV. M.D. van de Wetering, A.M.E. Bos, H.J. van der Pal, M.M. vd Heuvel-Eibrink and W.H. Wallace have nothing to disclose.

REFERENCES

1. Crawshaw M. Psychosocial oncofertility issues faced by adolescents and young adults over their lifetime: A review of the research. Hum Fertil 2013;16:59–63.
2. Armuand G, Wettergren L, Nilsson J, et al. Threatened fertility: A longitudinal study exploring experiences of fertility and having children after cancer treatment. Eur J Cancer Care (Engl) 2018;27:e12798.
3. van Dorp W, Haupt R, Anderson RA, et al. Reproductive function and outcomes in female survivors of childhood, adolescent, and young adult cancer: A review. J Clin Oncol 2018;36:2169–80.
4. Anderson RA, Mitchel RT, Kelsey TW, et al. Cancer treatment and gonadal function: Experimental and established strategies for fertility preservation in children and young adults. Lancet Diabetes Endocrinol 2015;3:556–67.
5. van den Berg MH, Overbeek A, Lambalk CB, et al. Long-term effects of childhood cancer treatment on hormonal and ultrasound markers of ovarian reserve. Hum Reprod 2018;33:1474–88.
6. van Dorp W, Mulder RL, Kremer LC, et al. Recommendations for premature ovarian insufficiency surveillance for female survivors of childhood, adolescent, and young adult cancer: A report from the International Late Effects of Childhood Cancer Guideline Harmonization Group in collaboration with the PanCareSurFup Consortium. J Clin Oncol 2016;34:3440–50.
7. Green DM, Nolan VG, Goodman PJ, et al. The Cyclophosphamide equivalent dose as an approach for quantifying alkylating agent exposure: A report from the childhood cancer Survivor Study. Pediatr Blood Cancer 2014;61:53–67.

8. Clement SC, Kraal KC, van Eck-Smit BL, et al. Primary ovarian insufficiency in children after treatment with 131I-metaiodobenzylguanidine for neuroblastoma: Report of the first two cases. J Clin Endocrinol Metab 2014;99:E112–6.

9. Clement SC, Peeters RP, Ronckers CM, et al. Intermediate and long-term adverse effects of radioiodine therapy for differentiated thyroid carcinoma - A systematic review. Cancer Treat Rev 2015;41:925–34.

10. van der Kooi ALF, Clemens E, Broer L, et al. Genetic variation in gonadal impairment in female survivors of childhood cancer: A PanCareLIFE study protocol. BMC Cancer 2018;18:930.

11. Wo JY, Viswanathan AN. Impact of Radiotherapy on Fertility, Pregnancy, and Neonatal Outcomes in Female Cancer Patients. Int J Radiat Oncol Biol Phys 2009;73:1304–12.

12. Dewailly D, Andersen CY, Balen A, et al. The physiology and clinical utility of anti-Müllerian hormone in women. Hum Reprod Update 2014;20:370–85.

13. Kelsey TW, Wright P, Nelson SM, et al. A validated model of serum Anti-Müllerian hormone from conception to menopause. PLoS One 2011;6:e22024.

14. van der Kooi AL, van den Heuvel-Eibrink MM, van Noortwijk A, et al. Longitudinal follow-up in female Childhood Cancer Survivors: no signs of accelerated ovarian function loss. Hum Reprod 2017;32:193–200.

15. van Dorp W, van den Heuvel-Eibrink MM, de Vries AC, et al. Decreased serum anti-Müllerian hormone levels in girls with newly diagnosed cancer. Hum Reprod 2014;29:337–42.

16. Anderson RA, Wallace WHB. Pregnancy and live birth after successful cancer treatment in young women: the need to improve fertility preservation and advice for female cancer patients. Expert Rev Anticancer Ther 2018;18:1–2.

17. Anderson RA, Wallace WHB, Telfer EE. Ovarian tissue cryopreservation for fertility preservation: clinical and research perspectives. Hum Reprod Open 2017;(1): hox001.

18. Armuand GM, Rodriguez-Wallberg KA, Wettergren L, et al. Sex differences in fertility-related information received by young adult cancer survivors. J Clin Oncol 2012;30:2147–53.

19. Rodriguez-Wallberg KA1, Oktay K. Fertility preservation medicine: options for young adults and children with cancer. J Pediatr Hematol Oncol 2010;32(5): 390–6.

20. Donnez J, Dolmans MM. Fertility preservation in women. N Engl J Med 2017; 377(17):1657–65.

21. Donnez J, Dolmans MM, Demylle D, et al. Livebirth after orthotopic transplantation of cryopreserved ovarian tissue. Lancet 2004;364:1405–10.

22. Ernst E, Kjærsgaard M, Birkebæk NH, et al. Case report: Stimulation of puberty in a girl with chemo- and radiation therapy induced ovarian failure by transplantation of a small part of her frozen/thawed ovarian tissue. Eur J Cancer 2013;49: 911–4.

23. Poirot C, Abirached F, Prades M, et al. Induction of puberty by autograft of cryopreserved ovarian tissue. Lancet 2012;379:588.

24. von Wolff M, Stute P, Flück C. Autologous transplantation of cryopreserved ovarian tissue to induce puberty—the endocrinologists' view. Eur J Pediatr 2016;175:2007–10.

25. Oktay K, Bedoschi G. Oocyte cryopreservation for fertility preservation in postpubertal female children at risk for premature ovarian failure due to accelerated follicle loss in turner syndrome or cancer treatments. J Pediatr Adolesc Gynecol 2014;27:342–6.

26. Critchley HOD, Wallace WHB. Impact of cancer treatment on uterine function. J Natl Cancer Inst Monogr 2005;64–8.
27. Kool EM, van der Graaf R, Bos AME, et al. Stakeholders views on the ethical aspects of oocyte banking for third-party assisted reproduction: a qualitative interview study with donors, recipients and professionals. Hum Reprod 2019;34: 842–50.
28. Oktem O, Kim SS, Selek U, et al. Ovarian and uterine functions in female survivors of childhood cancers. Oncologist 2018;23:214–24.
29. Anderson RA, Brewster DH, Wood R, et al. The impact of cancer on subsequent chance of pregnancy: a population based analysis. Hum Reprod 2018;33: 1281–90.
30. Armuand G, Skoog-Svanberg A, Bladh M, et al. Reproductive patterns among childhood and adolescent cancer survivors in Sweden: A population-based matched-cohort study. J Clin Oncol 2017;35:1577–83.
31. Barton SE, Najita JS, Ginsburg ES, et al. Infertility, infertility treatment, and achievement of pregnancy in female survivors of childhood cancer: A report from the Childhood Cancer Survivor Study cohort. Lancet Oncol 2013;14:873–81.
32. Kenney LB, Antal Z, Ginsberg JP, et al. Improving male reproductive health after childhood, adolescent, and young adult cancer: Progress and future directions for survivorship research. J Clin Oncol 2018;36:2160–8.
33. van der Kooi ALF, Brewster DH, Wood R, et al. Perinatal risks in female cancer survivors: A population-based analysis. PLoS One 2018;13(8):e0202805.
34. Burgos N, Cintron D, Latortue-Albino P, et al. Estrogen-based hormone therapy in women with primary ovarian insufficiency: a systematic review. Endocrine 2017; 58:413–25.
35. Crofton PM, Evans N, Bath LE, et al. Physiological versus standard sex steroid replacement in young women with premature ovarian failure: Effects on bone mass acquisition and turnover. Clin Endocrinol (Oxf) 2010;73:707–14.
36. Maclaran K, Panay N. Current concepts in premature ovarian insufficiency. Womens Health 2015;11:169–82.
37. Moskowitz CS, Chou JF, Sklar CA, et al. Radiation-associated breast cancer and gonadal hormone exposure: A report from the Childhood Cancer Survivor Study. Br J Cancer 2017;117:290–9.
38. HRT for menopause: A NICE treatment? Lancet 2015;385:1835–42.
39. Gravholt CH, Andersen NH, Conway GS, et al. Clinical practice guidelines for the care of girls and women with Turner syndrome: Proceedings from the 2016 Cincinnati International Turner Syndrome Meeting. Eur J Endocrinol 2017;177: G1–70.
40. Palmert MR, Dunkel L. Clinical practice. Delayed puberty. N Engl J Med 2012; 366:443–53.
41. Langrish JP, Mills NL, Bath LE, et al. Cardiovascular effects of physiological and standard sex steroid replacement regimens in premature ovarian failure. Hypertension 2009;53:805–11.
42. Skinner R, Mulder RL, Kremer LC, et al. Recommendations for gonadotoxicity surveillance in male childhood, adolescent, and young adult cancer survivors: a report from the International Late Effects of Childhood Cancer Guideline Harmonization Group in collaboration with the PanCareSurFup Consort. Lancet Oncol 2017;18:e75–90.
43. Stukenborg JB, Jahnukainen K, Hutka M, et al. Cancer treatment in childhood and testicular function: The importance of the somatic environment. Endocr Connect 2018;7:R69–87.

44. Chemaitilly W, Liu Q, van Iersel L, et al. Leydig cell function in male survivors of childhood cancer: a report from the st jude lifetime cohort study. J Clin Oncol 2019;37(32):3018–31.
45. Wigny KM, van Dorp W, van der Kooi AL, et al. Gonadal function in boys with newly diagnosed cancer before the start of treatment. Hum Reprod 2016;31: 2613–8.
46. Poganitsch-Korhonen M, Masliukaite I, Nurmio M, et al. Decreased spermatogonial quantity in prepubertal boys with leukaemia treated with alkylating agents. Leukemia 2017;31:1460–3.
47. Green DM, Liu W, Kutteh WH, et al. Cumulative alkylating agent exposure and semen parameters in adult survivors of childhood cancer: A report from the St Jude Lifetime Cohort Study. Lancet Oncol 2014;15:1215–23.
48. van Dorp W, van der Geest IM, Laven JS, et al. Gonadal function recovery in very long-term male survivors of childhood cancer. Eur J Cancer 2013;49:1280–6.
49. Kremer LC, Mulder RL, Oeffinger KC, et al. A worldwide collaboration to harmonize guidelines for the long-term follow-up of childhood and young adult cancer survivors: A report from the international late effects of Childhood Cancer Guideline Harmonization Group. Pediatr Blood Cancer 2013;60:543–9.
50. van Beek RD, Smit M, van den Heuvel-Eibrink MM, et al. Inhibin B is superior to FSH as a serum marker for spermatogenesis in men treated for Hodgkin's lymphoma with chemotherapy during childhood. Hum Reprod 2007;22:3215–22.
51. Green DM, Zhu L, Zhang N, et al. Lack of specificity of plasma concentrations of inhibin B and follicle-stimulating hormone for identification of azoospermic survivors of childhood cancer: A report from the St Jude lifetime cohort study. J Clin Oncol 2013;31:1324–8.
52. Rendtorff R, Beyer M, Müller A, et al. Low inhibin B levels alone are not a reliable marker of dysfunctional spermatogenesis in childhood cancer survivors. Andrologia 2012;44:219–25.
53. Kelsey TW, McConville L, Edgar AB, et al. Follicle Stimulating Hormone is an accurate predictor of azoospermia in childhood cancer survivors. PLoS One 2017; 12:e0181377.
54. Long CJ, Ginsberg JP, Kolon TF. Fertility Preservation in Children and Adolescents with Cancer. Urology 2016;91:190–6.
55. Adank MC, van Dorp W, Smit M, et al. Electroejaculation as a method of fertility preservation in boys diagnosed with cancer: A single-center experience and review of the literature. Fertil Steril 2014;102:199–205.
56. Green DM, Kawashima T, Stovall M, et al. Fertility of male survivors of childhood cancer: A report from the childhood cancer survivor study. J Clin Oncol 2010;28: 332–9.
57. Shalet SM. Radiation and hypothalamic pituitary function. Clin Pediatr Endocrinol 1994;3:1–10.
58. Prior M, Stewart J, McEleny K, et al. Fertility induction in hypogonadotropic hypogonadal men. Clin Endocrinol (Oxf) 2018;89:712–8.
59. Chemaitilly W, Li Z, Huang S, et al. Anterior hypopituitarism in adult survivors of childhood cancers treated with cranial radiotherapy: A report from the st jude lifetime cohort study. J Clin Oncol 2015;33:492–500.
60. Brignardello E, Felicetti F, Castiglione A, et al. Gonadal status in long-term male survivors of childhood cancer. J Cancer Res Clin Oncol 2016;142:1127–32.
61. Clement SC, Schouten-van Meeteren AY, Boot AM, et al. Prevalence and risk factors of early endocrine disorders in childhood brain tumor survivors: A nationwide, multicenter study. J Clin Oncol 2016;34:4362–70.

Renal and Hepatic Health After Childhood Cancer

Matthew J. Ehrhardt, MD, MS[a,b], Roderick Skinner, MB ChB, PhD, FRCPCH[c,d,*], Sharon M. Castellino, MD, MSc[e,f]

KEYWORDS

- Nephrotoxicity • Hepatotoxicity • Survivorship • Childhood cancer • Late effects

KEY POINTS

- Childhood cancer survivors are at risk for long-term toxicity from childhood cancer treatments, including renal and hepatic injury.
- Long-term renal toxicity is associated with prior exposure to ifosfamide, platinum agents, renal surgery, and radiotherapy and predominantly manifests as proximal tubular and glomerular injury.
- Long-term hepatotoxicity is associated with previous treatment with mercaptopurine, thioguanine, methotrexate, hepatic radiotherapy, transfusion-associated infectious hepatitis, and iron overload; it is often indolent in presentation, with the rare but most serious manifestation being cirrhosis.
- Prospective studies investigating long-term renal and hepatic injury are needed to better inform surveillance and interventions to alleviate further injury, and to guide the development of subsequent frontline cancer treatment protocols.

INTRODUCTION

Approximately two-thirds of childhood cancer survivors (CCSs) experience at least 1 chronic health condition,[1] among which are long-term and/or late-occurring renal and hepatic conditions (**Table 1**).

[a] Department of Oncology, St. Jude Children's Research Hospital, Memphis, TN, USA; [b] Department of Epidemiology and Cancer Control, St. Jude Children's Research Hospital, Memphis, TN, USA; [c] Department of Paediatric and Adolescent Haematology/Oncology, Great North Children's Hospital, Newcastle upon Tyne, UK; [d] Clinical and Translational Research Institute, Newcastle University Centre for Cancer, Newcastle University, Newcastle upon Tyne, UK; [e] Department of Pediatrics, Hematology-Oncology, Emory University School of Medicine, Atlanta, GA, USA; [f] Aflac Cancer and Blood Disorders Center, Children's Healthcare of Atlanta, Atlanta, GA, USA
* Corresponding author. Department of Paediatric and Adolescent Oncology, Great North Children's Hospital, Royal Victoria Infirmary, Newcastle upon Tyne Hospitals NHS Foundation Trust, Queen Victoria Road, Newcastle upon Tyne NE1 4LP, UK.
E-mail address: roderick.skinner@newcastle.ac.uk

Pediatr Clin N Am 67 (2020) 1203–1217
https://doi.org/10.1016/j.pcl.2020.07.011
0031-3955/20/© 2020 Elsevier Inc. All rights reserved.

pediatric.theclinics.com

Table 1
Long-term effects on renal and hepatic health in childhood cancer survivors

Cancer Treatment Risk Factor	Potential Late Effect	Additional Risk Factors	Potential Evaluation
Renal Late Effects			
Ifosfamide	CKD (glomerular)[4,8,9,12–15] Proximal tubular injury (hypophosphatemia, Fanconi syndrome)[6–10] Distal tubular injury (nephrogenic diabetes insipidus)[82,83]	Higher cumulative ifosfamide doses, concurrent nephrotoxic treatments (especially cisplatin), unilateral nephrectomy[8,9,81]	Blood pressure Urinalysis (protein/albumin, glucose) Serum creatinine, phosphate, calcium, alkaline phosphatase ± other electrolytes/minerals (eg, potassium) if Fanconi syndrome suspected GFR estimation (if creatinine level significantly increased) Calculate renal tubular threshold for phosphate (Tm_p/GFR)
Platinum agents (cisplatin, carboplatin)	CKD (glomerular)[4,21,23–25] Tubular injury (hypomagnesemia, hypocalcemia)[16–18]	Higher cumulative cisplatin dose or higher dose rate[17,22–25]	Blood pressure Urinalysis (protein/albumin) Serum creatinine, magnesium, calcium GFR estimation (if creatinine level significantly increased)
Renal RT	CKD (glomerular)[28–30] Proteinuria[28–30] Hypertension[22]	Higher renal RT dose[31]	Blood pressure Urinalysis (protein/albumin) Serum creatinine GFR measurement (if creatinine level significantly increased)
Renal surgery	Hyperfiltration[32] CKD (glomerular)[4,22] Proteinuria[33,34] Hypertension[35]	Amount of renal tissue removed[84]	Blood pressure Urinalysis (protein/albumin) Serum creatinine GFR measurement (if creatinine level significantly increased)

HSCT	CKD (glomerular)[36,37] Tubulopathy[36]	Multiple pre-HSCT and peri-HSCT factors, including prior treatment, conditioning treatment, serious early HSCT complications, supportive care treatments (eg, antimicrobials and immunosuppressive agents)[37]	Blood pressure Urinalysis (protein/albumin) Serum creatinine Other serum measurements may be indicated in patients who have received potentially nephrotoxic chemotherapy before HSCT GFR measurement (if creatinine level significantly increased)
Hepatic Late Effects			
Mercaptopurine or thioguanine	Hepatic dysfunction (fibrosis)[46,52] Sequelae of SOS[45,52]	Viral hepatitis, treatment before 1970, abdominal radiotherapy, prior SOS, siderosis, hepatosteatosis[45,46,52,69]	Abdominal examination (splenomegaly) Platelet count, serum ALT, serum GGT, serum bilirubin Other considerations for additional testing/intervention: serum prothrombin time, serum ferritin, screening for viral hepatitis Abdominal ultrasonography with portal flow, liver MRI, or FerriScan Screening for alcohol intake Immunization against hepatitis A, B
Methotrexate	Hepatic dysfunction[46,48-51]	Viral hepatitis, treatment before 1970, abdominal RT, prior SOS[46,69]	
Abdominal RT exposing the liver	Cholelithiasis[38] Hepatic fibrosis/cirrhosis[61] Focal nodular hyperplasia[43]	Viral hepatitis, higher RT dose (>40 Gy to at least one-third of liver; ≥20 Gy to entire liver), siderosis, chronic GVHD, chronic hepatitis, steatosis, multiple transfusions, prior antimetabolite therapy, alcohol use, obesity, family history of cholelithiasis, ileal conduit, abdominal surgery, HSCT, neuroblastoma, high cumulative alkylating agent dose[46,61,69]	
HSCT	Hepatic dysfunction[63] Chronic hepatitis[63] Cirrhosis[78] Iron overload[63,65,66]	RT involving liver, GVHD, history of SOS, alcohol use[63]	

Abbreviations: ALT, alanine transaminase; CKD, chronic kidney disease; GFR, glomerular filtration rate; GGT, glutamyltransferase; GVHD, graft-versus-host disease; HSCT, hematopoietic stem cell transplant, RT, radiotherapy; SOS, sinusoidal obstruction syndrome.

RENAL LATE EFFECTS
Epidemiology

The risk for long-term renal toxicity is associated with the cumulative dose and dose intensity of specific cancer treatment agents. The reported prevalence of renal late effects in CCSs ranges widely, from 0% to 84%,[2] largely because of heterogeneity in study populations, treatment exposures, follow-up duration, and outcome definitions and ascertainment methods. Although the true prevalence of renal outcomes remains uncertain, clear associations with specific treatment exposures exist.

In general, adverse renal events in CCSs arise from reduced glomerular filtration rate (GFR), and tubular injury. In a study of 1442 CCSs followed for a median of 12.1 years from diagnosis, 28.1% had at least 1 abnormality, including hypertension (14.8%), albuminuria (14.5%), low GFR (4.5%), hypomagnesemia (8.8%), and hypophosphatemia (3.0%). Low GFR was associated with nephrectomy with or without nephrotoxic chemotherapy (cisplatin, carboplatin, ifosfamide) and/or radiotherapy, higher cumulative ifosfamide doses, high dose cyclophosphamide (defined as greater than or equal to 1 g/m2/course). Hypomagnesemia was associated with cumulative cisplatin exposure and/or nephrectomy, albuminuria with cumulative ifosfamide dose, and hypertension with abdominal radiotherapy.[3] In a longitudinal study of GFR in 1122 adult 5-year CCSs, the risk of a reduced GFR 35 years posttreatment was highest in those treated with higher cumulative ifosfamide and/or cisplatin doses and with nephrectomy.[4]

Chemotherapy

Ifosfamide

Ifosfamide is associated with proximal and distal tubular, as well as glomerular, dysfunction. Proximal tubular damage presents as hypophosphatemia and Fanconi syndrome, whereas distal injury usually manifests as nephrogenic diabetes insipidus.[5] The most serious form of proximal injury, Fanconi syndrome, results in excessive renal losses of glucose, amino acids, phosphate, bicarbonate, uric acid, sodium, potassium, magnesium, and small-molecular-weight proteins.[6] Tubular toxicity often develops acutely during treatment, although it may present after treatment completion, ranging in severity from asymptomatic aminoaciduria to fulminant Fanconi syndrome and proximal renal tubular acidosis. Among 218 patients treated with ifosfamide at St. Jude Children's Research Hospital, only 1.3% developed Fanconi syndrome.[7]

Patients with Fanconi syndrome recover to varying degrees after treatment completion, and long-term persistence of the complete syndrome is rare; individual biochemical abnormalities (eg, hypophosphatemia) can persist. Oberlin and colleagues[8] reported the long-term nephrotoxicity of ifosfamide among 183 survivors of childhood sarcoma. At a median follow-up of 10 years, 10.5% had tubular dysfunction; however, most were subclinical (eg, glycosuria) and only 1% had hypophosphatemia. In multivariable analyses, the renal tubular threshold for phosphate (Tm_p/GFR) was significantly reduced in patients who had received the highest cumulative doses of ifosfamide ($P = .02$), but there were no cases of hypophosphatemic rickets or nephrogenic diabetes insipidus.[8] In contrast, Skinner and colleagues[9] reported the prevalence of hypophosphatemia in 29 survivors who received ifosfamide. Although 22% had hypophosphatemia at 1 year, only 8% persisted at 10 years, suggesting improvement over time. Musiol and colleagues[10] noted that 36% of 38 central nervous system tumor survivors developed hypophosphatemia at a median follow-up of 3.2 years; however, longitudinal assessments were unavailable to assess potential recovery.

Given similar methodologies used to assess tubular toxicity in these studies, the variable prevalence may reflect differences in underlying diagnoses and hence ifosfamide schedules and doses.

Acute glomerular damage manifesting as severe acute kidney injury (AKI) is uncommon in children but recognized in adults.[11] Rates of chronic kidney disease (CKD) depend on the recovery of AKI.[12,13] Stages 2 to 3 CKD have been reported in 20% to 50% of children and adolescent survivors and may only become apparent months after ifosfamide completion.[14,15] In 1122 adult survivors at least 5 years from cancer diagnosis, ifosfamide was associated with a lower estimated GFR in exposed versus unexposed individuals ($P<.001$).[4] In Oberlin and colleagues'[8] study, 21% and 0.5% experienced grade 1 or 2 reductions in GFR, respectively, after ifosfamide.[8] In a study by Skinner and colleages,[9] although the prevalence of reduced glomerular function varied over time following ifosfamide (26% had lower GFRs at the end of therapy, 70% at 1 year from cancer diagnosis, and 50% at 10 years), differences between end-of-therapy and 10-year assessments did not reach statistical significance ($P = .22$).

Platinum compounds (cisplatin and carboplatin)

Platinum chemotherapy has been clearly associated with the development of tubular dysfunction, manifest by electrolyte and mineral wasting that often develops acutely but can persist long term. Many studies have shown hypomagnesemia and hypocalcemia caused by platinum agents,[16–18] but Fanconi syndrome rarely occurs. Stohr and colleagues[16] prospectively assessed 650 sarcoma survivors for renal dysfunction, comparing those treated with versus without platinum agents. Hypomagnesemia was identified in 12.1% of individuals exposed to cisplatin and 15.6% of individuals exposed to carboplatin versus 4.5% of controls at a median of 23 months ($P = .008$). Hypomagnesemia improved over time such that nobody required long-term supplementation.[16] Hypocalcemia has also been observed acutely, probably largely secondary to hypomagnesemia with decreased parathyroid hormone secretion.[19] Hypocalcemia in association with hypocalciuria has been reported but is rarely clinically significant.[20]

Platinum compounds have also been associated with long-term glomerular dysfunction. Mulder and colleagues[4] reported associations between cisplatin ($P<.001$) and carboplatin ($P = .006$) exposure and decreased GFR. In a separate study of 134 survivors, decreased GFR was the most prevalent (17.7%) renal late effect. However, this effect was mitigated when adjusting for other treatment exposures and years from treatment ($P = .09$).[21]

Dekkers and colleagues[22] observed that, among 763 adult CCSs, GFR was lower in those treated with compared with without high doses (>450 mg/m^2) of cisplatin ($P = .004$). Cisplatin dose rates exceeding 40 mg/m^2/d have been associated with greater long-term glomerular and tubular toxicity ($P<.005$) compared with dose rates of 40 mg/m^2/d in children.[17] Although initial pediatric studies found no relationship between age at exposure and cisplatin nephrotoxicity, long-term follow-up studies report glomerular, and to a lesser extent tubular, toxicity to be more common when treated at an older age.[23–25]

Methotrexate

Acute renal toxicity associated with high-dose (HD) methotrexate is well recognized. However, in a large cohort study of 1122 adult CCSs followed for a median of 7.3 years, HD methotrexate was not associated with a reduced GFR ($P = .07$).[4] Similarly, in multivariable models performed by Dekkers and colleagues,[22] there was no difference in GFR in survivors exposed to methotrexate versus not exposed (P = .36).[22] Based on these data, methotrexate is currently not thought to contribute to long-term nephrotoxicity in CCSs.

Supportive Care

Several supportive care drugs, including aminoglycosides, amphotericin, and angiotensin-converting enzyme inhibitors, can contribute to AKI during cancer therapy. However, with contemporary AKI management, CKD seldom ensues, and virtually no studies suggest these exposures predict the occurrence or severity of chronic nephrotoxicity.[26] However, calcineurin inhibitors commonly used in hematopoietic stem cell transplant (HSCT) recipients may cause hypomagnesemia, increased serum creatinine level, and hypertension acutely; prolonged exposure may cause chronic nephropathy with characteristic arteriolopathy and tubulointerstitial histologic features.[27]

Radiotherapy

Radiotherapy has been shown to increase risk for proteinuria, tubulopathy, and glomerular dysfunction in CCSs.[28–30] Associations are dose dependent, with renal doses greater than 20 Gy resulting in highest risk.[31] In a study of 763 adult CCSs, adjusted models showed that spinal radiation was associated with a 12-fold increased risk for tubular dysfunction (P = .006), whereas abdominal radiation combined with nephrectomy was associated with a 3-fold increased risk for albuminuria (P = .05). Survivors exposed to abdominal radiotherapy, versus not exposed, were also more likely to be hypertensive (43% vs 22%; P = .003),[22] whereas total body irradiation (TBI) has been associated with lower GFR.[29]

Surgery

Partial or complete nephrectomy reduces the number of functioning nephrons, resulting in hyperfiltration in those remaining.[32] Although the impact of persistent hyperfiltration on renal function remains unproved, it is thought to cause progressive glomerular damage, initially manifest by proteinuria and microalbuminuria,[33,34] hypertension,[35] and subsequently CKD. Nephrectomy has been shown to be one of the principal causes of CKD in CCSs,[4] and is associated with a reduced GFR regardless of whether or not individuals received concurrent abdominal radiation exposure (P<.001).[22]

Hematopoietic Stem Cell Transplant

Renal toxicity following HSCT is multifactorial. Treatment of the underlying malignancy may contribute, whereas HSCT conditioning regimens may include high doses of nephrotoxic chemotherapy and/or TBI. Frequent and prolonged use of nephrotoxic supportive care agents is a factor. Compromised renal perfusion caused by acute transplant-related complications, including hemorrhage, sepsis, or hepatic sinusoidal obstruction syndrome (SOS, formerly termed veno-occlusive disease [VOD]), may cause nonreversible AKI. Therefore, it is unsurprising that chronic nephrotoxicity is frequent after HSCT and has been reported in up to 50% of survivors.[36] Glomerular toxicity is the most common renal injury following HSCT. TBI is the major contributor to nephrotoxicity after allogeneic HSCT, but the other aforementioned risk factors are often important.[37] Tubular impairment, less common and usually less severe, is likely caused by conditioning chemotherapy, often in the context of autologous HSCT for heavily pretreated children with relapsed or refractory solid tumors.[36]

HEPATIC LATE EFFECTS
Epidemiology

Acute and subacute hepatobiliary injury manifests as increased liver transaminase levels or hyperbilirubinemia and is associated with multiple chemotherapies, HSCT, and radiotherapy. However, the prevalence of and risks for long-term liver injury in CCSs are uncertain, and associations between acute and late toxicity are unclear. Among a self-report cohort, CCSs are twice as likely to report a hepatic-related health issue and nearly 9 times more likely to report cirrhosis compared with sibling controls.[38] In the Adult Life after Childhood Cancer in Scandinavia (ALiCCS) cohort of 31,132 CCSs with extended follow-up, there is a 3-fold higher risk of liver disease–related hospitalization compared with the general population.[39] A Cochrane Review of 33 studies reported associations between antineoplastic therapy and late hepatotoxicity (measured by liver enzymes, bilirubin, or coagulation times) in CCSs, and found that the prevalence varied from 0% to 84%.[40] In large cohort studies reporting the results of direct assessments, hepatocellular injury (abnormal alanine aminotransferase [ALT]) and biliary tract injury (abnormal glutamyltransferase [GGT]) were noted in 8.7% of 1362 CCSs a median of 12.4 years from diagnosis. In adjusted models, increased ALT and GGT levels were associated with hepatic radiotherapy, higher body mass index, higher alcohol intake, and longer follow-up time. Older age at diagnosis was only significantly associated with increased GGT levels.[41] St. Jude investigators observed an increased ALT in 41.3% of 2751 directly assessed adult CCSs. Notably, fewer than 10% of these were grade 2 or higher. Adjusted models identified that non-Hispanic white race/ethnicity, age at evaluation, being overweight or obese, metabolic syndrome, current statin treatment, hepatitis C virus (HCV) infection, prior treatment with busulfan or thioguanine, history of hepatic surgery, and the percentage of liver treated with greater than or equal to 10 Gy were associated with increased ALT level.[42]

The most common chemotherapies associated with acute hepatotoxicity include methotrexate, mercaptopurine, thioguanine, dactinomycin, and busulfan; however, attribution of late hepatotoxicity to specific agents has proved difficult because of multiagent and multimodal exposures in most CCSs. In addition, liver injury can be indolent, rendering it difficult to identify.

The most commonly observed hepatobiliary late effects in CCSs include asymptomatic transaminitis, cholelithiasis, focal nodular hyperplasia (FNH), nodular regenerative hyperplasia, microvesicular fatty change, infectious hepatitis, and transfusion-related iron overload.[43,44] Treatment-related injury is likely related to various combinations of cholestasis, hepatocellular necrosis, biliary ductal injury, steatosis, and SOS.[43] Hepatic fibrosis, in response to inflammation from chronic viral hepatitis, drug-induced injury, fatty infiltration, or siderosis, is a risk factor for subsequent cirrhosis, portal hypertension, and hepatocellular carcinoma.[45–47] Histologic findings of liver injury include periportal and concentric fibrosis and injury to sinusoidal endothelial cells.[43,44] In addition to cancer therapy itself, supportive care measures, including total parenteral nutrition and transfusion therapy, may contribute to liver injury in CCSs. The importance of comorbid conditions (eg, obesity, excessive alcohol consumption) has recently been highlighted.

Chemotherapy

Methotrexate
Acute and subacute methotrexate-induced hepatotoxicity is characterized by transient increases of serum transaminase or alkaline phosphatase levels.[48] The risk of

fibrosis or cirrhosis after daily oral methotrexate is more than 2-fold greater than that with intermittent parenteral administration.[49] Histologic studies of liver from children treated with methotrexate showed mild structural changes and a low incidence of portal fibrosis.[48,50] These findings suggest that methotrexate-induced fibrosis regresses or stabilizes after discontinuation and rarely produces end-stage liver disease in the absence of other antimetabolite therapy or comorbidities.[48] Two larger retrospective studies evaluating increased transaminase level and biliary tract injury provide moderate evidence of no long-term injury in CCSs.[41,42] Interestingly, there are no reports of long-term hepatotoxicity in osteosarcoma survivors who receive shorter-duration HD methotrexate despite increased transaminase levels during therapy; however, in leukemia survivors with viral hepatitis who received parenteral, oral, or HD-methotrexate regimens, evidence supports risk for progressive hepatic dysfunction that persists into adulthood.[46,51]

6-Mercaptopurine and 6-Thioguanine

The antimetabolites 6-thioguanine and 6-mercaptopurine have been associated with subacute hepatocellular and cholestatic disease[52] Genetic deficiency of thiopurine S-methyltransferase (TPMT) is thought to be a predisposing factor for skewed antimetabolite processing resulting in neutropenia and increased transaminase level, but there is inconsistent evidence associating TPMT variant genotypes with the more serious sequelae of SOS following thioguanine exposure.[53,54] SOS following antimetabolite therapy is typically more indolent than that occurring during HSCT. Although most children with thiopurine-associated SOS recover, a subset develop progressive hepatic fibrosis and nodular regenerative hyperplasia,[45,52] manifest as thrombocytopenia with varying degrees of portal hypertension.[55]

Actinomycin

Acute, dose-related, reversible SOS has been observed in children treated with dactinomycin for Wilms tumor or rhabdomyosarcoma.[56,57] However, the prevalence of chronic hepatopathy with extended follow-up is unknown, with no demonstrable risk for biliary tract injury noted at a median of 12 years.[41]

Radiotherapy

Radiotherapy-associated hepatopathy after contemporary treatment is uncommon in CCSs.[58–60] The risk of injury in children increases with radiation dose, volume of hepatic tissue in the radiation field, younger age at treatment, previous partial hepatectomy, and concomitant use of radiomimetic chemotherapy (eg, dactinomycin). In the National Wilms Tumor Study (NWTS) group cohort, development of portal hypertension was associated with right-flank radiation and a dose greater than 15 Gy.[61] The dose threshold for irreversible liver injury is uncertain but is currently under investigation.[62]

Hematopoietic Stem Cell Transplant

Hepatic dysfunction in long-term survivors of HSCT is largely related to graft-versus-host disease (GVHD). In addition, high transfusion requirements in these CCSs confer risks for chronic infection with hepatotropic viruses and for iron overload.[63] Liver GVHD is associated with hepatocellular necroinflammatory changes, paucity of interlobular bile ducts, and interhepatic cholestasis.[63] SOS, an acute event of HSCT, arises from endothelial injury and hepatocellular injury but differs in its severity and tempo from that of chemotherapy-associated SOS in the nontransplant setting. SOS in HSCT is largely attributed to transplant conditioning regimens; however, a recent genome-wide association study analysis of pediatric patients who received busulfan-based conditioning found genetic contributors to this risk. In adjusted models, polymorphisms in the *UGT2B10* and *KIAA1715* genes were noted to confer increased risk for SOS with some dependence on the conditioning regimen.[64] The long-term clinical outcomes of CCSs who survive HSCT-associated acute SOS are unknown. Recently an association has been noted between autologous HSCT and FNH.[64]

Specific Hepatic Late Effects

Transfusion-related iron overload

The prevalence and severity of transfusion-related iron overload, occurring independently or as a contributing factor to other liver injury in CCSs, remain incompletely characterized but approach 25.9% following HSCT.[65] In a multivariable analysis, cumulative packed red blood cell volume and older age at diagnosis predicted increased liver iron concentration.[66] Receipt of an allogeneic HSCT is also a significant risk factor.[65] A recent study identified hyperferritinemia (>500 ng/mL) in 2.6% of 116 CCSs, with red cell transfusion volume correlating with ferritin ($r = 0.74$, $P<.0001$). MRI (T2 MRI or FerriScan) has emerged as an accurate, noninvasive means for measuring liver iron content,[67] but further research is needed to better characterize CCSs at greatest risk and who will benefit from interventions to reduce iron burden and improve organ function.[68]

Transfusion-acquired hepatitis

Infectious hepatitis has been a major contributor to liver morbidity and mortality, especially in survivors transfused before the initiation of effective blood product screening for hepatitis B virus (HBV) and HCV in 1972 and 1993, respectively.[46,69–71] Survivors with chronic hepatitis are at risk for progressive fibrosis, cirrhosis, and hepatocellular carcinoma, with hepatocellular carcinoma largely attributable to chronic HBV and HCV infection.[47,72] The prevalence of transfusion-related HCV in historical CCS cohorts ranges from 5% to 50% depending on geographic location.[46,71] Coinfection with HBV and HCV might accelerate progression, as does concomitant immunosuppression or HSCT-associated hepatotoxicity.[47,71]

Focal nodular hyperplasia

FNH is a benign, incidental imaging finding in CCSs representing polyclonal proliferation of hepatocytes surrounding a central scar. It is characterized with specificity by MRI and rarely associated with complications or malignant transformation. The pathogenesis of FNH is poorly understood but thought to be a reaction to a localized vascular anomaly. Prior HSCT, VOD/SOS, hormonal therapy, diagnosis of neuroblastoma, radiation therapy exposing the liver, and HD alkylating agent exposure are all associated with FNH.[73] Biopsy or resection is usually unnecessary unless the lesions grow or the patient develops symptom warranting intervention.

Novel Agents and Unknown Risk for Renal and Hepatic Late Effects

Although several emerging, targeted anticancer drugs can be nephrotoxic or hepatotoxic, most published reports are from adult studies and do not inform long-term outcomes,[74] particularly in children. AKI with biopsy features of acute tubulointerstitial nephritis, and immune-mediated hepatitis, have been reported in up to 2% and 1% to 6%, respectively, of adults treated with immune checkpoint inhibitors.[75,76] Although most partially improve with steroids, ongoing surveillance is recommended given the potential for severe and lasting consequences, and studies in CCSs will be needed. Minimal change/focal segmental glomerulosclerosis and thrombotic microangiopathy have been associated with vascular endothelial growth factor inhibitors but seem to be reversible with drug discontinuation.[77] Growing recognition of the frequency and potential implications of a range of nephrotoxicity after exposure to new, as well as existing, anticancer agents has prompted the establishment of onconephrology, as well as a heightened awareness of the need to coordinate acute and late-onset nephrotoxicity data collection following novel treatments in both children and adults.

Previous treatment with the novel antibody drug conjugates gemtuzumab ozogamicin and inotuzumab ozogamicin are reported as risks for post-HSCT SOS in clinical trials.[78] Although tyrosine kinase inhibitors (TKIs) have become important agents for many cancers, most are reported to induce acute and subacute hepatic injury. Although such TKI-related damage is thought to be reversible, the risk of long-term cirrhosis is unknown and requires diligent surveillance.[79]

Survivorship Guidelines

Clinical practice guidelines by national organizations have increased early detection of and intervention for late adverse effects of cancer therapy. Guidelines are currently being harmonized to develop specific consensus recommendations regarding surveillance for specific late effects.[80] Adapting a similar approach to prior International Guideline Harmonization Group for Late Effects of Childhood Cancer efforts, renal toxicity and hepatic toxicity task forces are actively developing consensus guidelines based on a thorough review and grading of existing evidence.

SUMMARY

Several studies report an increased risk for late-occurring adverse renal and hepatic health effects in CCSs. Although clear associations exist, most existing studies are limited by small sample sizes, heterogeneity of underlying disease populations, and variable definitions of exposures and outcomes. In addition, many reflect older survivor cohorts that may not inform about potential late complications of contemporary and evolving treatment strategies and novel treatment agents. Despite these limitations, clinicians providing medical care to CCSs should have heightened awareness for late renal and liver toxicity, and future investigations will be critical to better quantifying risk, identifying key risk factors, and prioritizing interventions seeking to maximize health and quality care for CCSs.

REFERENCES

1. Oeffinger KC, Mertens AC, Sklar CA, et al. Chronic health conditions in adult survivors of childhood cancer. N Engl J Med 2006;355(15):1572–82.
2. Kooijmans EC, Bokenkamp A, Tjahjadi NS, et al. Early and late adverse renal effects after potentially nephrotoxic treatment for childhood cancer. Cochrane Database Syst Rev 2019;3:CD008944.
3. Knijnenburg SL, Jaspers MW, van der Pal HJ, et al. Renal dysfunction and elevated blood pressure in long-term childhood cancer survivors. Clin J Am Soc Nephrol 2012;7(9):1416–27.
4. Mulder RL, Knijnenburg SL, Geskus RB, et al. Glomerular function time trends in long-term survivors of childhood cancer: a longitudinal study. Cancer Epidemiol Biomarkers Prev 2013;22(10):1736–46.
5. Skinner R, Sharkey IM, Pearson AD, et al. Ifosfamide, mesna, and nephrotoxicity in children. J Clin Oncol 1993;11(1):173–90.
6. Foreman JW, Roth KS. Human renal Fanconi syndrome–then and now. Nephron 1989;51(3):301–6.

7. Pratt CB, Meyer WH, Jenkins JJ, et al. Ifosfamide, Fanconi's syndrome, and rickets. J Clin Oncol 1991;9(8):1495–9.
8. Oberlin O, Fawaz O, Rey A, et al. Long-term evaluation of Ifosfamide-related nephrotoxicity in children. J Clin Oncol 2009;27(32):5350–5.
9. Skinner R, Parry A, Price L, et al. Glomerular toxicity persists 10 years after ifosfamide treatment in childhood and is not predictable by age or dose. Pediatr Blood Cancer 2010;54(7):983–9.
10. Musiol K, Sobol-Milejska G, Nowotka L, et al. Renal function in children treated for central nervous system malignancies. Childs Nerv Syst 2016;32(8):1431–40.
11. Willemse PH, de Jong PE, Elema JD, et al. Severe renal failure following high-dose ifosfamide and mesna. Cancer Chemother Pharmacol 1989;23(5):329–30.
12. Loebstein R, Atanackovic G, Bishai R, et al. Risk factors for long-term outcome of ifosfamide-induced nephrotoxicity in children. J Clin Pharmacol 1999;39(5):454–61.
13. Friedlaender MM, Haviv YS, Rosenmann E, et al. End-stage renal interstitial fibrosis in an adult ten years after ifosfamide therapy. Am J Nephrol 1998;18(2):131–3.
14. Skinner R, Cotterill SJ, Stevens MC. Risk factors for nephrotoxicity after ifosfamide treatment in children: a UKCCSG Late Effects Group study. United Kingdom Children's Cancer Study Group. Br J Cancer 2000;82(10):1636–45.
15. Prasad VK, Lewis IJ, Aparicio SR, et al. Progressive glomerular toxicity of ifosfamide in children. Med Pediatr Oncol 1996;27(3):149–55.
16. Stohr W, Paulides M, Bielack S, et al. Nephrotoxicity of cisplatin and carboplatin in sarcoma patients: a report from the late effects surveillance system. Pediatr Blood Cancer 2007;48(2):140–7.
17. Skinner R, Pearson AD, English MW, et al. Cisplatin dose rate as a risk factor for nephrotoxicity in children. Br J Cancer 1998;77(10):1677–82.
18. Brock PR, Koliouskas DE, Barratt TM, et al. Partial reversibility of cisplatin nephrotoxicity in children. J Pediatr 1991;118(4 Pt 1):531–4.
19. Lajer H, Daugaard G. Cisplatin and hypomagnesemia. Cancer Treat Rev 1999;25(1):47–58.
20. Bianchetti MG, Kanaka C, Ridolfi-Luthy A, et al. Chronic renal magnesium loss, hypocalciuria and mild hypokalaemic metabolic alkalosis after cisplatin. Pediatr Nephrol 1990;4(3):219–22.
21. Mudi A, Levy CS, Geel JA, et al. Paediatric cancer survivors demonstrate a high rate of subclinical renal dysfunction. Pediatr Blood Cancer 2016;63(11):2026–32.
22. Dekkers IA, Blijdorp K, Cransberg K, et al. Long-term nephrotoxicity in adult survivors of childhood cancer. Clin J Am Soc Nephrol 2013;8(6):922–9.
23. Skinner R, Parry A, Price L, et al. Persistent nephrotoxicity during 10-year follow-up after cisplatin or carboplatin treatment in childhood: relevance of age and dose as risk factors. Eur J Cancer 2009;45(18):3213–9.
24. Daugaard G, Abildgaard U, Holstein-Rathlou NH, et al. Renal tubular function in patients treated with high-dose cisplatin. Clin Pharmacol Ther 1988;44(2):164–72.
25. Daugaard G, Rossing N, Rorth M. Effects of cisplatin on different measures of glomerular function in the human kidney with special emphasis on high-dose. Cancer Chemother Pharmacol 1988;21(2):163–7.
26. Patzer L. Nephrotoxicity as a cause of acute kidney injury in children. Pediatr Nephrol 2008;23(12):2159–73.

27. Fujinaga S, Kaneko K, Muto T, et al. Independent risk factors for chronic cyclosporine induced nephropathy in children with nephrotic syndrome. Arch Dis Child 2006;91(8):666–70.

28. Dawson LA, Kavanagh BD, Paulino AC, et al. Radiation-associated kidney injury. Int J Radiat Oncol Biol Phys 2010;76(3 Suppl):S108–15.

29. Frisk P, Bratteby LE, Carlson K, et al. Renal function after autologous bone marrow transplantation in children: a long-term prospective study. Bone Marrow Transplant 2002;29(2):129–36.

30. Luxton RW. Radiation nephritis. A long-term study of 54 patients. Lancet 1961; 2(7214):1221–4.

31. Cassady JR. Clinical radiation nephropathy. Int J Radiat Oncol Biol Phys 1995; 31(5):1249–56.

32. Tiburcio FR, Rodrigues KES, Belisario AR, et al. Glomerular hyperfiltration and beta-2 microglobulin as biomarkers of incipient renal dysfunction in cancer survivors. Future Sci OA 2018;4(8):FSO333.

33. Bailey S, Roberts A, Brock C, et al. Nephrotoxicity in survivors of Wilms' tumours in the North of England. Br J Cancer 2002;87(10):1092–8.

34. Levitt GA, Yeomans E, Dicks Mireaux C, et al. Renal size and function after cure of Wilms' tumour. Br J Cancer 1992;66(5):877–82.

35. Finklestein JZ, Norkool P, Green DM, et al. Diastolic hypertension in Wilms' tumor survivors: a late effect of treatment? A report from the National Wilms' Tumor Study Group. Am J Clin Oncol 1993;16(3):201–5.

36. Patzer L, Ringelmann F, Kentouche K, et al. Renal function in long-term survivors of stem cell transplantation in childhood. A prospective trial. Bone Marrow Transplant 2001;27(3):319–27.

37. Esiashvili N, Chiang KY, Hasselle MD, et al. Renal toxicity in children undergoing total body irradiation for bone marrow transplant. Radiother Oncol 2009;90(2): 242–6.

38. Goldsby R, Chen Y, Raber S, et al. Survivors of childhood cancer have increased risk of gastrointestinal complications later in life. Gastroenterology 2011;140(5): 1464–71.e1.

39. Asdahl PH, Winther JF, Bonnesen TG, et al. Gastrointestinal and liver disease in Adult Life After Childhood Cancer in Scandinavia: A population-based cohort study. Int J Cancer 2016;139(7):1501–11.

40. Mulder RL, Bresters D, Van den Hof M, et al. Hepatic late adverse effects after antineoplastic treatment for childhood cancer. Cochrane Database Syst Rev 2019;(4):CD008205.

41. Mulder RL, Kremer LC, Koot BG, et al. Surveillance of hepatic late adverse effects in a large cohort of long-term survivors of childhood cancer: prevalence and risk factors. Eur J Cancer 2013;49(1):185–93.

42. Green DM, Wang M, Krasin MJ, et al. Serum alanine aminotransferase elevations in survivors of childhood cancer: a report from the St. Jude Lifetime Cohort Study. Hepatology 2019;69(1):94–106.

43. Floyd J, Mirza I, Sachs B, et al. Hepatotoxicity of chemotherapy. Semin Oncol 2006;33(1):50–67.

44. Rodriguez-Frias EA, Lee WM. Cancer chemotherapy II: atypical hepatic injuries. Clin Liver Dis 2007;11(3):663–76, viii.

45. Broxson EH, Dole M, Wong R, et al. Portal hypertension develops in a subset of children with standard risk acute lymphoblastic leukemia treated with oral 6-thioguanine during maintenance therapy. Pediatr Blood Cancer 2005;44(3):226–31.

46. Castellino S, Lensing S, Riely C, et al. The epidemiology of chronic hepatitis C infection in survivors of childhood cancer: an update of the St Jude Children's Research Hospital hepatitis C seropositive cohort. Blood 2004;103(7):2460–6.

47. Strickland DK, Jenkins JJ, Hudson MM. Hepatitis C infection and hepatocellular carcinoma after treatment of childhood cancer. J Pediatr Hematol Oncol 2001; 23(8):527–9.

48. Parker D, Bate CM, Craft AW, et al. Liver damage in children with acute leukaemia and non-Hodgkin's lymphoma on oral maintenance chemotherapy. Cancer Chemother Pharmacol 1980;4(2):121–7.

49. Hutter RVP SF, Tan CTC, Murphy ML, et al. Hepatic fibrosis in children with acute leukemia: a complication of therapy. Cancer 1960;13:288–307.

50. Halonen P, Mattila J, Makipernaa A, et al. Erythrocyte concentrations of metabolites or cumulative doses of 6-mercaptopurine and methotrexate do not predict liver changes in children treated for acute lymphoblastic leukemia. Pediatr Blood Cancer 2006;46(7):762–6.

51. Farrow AC, Buchanan GR, Zwiener RJ, et al. Serum aminotransferase elevation during and following treatment of childhood acute lymphoblastic leukemia. J Clin Oncol 1997;15(4):1560–6.

52. De Bruyne R, Portmann B, Samyn M, et al. Chronic liver disease related to 6-thioguanine in children with acute lymphoblastic leukaemia. J Hepatol 2006;44(2): 407–10.

53. Lennard L, Richards S, Cartwright CS, et al. The thiopurine methyltransferase genetic polymorphism is associated with thioguanine-related veno-occlusive disease of the liver in children with acute lymphoblastic leukemia. Clin Pharmacol Ther 2006;80(4):375–83.

54. Wray L, Vujkovic M, McWilliams T, et al. TPMT and MTHFR genotype is not associated with altered risk of thioguanine-related sinusoidal obstruction syndrome in pediatric acute lymphoblastic leukemia: a report from the Children's Oncology Group. Pediatr Blood Cancer 2014;61(11):2086–8.

55. Vora A, Mitchell CD, Lennard L, et al. Toxicity and efficacy of 6-thioguanine versus 6-mercaptopurine in childhood lymphoblastic leukaemia: a randomised trial. Lancet 2006;368(9544):1339–48.

56. Green DM, Norkool P, Breslow NE, et al. Severe hepatic toxicity after treatment with vincristine and dactinomycin using single-dose or divided-dose schedules: a report from the National Wilms' Tumor Study. J Clin Oncol 1990;8(9):1525–30.

57. Sulis ML, Bessmertny O, Granowetter L, et al. Veno-occlusive disease in pediatric patients receiving actinomycin D and vincristine only for the treatment of rhabdomyosarcoma. J Pediatr Hematol Oncol 2004;26(12):843–6.

58. Dawson LA, Ten Haken RK. Partial volume tolerance of the liver to radiation. Semin Radiat Oncol 2005;15(4):279–83.

59. Milano MT, Constine LS, Okunieff P. Normal tissue tolerance dose metrics for radiation therapy of major organs. Semin Radiat Oncol 2007;17(2):131–40.

60. Pan CC, Kavanagh BD, Dawson LA, et al. Radiation-associated liver injury. Int J Radiat Oncol Biol Phys 2010;76(3 Suppl):S94–100.

61. Warwick AB, Kalapurakal JA, Ou SS, et al. Portal hypertension in children with Wilms' tumor: a report from the National Wilms' Tumor Study Group. Int J Radiat Oncol Biol Phys 2010;77(1):210–6.

62. Hall M, Bradley JA, Jackson A, et al. Dose response for veno-occlusive disease after whole-liver radiation therapy: a preliminary report from the Pediatric Normal Tissue Effects in the Clinic (PENTEC) group. Int J Radiat Oncol Biol Phys 2017; 101(4):1005.

63. McDonald GB. Hepatobiliary complications of hematopoietic cell transplantation, 40 years on. Hepatology 2010;51(4):1450–60.
64. Ansari M, Petrykey K, Rezgui MA, et al. Genetic susceptibility to hepatic sinusoidal obstruction syndrome in pediatric patients undergoing hematopoietic stem cell transplantation. Biol Blood Marrow Transplant 2020;26(5):920–7.
65. Schempp A, Lee J, Kearney S, et al. Iron overload in survivors of childhood cancer. J Pediatr Hematol Oncol 2016;38(1):27–31.
66. Ruccione KS, Wood JC, Sposto R, et al. Characterization of transfusion-derived iron deposition in childhood cancer survivors. Cancer Epidemiol Biomarkers Prev 2014;23(9):1913–9.
67. Vag T, Kentouche K, Krumbein I, et al. Noninvasive measurement of liver iron concentration at MRI in children with acute leukemia: initial results. Pediatr Radiol 2011;41(8):980–4.
68. Trovillion EM, Schubert L, Dietz AC. Iron overload in survivors of childhood cancer. J Pediatr Hematol Oncol 2018;40(5):396–400.
69. Locasciulli A, Testa M, Pontisso P, et al. Prevalence and natural history of hepatitis C infection in patients cured of childhood leukemia. Blood 1997;90(11):4628–33.
70. Locasciulli A, Testa M, Valsecchi MG, et al. Morbidity and mortality due to liver disease in children undergoing allogeneic bone marrow transplantation: a 10-year prospective study. Blood 1997;90(9):3799–805.
71. Paul IM, Sanders J, Ruggiero F, et al. Chronic hepatitis C virus infections in leukemia survivors: prevalence, viral load, and severity of liver disease. Blood 1999; 93(11):3672–7.
72. Fujisawa T, Komatsu H, Inui A, et al. Long-term outcome of chronic hepatitis B in adolescents or young adults in follow-up from childhood. J Pediatr Gastroenterol Nutr 2000;30(2):201–6.
73. Cattoni A, Rovelli A, Prunotto G, et al. Hepatic focal nodular hyperplasia after pediatric hematopoietic stem cell transplantation: The impact of hormonal replacement therapy and iron overload. Pediatr Blood Cancer 2019;67:e28137.
74. Porta C, Cosmai L, Gallieni M, et al. Renal effects of targeted anticancer therapies. Nat Rev Nephrol 2015;11(6):354–70.
75. Nadeau BA, Fecher LA, Owens SR, et al. Liver toxicity with cancer checkpoint inhibitor therapy. Semin Liver Dis 2018;38(4):366–78.
76. Perazella MA, Shirali AC. Nephrotoxicity of cancer immunotherapies: past, present and future. J Am Soc Nephrol 2018;29(8):2039–52.
77. Ollero M, Sahali D. Inhibition of the VEGF signalling pathway and glomerular disorders. Nephrol Dial Transplant 2015;30(9):1449–55.
78. Corbacioglu S, Jabbour EJ, Mohty M. Risk factors for development of and progression of hepatic veno-occlusive disease/sinusoidal obstruction syndrome. Biol Blood Marrow Transplant 2019;25(7):1271–80.
79. Shah RR, Morganroth J, Shah DR. Hepatotoxicity of tyrosine kinase inhibitors: clinical and regulatory perspectives. Drug Saf 2013;36(7):491–503.
80. Kremer LC, Mulder RL, Oeffinger KC, et al. A worldwide collaboration to harmonize guidelines for the long-term follow-up of childhood and young adult cancer survivors: a report from the International Late Effects of Childhood Cancer Guideline Harmonization Group. Pediatr Blood Cancer 2013;60(4):543–9.
81. Rossi R, Godde A, Kleinebrand A, et al. Unilateral nephrectomy and cisplatin as risk factors of ifosfamide-induced nephrotoxicity: analysis of 120 patients. J Clin Oncol 1994;12(1):159–65.
82. Skinner R, Pearson AD, English MW, et al. Risk factors for ifosfamide nephrotoxicity in children. Lancet 1996;348(9027):578–80.

83. Negro A, Regolisti G, Perazzoli F, et al. Ifosfamide-induced renal Fanconi syndrome with associated nephrogenic diabetes insipidus in an adult patient. Nephrol Dial Transplant 1998;13(6):1547–9.
84. Cost NG, Sawicz-Birkowska K, Kajbafzadeh AM, et al. A comparison of renal function outcomes after nephron-sparing surgery and radical nephrectomy for nonsyndromic unilateral Wilms tumor. Urology 2014;83(6):1388–93.

Hearing and Other Neurologic Problems

Check for updates

Wendy Landier, PhD, CRNP[a],*, Richard J. Cohn, MBBCh, FCP (SA), FRACP[b],
Marry M. van den Heuvel-Eibrink, MD, PhD[c]

KEYWORDS

- Ototoxicity • Antineoplastic therapy • Surveillance • Management • Otoprotection
- Peripheral neuropathy • Motor deficits • Seizures

KEY POINTS

- Childhood malignancies commonly treated with potentially ototoxic therapy include neuroblastoma; osteosarcoma; retinoblastoma; and hepatic, germ cell, and central nervous system tumors.
- Risk of hearing loss is increased for younger children, those with central nervous system tumors, and those treated with multiple ototoxic agents at higher doses.
- Early detection of and intervention for hearing impairment is particularly crucial for young children who are still developing language.
- There is considerable interindividual variability in hearing outcomes among survivors treated with similar ototoxic regimens, suggesting that genetic susceptibility may play a role.
- Peripheral neuropathy typically persists following completion of treatment and may be an important contributor to physical performance limitations.

INTRODUCTION

Ototoxicity (including hearing loss, tinnitus, vertigo, and impaired balance) and other neurologic toxicities (including peripheral sensory and motor neuropathies and seizures) are potential consequences of exposure to common therapeutic agents used to treat childhood cancer. Therapeutic agents commonly associated with ototoxicity

[a] Pediatric Hematology/Oncology, Institute for Cancer Outcomes and Survivorship, University of Alabama at Birmingham, 1600 7th Avenue South, Lowder 500, Birmingham, AL 35233, USA; [b] School of Women's and Children's Health, UNSW Sydney, Medicine, Clinical Oncology, Kids Cancer Centre, Sydney Children's Hospital, High Street, Randwick, Sydney, New South Wales 2031, Australia; [c] University of Utrecht, Princess Maxima Center for Pediatric Oncology, Prinses Maxima Centrum voor kinderoncologie, Postbus 113 – 3720 AC Bilthoven Heidelberglaan 25, 3584 CS Utrecht, Room number: 2-5 F3, The Netherlands
* Corresponding author.
E-mail address: wlandier@peds.uab.edu

Pediatr Clin N Am 67 (2020) 1219–1235
https://doi.org/10.1016/j.pcl.2020.07.012
0031-3955/20/© 2020 Elsevier Inc. All rights reserved.

and other neurologic toxicities include the platinum and vinca alkaloid classes of anti-neoplastic chemotherapy; supportive care agents, such as aminoglycoside antibiotics and loop diuretics; cranial radiation; and surgery involving structures critical to cochlear and neurologic function. Because these therapeutic exposures are commonly used in the treatment of a wide range of pediatric cancers, a large proportion of childhood cancer survivors are at risk for experiencing long-term ototoxic or neurologic toxicities. This article provides an overview of ototoxicity and other neurologic toxicities related to childhood cancer treatment, discusses the challenges that these toxicities may pose for survivors, and presents an overview of current recommendations for surveillance and clinical management of these potentially life-altering toxicities of childhood cancer treatment.

OTOTOXICITY
Hearing Loss

Hearing loss related to childhood cancer therapy can range from mild to profound in both its objective manifestation and in its impact on functional outcomes. The extent of hearing loss experienced by individual survivors of childhood cancer is contingent on numerous factors involving the type and magnitude of exposure to ototoxic agents, as well as characteristics of the host. Potential adverse outcomes include permanent severe to profound hearing loss, which often results in communication challenges and problems with social interaction and may impair cognitive performance and affect survivor health-related quality of life. In addition, in survivors who develop hearing loss at a young age, the development of language and social skills may also be impaired.[1,2]

This article reviews populations at risk and the prevalence, underlying pathophysiology, and clinical manifestations of hearing loss related to ototoxic exposures during childhood cancer therapy. It also describes recommendations for surveillance, grading systems for classifying the severity of deficits, interventions for management, and strategies for prevention and risk mitigation of hearing loss in childhood cancer survivors.

At-risk populations

Childhood malignancies commonly treated with platinum chemotherapy include neuroblastoma; osteosarcoma; retinoblastoma; and hepatic, germ cell, and central nervous system tumors. Platinum chemotherapy is also frequently used in salvage regimens to treat many types of recurrent and progressive childhood cancers.[3–6] In addition, loop diuretics and aminoglycoside antibiotics are widely used in supportive care regimens in order to manage medical complications encountered during childhood cancer treatment. Cranial radiation is often used in the treatment of childhood tumors involving the brain, head, and neck, and in some relapsed leukemias and lymphomas. Surgery to remove tumors of the head, neck, and brain that involve or are adjacent to auditory structures (including rhabdomyosarcomas, nasopharyngeal carcinomas, base of skull tumors, and brain tumors) may result in risk of direct surgical damage to the cochlea, auditory nerve, or surrounding structures.[7] Tumors that induce increased intracranial pressure by obstructing flow of cerebrospinal fluid through the lateral or third ventricles, such as large posterior fossa and spinal tumors, may require placement of ventriculoperitoneal (VP) shunts, which also increase subsequent risk for hearing loss.[8]

Prevalence

The prevalence of hearing loss in childhood cancer survivors who have been exposed to ototoxic agents depends on many factors, including the treatment regimen and course (ie, cumulative ototoxic exposures), age at exposure, follow-up time, intensity and magnitude of exposure, and survivor susceptibility to the ototoxic effects of the therapeutic agents. Given the wide variability in range and intensity of ototoxic exposures, and in survivor response to these exposures, it is perhaps not surprising that the reported prevalence of hearing loss in children exposed to potential ototoxic agents during their cancer treatment ranges from 4% to 90%.[5,9–16] Nevertheless, the prevalence of hearing loss increases with exposure to ototoxic therapy at a younger age,[10,11,13,17] and at higher cumulative doses.[10,11,17,18] In addition, the variability in reported prevalence suggests that genetic susceptibility (or lack thereof) may also be an important factor.[19–22] In addition, another factor contributing to the variability in reports of prevalence of hearing loss in childhood cancer survivors is the lack of agreement on a consistent grading system to measure and report hearing loss in this population (**Fig. 1**).[10,15]

Pathophysiology
Although the ears are completely formed at birth, maturation of the auditory cortex and neuronal pathways continues throughout infancy and into early childhood, and the interhemispheric sensory transfer through the corpus callosum does not mature for several years.[23] Thus, infants and young children are especially vulnerable to the damaging effects of potentially ototoxic therapy.

Hearing loss is generally classified as one of 3 types: conductive (caused by a pathologic process involving the outer or middle ear), sensorineural (resulting from a pathologic process involving the cochlea or auditory nerve), or mixed (a combination of both conductive and sensorineural components). Hearing loss as a consequence of pharmacologic therapy during childhood cancer treatment is typically sensorineural, whereas hearing loss resulting from radiation, surgery, and/or tumor-related injury is often mixed in origin.

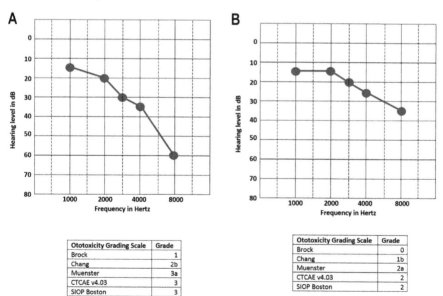

A

Ototoxicity Grading Scale	Grade
Brock	1
Chang	2b
Muenster	3a
CTCAE v4.03	3
SIOP Boston	3

B

Ototoxicity Grading Scale	Grade
Brock	0
Chang	1b
Muenster	2a
CTCAE v4.03	2
SIOP Boston	2

Fig. 1. Audiograms of children with (A) cisplatin-induced hearing loss; and (B) radiation-related hearing loss; variability in grades of hearing loss is present across the ototoxicity grading scales commonly used in pediatric oncology. CTAE, Common Terminology Criteria for Adverse Events; SIOP, International Society of Pediatric Oncology.

Hearing loss related to pharmacologic agents The platinum-based chemotherapy agents used in childhood cancer treatment (cisplatin, carboplatin, and oxaliplatin) have different chemical structures and adverse effect profiles. Irreversible sensorineural hearing loss is a well-recognized adverse effect of treatment with cisplatin[24,25]; risk is increased for younger children (particularly those ≤5 years of age at treatment), those with central nervous system tumors, and those treated with higher doses and multiple ototoxic agents (eg, platinum chemotherapy combined with cranial radiation).[25–27] Hearing loss is typically not seen with lower doses of carboplatin; however, the risk increases with myeloablative doses.[10,28] Ototoxicity related to oxaliplatin is rarely reported, and is isolated to case reports.[29] Ifosfamide, an alkylating agent without known ototoxic effects, may play a role in increasing the risk for hearing loss in patients treated concomitantly with cisplatin.[30] Gentamicin[31] and furosemide[32] are common potentially ototoxic supportive care agents used to treat infectious and metabolic complications arising during antineoplastic therapy.

The mechanism of action underlying platinum-related and aminoglycoside-related ototoxicity is the production of toxic levels of reactive oxygen species (ie, oxidative stress) in the cochlea. This mechanism results in destruction of cochlear hair (sensory) cells,[33,34] and damage to the stria vascularis and spiral ganglion cells.[34] In addition, cisplatin is retained in the cochlea for months to years following chemotherapy, likely resulting in cochlear hair cells receiving higher cumulative exposure to cisplatin, compared with other tissues.[35] The specialized cochlear hair cells are arranged tonotopically (from high to low frequency) along the organ of Corti, and each hair cell is sensitive to only a limited frequency range.[36] The initial hair cell loss resulting from exposure to ototoxic pharmacologic agents typically occurs at the base of the cochlea, where hair cells sensitive to high-frequency sounds (>2000 Hz) are located. However, as cumulative exposure to ototoxic pharmacologic agents increases, hair cells sensitive to lower-pitch sounds within the speech frequencies (500–2000 Hz), located toward the apex of the cochlea, are also affected.[37] Humans are born with a full complement of cochlear hair cells, which do not regenerate; therefore, sensorineural hearing loss related to therapy with platinum and/or aminoglycosides is typically bilateral and irreversible,[13,38] and can also be accompanied by tinnitus and vertigo.[25]

The mechanism of action underlying ototoxicity related to loop diuretics is thought to be associated with fluid and electrolyte shifts within the inner ear, resulting in edema of cochlear tissue.[32] Thus, the hearing loss associated with loop diuretics is typically reversible.[32] Nevertheless, concomitant administration of loop diuretics may potentiate the ototoxic effects of aminoglycosides or platinum chemotherapy.[31,39]

Hearing loss related to radiation Hearing loss resulting from radiation to the auditory structures is multifactorial and dose related. Radiation delivered to the temporal bone in high doses (ie, ≥30 Gy) is particularly likely to place children at risk for sensorineural hearing loss,[40–42] although newer radiation techniques, including conformal and proton-beam therapy, may limit cochlear exposure and reduce the risk.[41,43,44] The exact mechanism of radiation-related sensorineural hearing loss is unknown but is thought to be related to injury of the cochlear apparatus and/or small vessels, leading to hypoxia involving inner ear structures.[45] Radiation-related sensorineural hearing loss is generally irreversible, progresses from high to low frequencies as cumulative exposure increases, and may worsen over time.[46] Treatment with radiation to the auditory structures at doses greater than or equal to 30 Gy is also associated with conductive hearing loss caused by tympanosclerosis, otosclerosis, and mucociliary or eustachian tube dysfunction.[47] Radiation delivered to the mastoid bone and posterior nasopharynx increases the risk for conductive hearing loss associated with chronic serous otitis media.[48] Radiation that involves the external auditory canal may also lead to conductive hearing loss associated with excessive and/or dry cerumen production and chronic soft tissue infections.[45] Children who receive multimodality ototoxic therapy, such as platinum chemotherapy combined with radiation to auditory structures, have an increased risk for developing ototoxicity.[49,50]

Hearing loss related to surgery/tumor Tumors that are located near the cochlea, auditory nerve, or other auditory structures may cause hearing loss as a result of pressure on, or infiltration of, critical structures. Children who undergo surgical procedures to resect head, neck, or brain tumors near or involving the cochlea, auditory nerve, or surrounding structures may experience injury to these structures that results in hearing loss.[7,51] For children with posterior fossa tumors, such as cerebellar astrocytoma, medulloblastoma, or ependymoma, that may be adjacent to or infiltrate the auditory nerve, intraoperative neurophysiologic monitoring may help to limit damage.[7] In addition, hearing loss is associated with rapid changes in intracranial pressure that can occur during tumor resection, profound blood loss, lumbar puncture, or with placement of a ventriculostomy or VP shunt for management of hydrocephalus.[8,52] The underlying mechanism for hearing loss related to rapid changes in intracranial pressure is thought to involve the anatomic connection (cochlear aqueduct) between the cochlear perilymph and the cerebrospinal fluid.

Clinical manifestations of hearing loss

Sensorineural hearing loss related to pharmacologic agents is typically bilateral, symmetric, and irreversible, and is usually rapid in onset (occurring within days to weeks of exposure). In contrast, radiation-related sensorineural hearing loss may not become apparent for months to years following exposure. Children who experience hearing loss as a result of shunting of cerebrospinal fluid for management of hydrocephalus may have temporary or permanent loss, and some also experience heightened sensitivity to sound (hyperacusis). Surgery-related hearing loss is often permanent, but it may improve following surgery in a limited number of cases.

Severe to profound hearing loss affecting the classic speech frequencies (500–2000 Hz) is often clinically evident because of readily identifiable communication impairment in the survivor. High-frequency hearing loss (affecting frequencies >2000 Hz) may be asymptomatic or may be associated with tinnitus or vertigo, as well as difficulty hearing in the presence of background noise.

Manifestations of hearing loss in very young children may include difficulty with language acquisition and communication skills, even if the hearing loss is of mild to moderate severity and limited to the high-frequency ranges, because language acquisition depends on the high-frequency fricative sounds (ie, consonant sounds such as s, th, f, and k), which are critical for speech discrimination.[53] Young children unable to hear these high-frequency sounds may be unable to distinguish the meaning of words, severely impairing development of language as well as social and cognitive skills. Older children who have acquired language before sustaining high-frequency hearing loss may experience the perception of hearing but not understanding, particularly when the speaker's voice is high pitched (eg, among women and children). Thus, the clinical implications of even mild high-frequency hearing loss are significant and can adversely affect cognitive and social development and quality of life in childhood cancer survivors.[54]

Surveillance/grading systems

Audiologic assessment Hearing is typically assessed via an audiologic assessment conducted by an audiologist. Central to this assessment is pure-tone audiometry,[55] which tests the ability to hear sound at different frequencies or pitches (measured in Hertz) and at different intensities or degrees of loudness (measured in decibels). Sounds are generally presented across a range of frequencies (at minimum, in octaves ranging from 500–8000 Hz) and at varying intensities. The pure-tone threshold is the lowest level of intensity at which the sound can first be heard 50% of the time; a normal threshold is usually considered to be less than or equal to 20 dB.[56] In childhood cancer survivors who have experienced sensorineural hearing loss, changes in hearing thresholds are typically observed initially in the high-frequency ranges, and progress to the lower frequencies with additional exposures and over time.[15,57] Most survivors who are 4 to 5 years of age or older are able to undergo conventional audiologic assessment in a sound-attenuating booth. Adaptations to pure-tone audiologic testing are made for young children using play audiometry or visual reinforcement techniques.[58] Survivors unable to cooperate with behavioral testing because of young age or impaired cognition can be tested using electrophysiologic techniques, such as auditory brainstem response.[55] Additional testing that may be incorporated in an audiologic assessment include extended high-frequency audiometry, which assesses thresholds above the conventional range (ie, 9000–20,000 Hz) and may be used for detecting early hearing loss and loss affecting the ability to hear in noisy environments; testing of interoctave frequencies (750, 1500, 300, and 6000 Hz); and testing of distortion product otoacoustic emissions, which test cochlear response to sound.[59]

Surveillance recommendations The frequency of surveillance for changes in auditory function depends on the survivor's age and exposure to ototoxic therapy. Although there has been variability in recommendations for surveillance across organizations that develop guidelines for survivorship care,[60–62] an international guidelines harmonization panel recently reviewed the available evidence and recommended that survivors completing cancer therapy, who have received cisplatin with or without high-dose carboplatin (>1500 mg/m^2) and/or head/brain radiation therapy at cumulative doses of greater than or equal to 30 Gy, undergo an auditory assessment at the end of therapy and then annually for children less than 6 years of age, every other year for children between 6 and 12 years of age, and every 5 years for survivors aged 13 years and older, because hearing loss may progress over time. The panel also recommended that surveillance every 5 years may be reasonable for survivors who have undergone placement of ventricular shunts. The auditory assessment should consist of, at minimum, pure-tone audiometry at frequencies between 1000 and 8000 Hz for survivors aged 6 years and older (with referral to an audiologist if loss >15 dB is detected at any frequency), and a full annual audiological evaluation by an audiologist for all survivors younger than 6 years. The panel also recommended that any survivor who has developed hearing loss should remain under the routine care of an audiologist.[42]

Grading of hearing loss Several grading scales (**Table 1**) are currently used to classify hearing loss; variability in classification has implications for clinical care and for comparison of clinical trial outcomes.[63] Ototoxicity grading scales used in pediatric oncology generally assign a toxicity rating ranging from 0 (normal hearing or clinically insignificant loss) to 4 (severe to profound hearing loss). A recent comparison of 5 commonly used grading scales applied to nearly 3800 audiograms of patients with childhood cancer treated with platinum-based chemotherapy found that the prevalence of deleterious hearing loss (defined as grade 2 or higher) across scales ranged from 40.3% to 59.3%.[15]

Table 1
Ototoxicity grading scales commonly used in pediatric oncology

Grading Scale	Description	Scoring
Brock[57]	Designed to capture the progression of hearing loss from high to low frequencies commonly seen with sensorineural hearing loss associated with platinum chemotherapy; captures hearing loss >40 dB	5-point scale 0 (<40 dB at all frequencies) 1 (≥40 dB at 8000 Hz) 2 (≥40 dB at ≥4000 Hz) 3 (≥40 dB at ≥2000 Hz) 4 (≥40 dB at ≥1000 Hz)
Chang[88]	Modified Brock scale; includes interval frequencies (ie, 3000 and 6000 Hz); captures hearing loss >20 dB	7-point scale 0 (≤20 dB at 1000, 2000, and 4000 Hz) 1a (≥40 dB at 6000–12,000 Hz) 1b (>20 and <40 dB at 4000 Hz) 2a (≥40 dB at ≥4000 Hz) 2b (>20 and <40 dB at <4000 Hz) 3 (≥40 dB at ≥2000 or ≥3000 Hz) 4 (≥40 dB at ≥1000 Hz)
Muenster[89]	Designed for early detection of hearing loss; captures hearing loss >10 dB (allows detection of minimal hearing loss >10–20 dB); captures tinnitus	8-point scale 0 (<10 dB at all frequencies) 1 (>10 to ≤20 dB at ≥1 frequency or tinnitus) 2a (>20 to ≤40 dB at ≥4000 Hz) 2b (>40 to ≤60 dB at ≥4000 Hz) 2c (>60 dB at ≥4000 Hz) 3a (>20 to ≤40 dB at <4000 Hz) 3b (>40 to ≤60 dB at <4000 Hz) 3c (>60 to <80 dB at <4000 Hz) 4 (≥80 dB at <4000 Hz)

(continued on next page)

Table 1
(continued)

Grading Scale	Description	Scoring
NCI CTCAE, Version 4.03 (2010)[90]	Requires baseline assessment; captures change from baseline and not absolute hearing loss; includes some subjective assessments at higher grades	4-point scale 1 (threshold shift >20 dB at 8000 Hz in at least 1 ear) 2 (threshold shift >20 dB at ≥4000 Hz in at least 1 ear) 3 (threshold sift >20 dB at ≥3000 Hz in at least 1 ear; hearing loss sufficient to indicate therapeutic intervention, including hearing aids; additional speech-language–related services indicated) 4 (indication for cochlear implant and additional speech-language–related services)
SIOP Boston (2012)[19]	Grades progression of hearing loss from high to low frequencies; uses absolute hearing levels; captures hearing loss >20 dB	5-point scale 0 (≤20 dB at all frequencies) 1 (>20 dB at >4000 Hz) 2 (>20 dB at ≥4000 Hz) 3 (>20 dB at ≥2000 Hz or ≥3000 Hz) 4 (>40 dB at ≥2000 Hz)

Abbreviations: NCI CTCAE, National Cancer Institute Common Terminology Criteria for Adverse Events; SIOP, International Society of Pediatric Oncology.

Management of hearing loss

Intervention for identified hearing loss is crucial for survivor well-being and quality of life.[54] Early detection and management of hearing impairment is particularly crucial for very young children who are still developing language. Hearing aids are an important tool in managing hearing loss; however, even with improving technology, survivors with significant hearing loss may still have a reduced ability to understand speech, particularly in noisy environments. Additional accommodations are often necessary for survivors with hearing loss, including the use of assistive devices (eg, remote microphone technology that enhances sound transmission over distance, telephone amplifiers, and alternate communication methods such as text), compensatory communication strategies, speech and language therapy, preferential classroom seating, and in some cases specialized classrooms for the hearing impaired.[64] For survivors with severe to profound hearing loss who do not derive benefit from well-fitted hearing aids, a cochlear implant or electroacoustic stimulation (integration of hearing aid and cochlear implant technology) may offer additional options. In all cases, referral to a skilled audiologist for ongoing management of hearing loss is crucial for success.[65]

Prevention/genetic predisposition

Otoprotection At present, there are no FDA-approved otoprotectants available for use in pediatric oncology; however, interest in 2 potentially otoprotective agents has resulted in several clinical trials that aimed to reduce hearing loss in children receiving cisplatin.[66] Evidence for efficacy of these agents has recently been reviewed by the Cochrane group.[67] Amifostine, a reactive oxygen scavenger originally developed as a radiation protectant,[68] has been tested in clinical studies as an otoprotectant for children receiving cisplatin for hepatoblastoma[69] and germ cell tumors,[70] but has failed to demonstrate otoprotection. A nonrandomized trial of amifostine in children with medulloblastoma showed that amifostine was otoprotective in children with average-risk disease but not in those with high-risk disease.[71] In a randomized clinical trial evaluating sodium thiosulfate, another free radical scavenger, in children treated with cisplatin for localized hepatoblastoma, a 48% reduction in hearing loss was seen in the sodium thiosulfate arm, with no impact on survival.[72] However, in another randomized trial of sodium thiosulfate among children receiving cisplatin for a variety of cancers, concern was raised regarding reduced event-free and overall survival among children with disseminated (but not localized) disease randomized to receive sodium thiosulfate.[73] Although hearing protection was significant in the group randomized to sodium thiosulfate, the possibility that sodium thiosulfate may have had a tumor-protective effect among children with disseminated disease remained a concern.

Additional strategies for otoprotection include counseling of all survivors at risk for hearing loss to avoid further exposure to ototoxic agents (eg, chelating agents, salicylates) whenever possible, and to avoid loud noises (especially $\geq$85 dB) and use protective measures (eg, ear plugs) in noisy environments in order to preserve hearing.[42,74]

Genetic predisposition There is considerable interindividual variability in the range of hearing outcomes (normal hearing to profound loss) among survivors treated with similar ototoxic regimens.[4,10,75] It is likely that this variability in outcomes is explained, at least partially, by differences in genetic susceptibility to the ototoxic effects of therapy.[19,21] As pharmacogenomics continues to rapidly evolve,[76] development of prediction models to identify individuals at high risk for platinum-related or radiation-related ototoxicity will help to inform future ototoxicity prevention strategies.[77] At this time, genes that have been identified as having a potential role in susceptibility to platinum-related hearing loss in childhood include thiopurine S-methyltranferase (*TPMT*; mechanism unknown),[75] catechol-*O*-methyltransferase (*COMT*; mechanism unknown),[75] acylphosphatase-2 (ACYP2; involved in calcium and magnesium transport),[78] and excision repair cross-complementation groups 1 and 2 (*ERCC1*, *ERCC2*; involved in repair of drug-induced damage).[79] Glutathione S-transferases (*GSTs*) are thought to play a role in susceptibility to radiation-related hearing loss in childhood as a result of cellular detoxification,[80] whereas mitochondrial gene mutations, through their role as mediators for some apoptotic pathways, are thought to have a potential role in susceptibility to aminoglycoside-related hearing loss in children.[81]

Tinnitus

Tinnitus is characterized by constant ringing or buzzing in the ear, and is thought to be a consequence of a mismatch between excitatory and inhibitory networks in the central auditory system that results in an overabundance of spontaneous neuronal activity involving sound perception.[82] Tinnitus is often associated with hearing loss, and may be the brain's attempt to fill the void in the absence of sound transmission. Although there are few studies of tinnitus in childhood cancer survivors, a recent systematic review indicates that the frequency rate of tinnitus ranges from 3% to 17% among survivors, which is higher than observed in healthy peers, and that the risk for tinnitus is independently associated with exposure to platinum-based chemotherapy, cranial radiation therapy at doses greater than 30 Gy, and a diagnosis of central nervous system tumor.[83] Although little is known about the impact of tinnitus on quality of life in childhood cancer survivors, studies of other populations affected by tinnitus indicate that this disorder is often associated with problems with sleep and concentration, depression, anxiety, and mental distress.[83] Management strategies include referral to an audiologist for hearing aids and/or sound therapy, cognitive behavior therapy, counseling, and education.[42]

Vertigo/Balance Problems

Vertigo, a spinning sensation that may be associated with vestibular disorder, which manifests as complaints of dizziness and balance problems, may result from several underlying disorders and has been poorly studied in childhood cancer survivors. In a Childhood Cancer Survivor Study survey of 1876, 5-year survivors of central nervous system tumors, the cumulative incidence of vertigo was 9% and 17% at 5 and 30 year after diagnosis, respectively; however, the association with hearing loss was not reported.[84] Further research is needed to understand the associations between ototoxic exposures and subsequent problems with vertigo and balance in childhood cancer survivors across diagnostic groups.

OTHER NEUROLOGIC TOXICITIES
Peripheral Neuropathy

Peripheral sensory or motor neuropathy as a consequence of chemotherapy used in treatment of childhood cancer is principally related to exposure to vinca alkaloids, cisplatin, and carboplatin. Risk factors considered to contribute to the variability in the reported incidence and natural history of chemotherapy-induced peripheral neuropathy (CIPN) include challenges in assessment and diagnosis, drug dose, duration, and concomitant medication, and patient factors such as age and inherited susceptibility.[85] In a recent study of 121 survivors of childhood extracranial malignancies (including liquid tumors), at a median (range) of 85 years (1.5–29 years) after treatment completion, 53% were found to have clinical abnormalities consistent with peripheral neuropathy, compared with 14% of healthy controls.[86] Functional deficits were identified in manual dexterity, distal sensation, and balance; long-term neurotoxicity was seen more frequently in survivors who received cisplatin, compared with vinca alkaloids.[86] In another recent study of 531 survivors of extracranial solid tumors of childhood, the prevalence of sensory and motor impairment was 20% and 17.5%, respectively, at a median of 25 years following diagnosis; exposure to vinca alkaloids was associated with motor impairment, whereas cisplatin exposure was associated with sensory impairment.[87] Nerve conduction studies are difficult in children because of the discomfort experienced, but may be useful to determine the pattern of nerve involvement and in excluding differential diagnoses, which include vitamin deficiencies, critical illness neuropathy, steroid myopathy, nerve root infiltration, and inherited neuropathies. No preventive or treatment strategies have proved to be of value for CIPN in children.[85] Because peripheral neuropathy typically persists following completion of childhood cancer treatment, it may be an important contributor to physical performance limitations, which may influence lifestyle choices and increase the risk of conditions such as obesity, diabetes, and osteoporosis in survivors of childhood cancers.[85] Screening of survivors at risk is imperative in order to provide effective and timely interventions, which may include physical and occupational therapy to minimize limitation in range of movement, as well as medications for management of neuropathic pain.

Motor Deficits and Seizures

Motor deficits (eg, weakness, paralysis, movement disorders, and ataxia) and seizures are observed in subsets of childhood cancer survivors, and may be related to injury sustained as a result of tumor infiltration and/or tumor-directed therapy (eg, surgery, chemotherapy and/or radiation). Although some motor deficits and seizures are seen at diagnosis and persist into survivorship, others may be late in onset and progressive. In a study of 1876 5-year survivors of central nervous system tumors, the cumulative incidence of late-onset (>5 years after diagnosis) motor impairment was 21% and 35% at 5 and 30 year after diagnosis, respectively, and seizures increased from 27% to 41%, respectively. The risk for motor impairment and seizures was significantly higher among survivors exposed to radiation doses greater than or equal to 50 Gy to the frontal region, and among those who had a history of tumor recurrence or stroke; whereas the risk for seizures was also higher among those with a history of meningioma and temporal lobe radiation (in a dose-dependent fashion).[84] Survivors with persistent symptoms require care by a (pediatric) neurologist, and may also benefit from evaluation by a (pediatric) physiatrist or rehabilitation medicine specialist and referral to speech, physical, and/or occupational therapy.

SUMMARY

This article provides an overview of ototoxicity and other neurologic toxicities related to treatment with platinum and vinca alkaloid chemotherapy, cranial radiation, and surgery for childhood cancer; examines the challenges that these toxicities may pose for survivors; and presents an overview of current recommendations for surveillance and clinical management of these potentially life-altering toxicities in survivors of childhood cancers.

Hearing loss in survivors of childhood cancer can profoundly affect the survivor's social, emotional, and cognitive functioning, as well as health-related quality of life. The extent of hearing loss that a survivor experiences, and its impact on the survivor's quality of life, is contingent on a range of factors, including age at exposure, magnitude of exposure, genetic predisposition, timeliness of surveillance, early identification of hearing loss, and the rapidity with which interventions are used to mitigate the impact of hearing loss on social and educational outcomes. Although otoprotective pharmacologic agents and risk-prediction models hold promise for the future, these strategies are not accessible to most children currently being treated for cancer. Tinnitus, and vertigo with associated balance problems, are also potential long-term effects associated with exposure to ototoxic therapy during childhood. In addition, peripheral neuropathy, motor deficits, and seizures are potential neurologic toxicities that may be associated with vinca alkaloids, platinum chemotherapy, and radiation and surgery involving critical structures of the nervous system. Awareness of these potential long-term adverse effects among clinicians who care for childhood cancer survivors, and implementation of effective strategies for their surveillance and management, are key components of the provision of quality survivorship care.

DISCLOSURE

The authors have nothing to disclose.

REFERENCES

1. Davis JM, Elfenbein J, Schum R, et al. Effects of mild and moderate hearing impairments on language, educational, and psychosocial behavior of children. J Speech Hear Disord 1986;51(1):53–62.
2. Bess FH, Dodd-Murphy J, Parker RA. Children with minimal sensorineural hearing loss: prevalence, educational performance, and functional status. Ear Hear 1998; 19(5):339–54.
3. Hale GA, Marina NM, Jones-Wallace D, et al. Late effects of treatment for germ cell tumors during childhood and adolescence. J Pediatr Hematol Oncol 1999; 21(2):115–22.
4. Kushner BH, Budnick A, Kramer K, et al. Ototoxicity from high-dose use of platinum compounds in patients with neuroblastoma. Cancer 2006;107(2):417–22.
5. Lewis MJ, DuBois SG, Fligor B, et al. Ototoxicity in children treated for osteosarcoma. Pediatr Blood Cancer 2009;52(3):387–91.
6. Orgel E, Jain S, Ji L, et al. Hearing loss among survivors of childhood brain tumors treated with an irradiation-sparing approach. Pediatr Blood Cancer 2012; 58(6):953–8.
7. Simon MV. Neurophysiologic intraoperative monitoring of the vestibulocochlear nerve. J Clin Neurophysiol 2011;28(6):566–81.
8. Guillaume DJ, Knight K, Marquez C, et al. Cerebrospinal fluid shunting and hearing loss in patients treated for medulloblastoma. J Neurosurg Pediatr 2012;9(4): 421–7.
9. Gupta AA, Capra M, Papaioannou V, et al. Low incidence of ototoxicity with continuous infusion of cisplatin in the treatment of pediatric germ cell tumors. J Pediatr Hematol Oncol 2006;28(2):91–4.
10. Landier W, Knight K, Wong FL, et al. Ototoxicity in children with high-risk neuroblastoma: prevalence, risk factors, and concordance of grading scales–a report from the Children's Oncology Group. J Clin Oncol 2014;32(6):527–34.
11. Knight KR, Kraemer DF, Neuwelt EA. Ototoxicity in children receiving platinum chemotherapy: underestimating a commonly occurring toxicity that may influence academic and social development. J Clin Oncol 2005;23(34):8588–96.

12. Nitz A, Kontopantelis E, Bielack S, et al. Prospective evaluation of cisplatin- and carboplatin-mediated ototoxicity in paediatric and adult soft tissue and osteosarcoma patients. Oncol Lett 2013;5(1):311–5.
13. Schell MJ, McHaney VA, Green AA, et al. Hearing loss in children and young adults receiving cisplatin with or without prior cranial irradiation. J Clin Oncol 1989;7(6):754–60.
14. Dean JB, Hayashi SS, Albert CM, et al. Hearing loss in pediatric oncology patients receiving carboplatin-containing regimens. J Pediatr Hematol Oncol 2008;30(2):130–4.
15. Clemens E, Brooks B, de Vries ACH, et al. A comparison of the Muenster, SIOP Boston, Brock, Chang and CTCAEv4.03 ototoxicity grading scales applied to 3,799 audiograms of childhood cancer patients treated with platinum-based chemotherapy. PLoS One 2019;14(2):e0210646.
16. Clemens E, de Vries AC, Pluijm SF, et al. Determinants of ototoxicity in 451 platinum-treated Dutch survivors of childhood cancer: A DCOG late-effects study. Eur J Cancer 2016;69:77–85.
17. Li Y, Womer RB, Silber JH. Predicting cisplatin ototoxicity in children: the influence of age and the cumulative dose. Eur J Cancer 2004;40(16):2445–51.
18. Stohr W, Langer T, Kremers A, et al. Cisplatin-induced ototoxicity in osteosarcoma patients: a report from the late effects surveillance system. Cancer Invest 2005;23(3):201–7.
19. Brock PR, Knight KR, Freyer DR, et al. Platinum-induced ototoxicity in children: a consensus review on mechanisms, predisposition, and protection, including a new International Society of Pediatric Oncology Boston ototoxicity scale. J Clin Oncol 2012;30(19):2408–17.
20. Travis LB, Fossa SD, Sesso HD, et al. Chemotherapy-induced peripheral neurotoxicity and ototoxicity: new paradigms for translational genomics. J Natl Cancer Inst 2014;106(5):dju044.
21. Bhatia S. Role of genetic susceptibility in development of treatment-related adverse outcomes in cancer survivors. Cancer Epidemiol Biomarkers Prev 2011;20(10):2048–67.
22. Mukherjea D, Rybak LP. Pharmacogenomics of cisplatin-induced ototoxicity. Pharmacogenomics 2011;12(7):1039–50.
23. Sininger YS, Doyle KJ, Moore JK. The case for early identification of hearing loss in children. Auditory system development, experimental auditory deprivation, and development of speech perception and hearing. Pediatr Clin North Am 1999;46(1):1–14.
24. Rybak LP, Mukherjea D, Jajoo S, et al. Cisplatin ototoxicity and protection: clinical and experimental studies. Tohoku J Exp Med 2009;219(3):177–86.
25. Langer T, Am Zehnhoff-Dinnesen A, Radtke S, et al. Understanding platinum-induced ototoxicity. Trends Pharmacol Sci 2013;34(8):458–69.
26. Ruggiero A, Trombatore G, Triarico S, et al. Platinum compounds in children with cancer: toxicity and clinical management. Anticancer Drugs 2013;24(10):1007–19.
27. Grewal S, Merchant T, Reymond R, et al. Auditory late effects of childhood cancer therapy: a report from the Children's Oncology Group. Pediatrics 2010;125(4):e938–50.
28. Punnett A, Bliss B, Dupuis LL, et al. Ototoxicity following pediatric hematopoietic stem cell transplantation: a prospective cohort study. Pediatr Blood Cancer 2004;42(7):598–603.

29. Oh SY, Wasif N, Garcon MC, et al. Ototoxicity associated with oxaliplatin in a patient with pancreatic cancer. JOP 2013;14(6):676–9.

30. Meyer WH, Ayers D, McHaney VA, et al. Ifosfamide and exacerbation of cisplatin-induced hearing loss. Lancet 1993;341(8847):754–5.

31. Bates DE. Aminoglycoside ototoxicity. Drugs Today (Barc) 2003;39(4):277–85.

32. Rybak LP. Ototoxicity of loop diuretics. Otolaryngol Clin North Am 1993;26(5):829–44.

33. Schacht J, Talaska AE, Rybak LP. Cisplatin and aminoglycoside antibiotics: hearing loss and its prevention. Anat Rec (Hoboken) 2012;295(11):1837–50.

34. Ding D, Allman BL, Salvi R. Review: ototoxic characteristics of platinum antitumor drugs. Anat Rec (Hoboken) 2012;295(11):1851–67.

35. Breglio AM, Rusheen AE, Shide ED, et al. Cisplatin is retained in the cochlea indefinitely following chemotherapy. Nat Commun 2017;8(1):1654.

36. Mann ZF, Kelley MW. Development of tonotopy in the auditory periphery. Hear Res 2011;276(1–2):2–15.

37. Roland JT, Cohen NL. Vestibular and auditory ototoxicity. In: Cummings CW, Fredrickson JM, Harker LA, et al, editors. Otolaryngology head and neck surgery. 3rd edition. St Louis (MO): Mosby; 1998. p. 3186–97.

38. McHaney VA, Thibadoux G, Hayes FA, et al. Hearing loss in children receiving cisplatin chemotherapy. J Pediatr 1983;102(2):314–7.

39. Stringer SP, Meyerhoff WL, Wright CG. Ototoxicity. In: Paparella MM, Shumrick DA, editors. Otolaryngology. 3rd edition. Philadelphia: Saunders; 1991. p. 1653–69.

40. Hua C, Bass JK, Khan R, et al. Hearing loss after radiotherapy for pediatric brain tumors: effect of cochlear dose. Int J Radiat Oncol Biol Phys 2008;72(3):892–9.

41. Merchant TE, Gould CJ, Xiong X, et al. Early neuro-otologic effects of three-dimensional irradiation in children with primary brain tumors. Int J Radiat Oncol Biol Phys 2004;58(4):1194–207.

42. Clemens E, van den Heuvel-Eibrink MM, Mulder RL, et al. Recommendations for ototoxicity surveillance for childhood, adolescent, and young adult cancer survivors: a report from the International Late Effects of Childhood Cancer Guideline Harmonization Group in collaboration with the PanCare Consortium. Lancet Oncol 2019;20(1):e29–41.

43. Bass JK, Hua CH, Huang J, et al. Hearing Loss in Patients Who Received Cranial Radiation Therapy for Childhood Cancer. J Clin Oncol 2016;34(11):1248–55.

44. Merchant TE, Hua CH, Shukla H, et al. Proton versus photon radiotherapy for common pediatric brain tumors: comparison of models of dose characteristics and their relationship to cognitive function. Pediatr Blood Cancer 2008;51(1):110–7.

45. Parsons JA. The effect of radiation on normal tissues of the head and neck. In: Million RR, Cassisi NJ, editors. Management of head and neck cancer. A multidisciplinary approach. Philadelphia: Lippincott; 1984. p. 173–207.

46. Mujica-Mota M, Waissbluth S, Daniel SJ. Characteristics of radiation-induced sensorineural hearing loss in head and neck cancer: a systematic review. Head Neck 2013;35(11):1662–8.

47. Young YH, Lu YC. Mechanism of hearing loss in irradiated ears: a long-term longitudinal study. Ann Otol Rhinol Laryngol 2001;110(10):904–6.

48. Walker GV, Ahmed S, Allen P, et al. Radiation-induced middle ear and mastoid opacification in skull base tumors treated with radiotherapy. Int J Radiat Oncol Biol Phys 2011;81(5):e819–23.

49. Warrier R, Chauhan A, Davluri M, et al. Cisplatin and cranial irradiation-related hearing loss in children. Ochsner J 2012;12(3):191–6.
50. Rivelli TG, Mak MP, Martins RE, et al. Cisplatin based chemoradiation late toxicities in head and neck squamous cell carcinoma patients. Discov Med 2015; 20(108):57–66.
51. Schoot RA, Theunissen EA, Slater O, et al. Hearing loss in survivors of childhood head and neck rhabdomyosarcoma; a long-term follow-up study. Clin Otolaryngol 2016;41(3):276–83.
52. Wang AC, Chinn SB, Than KD, et al. Durability of hearing preservation after microsurgical treatment of vestibular schwannoma using the middle cranial fossa approach. J Neurosurg 2013;119(1):131–8.
53. Stelmachowicz PG, Pittman AL, Hoover BM, et al. The importance of high-frequency audibility in the speech and language development of children with hearing loss. Arch Otolaryngol Head Neck Surg 2004;130(5):556–62.
54. Gurney JG, Tersak JM, Ness KK, et al. Hearing loss, quality of life, and academic problems in long-term neuroblastoma survivors: a report from the Children's Oncology Group. Pediatrics 2007;120(5):e1229–36.
55. Brooks B, Knight K. Ototoxicity monitoring in children treated with platinum chemotherapy. Int J Audiol 2018;57(sup4):S34–40.
56. Stach BA. Clinical audiology: an introduction. San Diego (CA): Singular; 1998.
57. Brock PR, Bellman SC, Yeomans EC, et al. Cisplatin ototoxicity in children: a practical grading system. Med Pediatr Oncol 1991;19(4):295–300.
58. Smits C, Swen SJ, Theo Goverts S, et al. Assessment of hearing in very young children receiving carboplatin for retinoblastoma. Eur J Cancer 2006;42(4): 492–500.
59. Knight KR, Kraemer DF, Winter C, et al. Early changes in auditory function as a result of platinum chemotherapy: use of extended high-frequency audiometry and evoked distortion product otoacoustic emissions. J Clin Oncol 2007; 25(10):1190–5.
60. Children's Oncology Group. Children's Oncology Group long-term follow-up guidelines for survivors of childhood, adolescent, and young adult cancers, version 4.0. Monrovia (CA): Children's Oncology Group; 2013.
61. Dutch Childhood Oncology Group. Guidelines for follow-up in survivors of childhood cancer 5 years after diagnosis. Amsterdam (the Netherlands): SKION; 2010.
62. United Kingdom Children's Cancer Study Group Late Effects Group. Therapy based long-term follow-up practice statement. London: United Kingdom Children's Cancer Study Group; 2011.
63. Neuwelt EA, Brock P. Critical need for international consensus on ototoxicity assessment criteria. J Clin Oncol 2010;28(10):1630–2.
64. Brookhouser PE, Beauchaine KL, Osberger MJ. Management of the child with sensorineural hearing loss. Medical, surgical, hearing aids, cochlear implants. Pediatr Clin North Am 1999;46(1):121–41.
65. Landier W. Ototoxicity and cancer therapy. Cancer 2016;122(11):1647–58.
66. Freyer DR, Brock P, Knight K, et al. Interventions for cisplatin-induced hearing loss in children and adolescents with cancer. Lancet Child Adolesc Health 2019;3(8):578–84.
67. van As JW, van den Berg H, van Dalen EC. Medical interventions for the prevention of platinum-induced hearing loss in children with cancer. Cochrane Database Syst Rev 2016;(9):CD009219.

68. Rybak LP, Whitworth CA, Mukherjea D, et al. Mechanisms of cisplatin-induced ototoxicity and prevention. Hear Res 2007;226(1–2):157–67.

69. Katzenstein HM, Chang KW, Krailo M, et al. Amifostine does not prevent platinum-induced hearing loss associated with the treatment of children with hepatoblastoma: a report of the Intergroup Hepatoblastoma Study P9645 as a part of the Children's Oncology Group. Cancer 2009;115(24):5828–35.

70. Marina N, Chang KW, Malogolowkin M, et al. Amifostine does not protect against the ototoxicity of high-dose cisplatin combined with etoposide and bleomycin in pediatric germ-cell tumors: a Children's Oncology Group study. Cancer 2005; 104(4):841–7.

71. Gurney JG, Bass JK, Onar-Thomas A, et al. Evaluation of amifostine for protection against cisplatin-induced serious hearing loss in children treated for average-risk or high-risk medulloblastoma. Neuro Oncol 2014;16(6):848–55.

72. Brock PR, Maibach R, Childs M, et al. Sodium thiosulfate for protection from cisplatin-induced hearing loss. N Engl J Med 2018;378(25):2376–85.

73. Freyer DR, Chen L, Krailo MD, et al. Effects of sodium thiosulfate versus observation on development of cisplatin-induced hearing loss in children with cancer (ACCL0431): a multicentre, randomised, controlled, open-label, phase 3 trial. Lancet Oncol 2017;18(1):63–74.

74. Gratton MA, Kamen BA. Potentiation of cisplatin ototoxicity by noise. J Clin Oncol 1990;8(12):2091–2.

75. Ross CJ, Katzov-Eckert H, Dube MP, et al. Genetic variants in TPMT and COMT are associated with hearing loss in children receiving cisplatin chemotherapy. Nat Genet 2009;41(12):1345–9.

76. Clemens E, van der Kooi ALF, Broer L, et al. The influence of genetic variation on late toxicities in childhood cancer survivors: A review. Crit Rev Oncol Hematol 2018;126:154–67.

77. Clemens E, Meijer AJ, Broer L, et al. Genetic determinants of ototoxicity during and after childhood cancer treatment: protocol for the PanCareLIFE Study. JMIR Res Protoc 2019;8(3):e11868.

78. Xu H, Robinson GW, Huang J, et al. Common variants in ACYP2 influence susceptibility to cisplatin-induced hearing loss. Nat Genet 2015;47(3):263–6.

79. Caronia D, Patino-Garcia A, Milne RL, et al. Common variations in ERCC2 are associated with response to cisplatin chemotherapy and clinical outcome in osteosarcoma patients. Pharmacogenomics J 2009;9(5):347–53.

80. Rednam S, Scheurer ME, Adesina A, et al. Glutathione S-transferase P1 single nucleotide polymorphism predicts permanent ototoxicity in children with medulloblastoma. Pediatr Blood Cancer 2013;60(4):593–8.

81. Xing G, Chen Z, Wei Q, et al. Mitochondrial 12S rRNA A827G mutation is involved in the genetic susceptibility to aminoglycoside ototoxicity. Biochem Biophys Res Commun 2006;346(4):1131–5.

82. Zeng FG. An active loudness model suggesting tinnitus as increased central noise and hyperacusis as increased nonlinear gain. Hear Res 2013;295:172–9.

83. Meijer AJM, Clemens E, Hoetink AE, et al. Tinnitus during and after childhood cancer: A systematic review. Crit Rev Oncol Hematol 2019;135:1–7.

84. Wells EM, Ullrich NJ, Seidel K, et al. Longitudinal assessment of late-onset neurologic conditions in survivors of childhood central nervous system tumors: a Childhood Cancer Survivor Study report. Neuro Oncol 2018;20(1):132–42.

85. Kandula T, Park SB, Cohn RJ, et al. Pediatric chemotherapy induced peripheral neuropathy: A systematic review of current knowledge. Cancer Treat Rev 2016; 50:118–28.

86. Kandula T, Farrar MA, Cohn RJ, et al. Chemotherapy-induced peripheral neuropathy in long-term survivors of childhood cancer: clinical, neurophysiological, functional, and patient-reported outcomes. JAMA Neurol 2018;75(8):980–8.

87. Ness KK, Jones KE, Smith WA, et al. Chemotherapy-related neuropathic symptoms and functional impairment in adult survivors of extracranial solid tumors of childhood: results from the St. Jude Lifetime Cohort Study. Arch Phys Med Rehabil 2013;94(8):1451–7.

88. Chang KW, Chinosornvatana N. Practical grading system for evaluating cisplatin ototoxicity in children. J Clin Oncol 2010;28(10):1788–95.

89. Schmidt CM, Bartholomaus E, Deuster D, et al. [The "Muenster classification" of high frequency hearing loss following cisplatin chemotherapy]. HNO 2007; 55(4):299–306.

90. National Cancer Institute. Common terminology criteria for adverse events, version 4.03 2010. Available at: http://evs.nci.nih.gov/ftp1/CTCAE/CTCAE_4.03/. Accessed October 28, 2019.

The Future of Childhood Cancer Survivorship
Challenges and Opportunities for Continued Progress

Stephanie B. Dixon, MD, MPH[a],*, Eric J. Chow, MD, MPH[b],
Lars Hjorth, MD[c,d], Melissa M. Hudson, MD[e],
Leontien C.M. Kremer, MD[f,g], Lindsay M. Morton, PhD[h],
Paul C. Nathan, MD, MSc[i], Kirsten K. Ness, PhD[j],
Kevin C. Oeffinger, MD[k], Gregory T. Armstrong, MD, MSCE[j]

KEYWORDS

- Adolescent • Cancer • Child • Delivery of health care • Neoplasms • Survivor
- Treatment outcome

KEY POINTS

- Childhood cancer survivorship research has made substantial advances toward improving understanding of treatment-related toxicities.
- Future efforts should
  - Emphasize collaborative approaches, including pooling of data across studies, to address a range of research questions.

Continued

[a] Department of Oncology, St. Jude Children's Research Hospital, MS 735, 262 Danny Thomas Place, Memphis, TN 38105, USA; [b] Fred Hutchinson Cancer Research Center, University of Washington, 1100 Fairview Avenue North, M4-C308, Seattle, WA 98109, USA; [c] Department of Paediatrics, Skane University Hospital, Lund, Sweden; [d] Clinical Sciences Lund, Lund University, Lund 221 85, Sweden; [e] Division of Cancer Survivorship, Department of Oncology, St. Jude Children's Research Hospital, MS 735, 262 Danny Thomas Place, Memphis, TN 38105, USA; [f] Princess Maxima Center, Heidelberglaan 25, Utrecht 3584 CS, Netherlands; [g] Emma Children's Hospital, Amsterdam UMC, Amsterdam, Netherlands; [h] Radiation Epidemiology Branch, Division of Cancer Epidemiology and Genetics, Department of Health and Human Services, National Cancer Institute, National Institutes of Health, 9609 Medical Center Drive, MSC 9778, Bethesda, MD 20892-9778, USA; [i] Division of Hematology/Oncology, The Hospital for Sick Children, 555 University Avenue, Room 9402 Black Wing, Toronto, ON M5G 1X8, Canada; [j] Department of Epidemiology and Cancer Control, St. Jude. Children's Research Hospital, MS 735, 262 Danny Thomas Place, Memphis, TN 38105, USA; [k] Duke Center for Onco-Primary Care, Duke Cancer Institute, 2424 Erwin Drive, Suite 601, Durham, NC 27705, USA
* Corresponding author.
E-mail address: stephanie.dixon@stjude.org

Pediatr Clin N Am 67 (2020) 1237–1251
https://doi.org/10.1016/j.pcl.2020.07.013

Continued

o Integrate individualized approaches to risk prediction, including integration of genomic data, to provide opportunities to prevent late effects in survivors.
o Maximize knowledge of late effects of novel therapies, intervention strategies, aging and accelerated aging, health services utilization, and dissemination and implementation science to better promote adoption of survivorship care recommendations by aging adult survivors and their providers.

INTRODUCTION

In 1975, Giulio D'Angio[1] stated that "cure is not enough" and late effects research was declared an essential priority. As detailed in the preceding articles in this issue, there is a growing, global population of childhood cancer survivors who face unique health and psychosocial challenges in adulthood as a result of their prior cancer treatment. Decades of studies have described the long-term and late health outcomes experienced by survivors including risks conferred by specific therapy exposures, and demographic and lifestyle factors.[2–6] However, the future of cancer survivorship research must focus on novel approaches to identify, prevent, and mitigate adverse effects of cancer therapy. Attention also should be paid to disseminate and implement uniform and cost-effective patient-centered survivorship care within diverse clinical settings. To do this, future research priorities must include multidisciplinary and internationally collaborative approaches to better understand the toxicity of novel agents, contribution of genetic factors and aging to late effects, targets for intervention, and the role of health services research and implementation science to ensure universal access to evidence-based and comprehensive survivorship care.

LARGE COHORT COLLABORATION: POOLING OF DATA TO ANSWER THE UNANSWERED QUESTIONS

Despite growing numbers of survivors, childhood cancer remains a rare disease, and although most survivors experience early and late complications of disease and treatment, identification of low prevalence, yet clinically important late effects, such as rare subsequent neoplasms, are difficult to ascertain due to the small number of events. Multiple institutions and cooperative groups have developed and followed childhood cancer survivors in large cohorts.[5,7–9] Still, the numbers of childhood cancer survivors with a given combination of treatment exposures or specific late effects are often not large enough to answer key research questions regarding risk for toxicity. Optimally, the pooling of data across groups and projects could address this issue.

Combining data from various cohorts can facilitate early identification of late complications, both known and novel, and updating of surveillance recommendations in long-term follow-up clinical practice guidelines. Two examples of recently completed studies highlight the power of using pooled cohort data to more accurately define late effect risks of specific therapeutic exposures as well as model an individual's risk for a specific late effect. In the first, demographic, treatment, and late-outcomes data from the Childhood Cancer Survivor Study (CCSS), the Dutch Children's Oncology Group's (DCOG) LATER study, and the St Jude Lifetime (SJLIFE) study were used to evaluate the assumption that the long-term cardiotoxicity of anthracycline and anthraquinone agents was equivalent to their established hematological toxicity profile.[10,11] This analysis, including data from nearly 30,000 childhood cancer survivors, demonstrated that daunorubicin, previously thought to be roughly isoequivalent to doxorubicin, was only half as cardiotoxic when cardiomyopathy was used as an endpoint, whereas mitoxantrone was at least 10 times as cardiotoxic as doxorubicin.[10,11] These findings prompted a change in the previous doxorubicin equivalent conversion of 1:1 for daunorubicin and reconsideration of the prior conversion of 4:1 for mitoxantrone. These findings will certainly impact the screening recommendations for individuals who received mitoxantrone or daunorubicin by modifying their cumulative anthracycline exposure and will also inform future frontline and relapse protocol development. In the second example, data from the CCSS, SJLIFE, and Emma Children's Hospital/Academic Medical Center were used to develop and validate a risk-prediction model for heart failure, ischemic heart disease, and stroke among 5-year childhood cancer survivors through age 50.[12–14] These models allow for individualized risk prediction based on demographic factors, chemotherapy and radiation doses, and traditional cardiovascular risk factors (hypertension, diabetes, dyslipidemia) that may assist in patient education as well as clinical decision making regarding potentially risk-reducing interventions.

Finally, if a late complication of cancer treatment has occurred, care should focus on ameliorating the effects and providing the necessary support to the survivor. By pooling cohort data, we are more likely to understand the magnitude and severity of late complications that should inform better understanding of the interventions and support services that may benefit the affected survivor. Optimizing care for childhood cancer survivors requires new collaborations across cooperative groups, institutional studies, and national and continental borders.

DEFINING GENETIC CONTRIBUTIONS TO LATE EFFECTS RISK

Research in the general population has demonstrated that genetic factors contribute to many of the conditions for which childhood cancer survivors have elevated risks, such as subsequent malignancies, cardiovascular disease, obesity, and hearing loss.[15] Advances in technology and concurrent reductions in genotyping and sequencing costs have facilitated research in large study populations, which has enabled the identification of both common and rare genetic risk variants in novel biological pathways that underlie these conditions in the general population.[16,17]

The contribution of inherited factors to the development of selected conditions in childhood cancer survivors is currently unknown.[18,19] However, as the technological advances used in the general population are leveraged to study cancer survivors, the future holds tremendous promise for defining the genetic contributions to a range of disease risks after childhood cancer. Preliminary evidence suggests that certain rare and common genetic factors act similarly in both the general population and among survivors,[20–22] although further research is needed to understand whether the joint effect of genetic susceptibility and treatment-related risks is additive or multiplicative. Other studies have identified novel genetic risk factors among survivors,[23] suggesting that the pathophysiology underlying treatment-related conditions may differ from that seen in the general population.

To comprehensively define the genetic contributions to disease risk after childhood cancer, international, interdisciplinary collaborations will be required to create studies with sufficient sample sizes and diversity of patient characteristics (eg, specific treatment exposures, race/ethnicity, and ages). As demonstrated in the general population, large sample sizes that enable replication of results in independent populations are especially important in genomics research to protect against false positive reports. However, the challenges of developing such collaborations are dwarfed by the importance of discovering the biological pathways that underlie these conditions, thereby providing clues to prevention approaches and informing clinical decision making for frontline treatment recommendations and long-term surveillance. The coming years should see a dramatic expansion in the consideration of genetic susceptibility in survivorship after childhood cancer.

IDENTIFYING LATE EFFECTS OF NOVEL THERAPIES

In recent years, improved understanding of the biology of many pediatric cancers has led to the development of multiple new agents that offer the promise of more effective and less toxic treatment (**Table 1**). For example, an initial success came with Philadelphia-positive acute lymphoblastic leukemia, in which the tyrosine kinase inhibitor, imatinib, plus chemotherapy, transformed 3-year event-free survival from less than 50% to ~80%.[24] The addition of other molecularly targeted agents to conventional chemotherapy is now routine in subsets of patients with acute myeloid leukemia, lymphoma, and sarcoma in whom specific tumor mutations appear amenable to such inhibitors (eg, FLT3-internal tandem duplications, anaplastic large cell kinase mutations, NTRK fusions, respectively).[25–27] The addition of antibody-based therapies to conventional chemotherapy has also improved outcomes for many pediatric malignancies. For example, dinutuximab, rituximab, brentuximab, and gemtuzumab are already considered standard of care for certain newly diagnosed or relapsed neuroblastomas, lymphomas, and leukemias, respectively.[28–31] Ongoing trials are testing the efficacy of other promising antibodies such as blinatumomab and inotuzumab,[32,33] and the optimal role of immune checkpoint inhibitors and genetically engineered chimeric antigen receptor (CAR) T cells.[34,35] For local control, surgery and radiotherapy have also evolved to become less invasive, or feature new techniques and particles (eg, protons) that more precisely target the tumor and limit dose to normal tissues.[36]

Nevertheless, "targeted" agents, like conventional chemotherapy, radiotherapy, and surgery, may have off-target effects.[36] For example, growth issues have been reported in children treated long-term with imatinib.[37,38] Although not yet reported in children, rare but serious immune-related toxicities (eg, autoimmune myocarditis) have been observed in adults, including young adults, treated with immune checkpoint inhibitors.[39] As experience with new agents and modalities grows, the established paradigm of requiring large phase 2 or 3 trials to establish efficacy before an agent becoming standard of care may no longer be feasible in all situations.[40] Given that pediatric cancer is relatively rare and, hopefully, that delayed but serious off-target toxicities are even less frequent, longitudinal systematic follow-up of children treated with novel emerging therapies is critical to determining whether these therapies are truly associated with improved long-term outcomes compared with historical treatments. Decades of follow-up are required to demonstrate improvements in long-term pediatric cancer outcomes.[41,42] To facilitate this, a joint effort by the pharmaceutical industry, government, and nongovernmental professional societies to organize infrastructure that enables such long-term follow-up is recommended. Such infrastructure should include, at minimum, the creation of a registry that allows for later linkage and ability to re-contact patients or families for follow-up information, or if possible, a more resource-intensive prospective cohort.

IDENTIFYING FRAILTY AND ACCELERATED AGING

Studies conducted in past decades identified increased risk for chronic health conditions, multiple health conditions, and mortality compared with the general population

Table 1
Molecularly targeted agents being used or under consideration for pediatric cancers

Target(s)	Drug(s)	Notable Toxicities[a]
ALK/ROS	Ceritinib Crizotinib Ensartinib Lorlatinib	Arrhythmia Dyslipidemia (lorlatinib) Hyperglycemia (ceritinib) Hallucinations/psychiatric (lorlatinib) Neuropathy/neuromuscular Pulmonary embolism (crizotinib) Respiratory Vision changes

BCR/ABL,
  KIT, PDGFR
	Dasatinib
	Imatinib
	Nilotinib
	Ponatinib
		Cardiac dysfunction
		Edema, effusions
		Growth and stature[a]
		Pulmonary hypertension (dasatinib)
		Thyroid dysfunction
		Vascular events, including
		  myocardial ischemia, peripheral arterial
		  occlusion, and stroke (ponatinib)

BRAF	Dabrafenib Vemurafenib	Hyperglycemia (dabrafenib) New acute development of skin cancers QT-prolongation (vemurafenib) Radiation sensitivity
CD3	Blinatumomab	B cell aplasia (Chimeric antigen receptor [CAR] T cells)[a] Cytokine release syndrome Neurotoxicity
CD19	Blinatumomab CAR T cells	Same as with CD3-targeted agents above
CD20	Rituximab	B cell aplasia
CD30	Brentuximab vedotin	Neuropathy Progressive multifocal leukoencephalopathy
CD33	Gemtuzumab ozogamicin	Hepatotoxicity, sinusoidal obstruction syndrome
CDK/cyclin (cell cycle)	Palbociclib Ribociclib	QT-prolongation (ribociclib)
EZH2	Tazemetostat	Limited experience to date
GD2	Dinutuximab Hu3F8 Hu14.18K322A	Capillary leak syndrome Neuropathic pain Reversible posterior leukoencephalopathy

HDAC (histone
  deacetylase)
	Entinostat
	Fimepinostat
	Panobinostat
	Romidepsin
	Vorinostat
		Arrhythmia/myocardial infarction
		Pulmonary embolus (vorinostat)
		*Limited experience for entinostat,
		  fimepinostat*

MEK/MAPK	Binimetinib Cobimetinib Selumetinib Trametinib	Cardiac dysfunction Skin toxicity Vision changes, retinopathy

(continued on next page)

Table 1 (continued)		
Target(s)	Drug(s)	Notable Toxicities[a]
mTOR	Everolimus Sirolimus Temsirolimus ABI-009 (Nab-Rapamycin) LY3023414	Dyslipidemia Hyperglycemia

PD-1, PDL-1, CTL4 (immune checkpoint)	Atezolizumab
	Avelimumab
	Cemiplimab
	Durvalumab
	Ipilimumab
	Nivolumab
	Pembrolizumab
		Autoimmune/inflammatory, including
		  Endocrinopathies
		  Myocarditis
		  Neurotoxicity
		  Pneumonitis

PI3K	Fimepinostat LY3023414	Hyperglycemia
TRK	Entrectinib Larotrectinib	Limited experience to date
VEGF, VEGFR, PDGFR, RET	Axitinib Bevacizumab Cabozantinib Lenvantinib Pazopanib Sorafenib Vandetanib	Cardiac dysfunction Hemorrhage, impaired wound healing Hepatotoxicity (pazopanib) Hypertension, proteinuria Intestinal perforation/fistula (bevacizumab) Thromboembolism Thyroid dysfunction (axitinib, pazopanib, sorafenib)

Abbreviations: MAPK, mitogen-activated protein kinase; mTOR, mammalian target of rapamycin; PD-1, programmed cell death 1; PDGFR, platelet-derived growth factor receptor; sPDL-1, PD-1 ligand; ROS, reactive oxygen species; VEGF, vascular endothelial growth factor; VEGFR, VEGF receptor.

[a] Toxicities that may persist well after cessation of therapy or develop later.

Adapted from Chow EJ, Antal Z, Constine LS, et al. New agents, emerging late effects, and the development of precision survivorship. J Clin Oncol. 2018;36(21):2231-2240; with permission.

and have suggested a process of accelerated aging among adult childhood cancer survivors.[2,3] More recently, measures generally used in geriatric populations, such as frailty, characterized by decreased physiologic reserve, have been identified as a prevalent condition among young adult childhood cancer survivors. At a median age of 33 years, survivors were observed to have rates of frailty higher than those observed in the general population in their seventh decade of life (**Fig. 1**).[43,44] Frailty, in the general population, identifies individuals who are at risk for poor health outcomes including early mortality.[43] Aging may be accelerated among childhood cancer survivors due to chemotherapy-induced and radiation-induced damage to normal, nonmalignant cells. Some evidence suggests that molecular mechanisms associated with physiologic aging in the general population may potentiate premature aging among survivors, including cellular senescence, telomere attrition, changes in DNA methylation patterns, accumulation of somatic DNA mutations, and loss of mitochondrial fidelity (**Fig. 2**).[45,46] However, few studies have evaluated specific associations of these mechanisms with accelerated aging in childhood cancer survivors.

Although better understanding of the underlying mechanisms is needed, existing data may also be used to guide effective clinical trial development. Markers of aging have been shown to be responsive to exercise in the general population.[46] Among

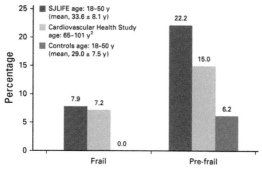

Fig. 1. Percentage of survivors in the SJLIFE who meet the criteria for frailty compared with participants in the Cardiovascular Health Study and healthy controls. N = 1922 (50.3% male); mean time since diagnosis, 25.5±7.7 years; mean age at diagnosis, 8.2±5.6 years; 43% leukemia; 33% with cranial radiation exposure. (*From* Ness KK, Kirkland JL, Gramatges MM, et al. Premature Physiologic Aging as a Paradigm for Understanding Increased Risk of Adverse Health Across the Lifespan of Survivors of Childhood Cancer. *J Clin Oncol.* 2018;36(21):2206-2215; with permission.)

childhood cancer survivors, exercise intervention led to increased lean mass, strength, and walking speed[47]; however, future research is needed to specifically measure the impact of exercise on biomarkers of aging. Senolytic agents selectively eliminate senescent cells that are no longer dividing and have demonstrated efficacy in the treatment of multiple chronic diseases in animal models including frailty and radiation-induced muscle wasting.[48,49] Clinical trials are needed to assess the impact of these and other pharmacologic agents on delaying or reversing markers of aging.

However, as premature aging among survivors differs from physiologic aging in the general population, improving not only the lifespan but also the health span of an aging population of adult childhood cancer survivors necessitates a better understanding of the molecular mechanisms most critical in potentiating early aging. With this knowledge, identification of specific subgroups of survivors at highest risk and subsequent development of novel pharmacologic and lifestyle interventions that target biologic pathways to prevent, or delay, aging associated with cancer and cancer treatment will be possible in the future.

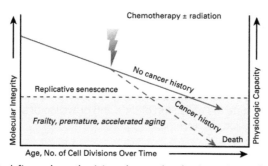

Fig. 2. Extrapolated figure hypothesizing that molecular integrity and associated physiologic capacity provoked by exposure to chemotherapy and/or radiation may be associated with excess risk and advanced onset of age-related diseases and frailty. (*From* Ness KK, Kirkland JL, Gramatges MM, et al. Premature Physiologic Aging as a Paradigm for Understanding Increased Risk of Adverse Health Across the Lifespan of Survivors of Childhood Cancer. *J Clin Oncol.* 2018;36(21):2206-2215; with permission.)

INTERVENTION AND PRECISION PREVENTION OF LATE EFFECTS

The National Institutes of Health has defined precision medicine as *"an emerging approach for disease prevention and treatment that takes into account people's individual variation in genes, environment, and lifestyle."* The use of cancer therapies targeted at specific molecular abnormalities in tumors has led to a revolution in the precision medicine approach to treating cancer. However, development of precision approaches to preventing or treating the late effects that can arise from cancer therapies has lagged. *Precision survivorship*[36] integrates the genomic features of a patient with cancer with traditional risk factors such as demographics (eg, age, sex, race/ethnicity) and treatment exposures (eg, cumulative chemotherapy doses, radiation) to more precisely predict late effects risk. Better risk prediction can be applied at the time of cancer therapy[50] to improve counseling or inform the use of protective agents or modification of chemotherapy dose or type, or in follow-up to guide the efficient use of surveillance, prophylaxis, or early therapy of subclinical late effects. This can be enhanced by integrating individual data about lifestyle, comorbid health conditions, and other chronic disease risk factors.[13] As other elements of a survivor's -omics profile become available (eg, proteomics, metabolomics),[51] risk-prediction models could be further enriched.

Most of the intervention studies aimed at improving survivor outcomes have focused on the completion of recommended late effects surveillance.[52–54] Despite this, adherence to published late effects guidelines is generally poor.[55] Similarly, trials of secondary chemoprevention of late effects (eg, use of low-dose tamoxifen to reduce breast cancer risk in irradiated survivors) have generally struggled to accrue patients, in part because of the lack of precision in determining at-risk survivors and survivors' reluctance to take medications with adverse side-effect profiles to prevent a late effect that they may or may not develop. More precise classification of "at-risk" status can improve the focus of interventions on those survivors at particularly elevated risk, potentially improving survivors' willingness to participate in such trials. In addition, true precision prevention acknowledges that interventions may need to be tailored to specific survivor phenotypes. For example, a recent study identified that survivors are at increased risk for exercise intolerance for many reasons (cardiac, pulmonary, neuropathic, and muscular impairments, among others).[56] Based on these findings, survivors will need interventions tailored to their specific deficits to improve their exercise tolerance.

Mobile health (mHealth) interventions offer an opportunity for better targeting of risk-based survivor care. In the survivorship context, mHealth platforms will allow for easier, real-time communication between survivors and their care providers, and remote collection of biometric data (eg, blood pressure), medical data (eg, teledermatology),[57] or patient-reported outcome measures (eg, pain). "Real-time" access to such individualized patient data will guide the provision of appropriate survivor care, even remotely. Thus, the combination of more precise predictors of long-term risk and new tools to facilitate the collection of data and provision of survivor care will herald a new era of precision survivorship.

THE FUTURE OF HEALTH SERVICES RESEARCH FOR CHILDHOOD CANCER SURVIVORS

Previous health service research in childhood cancer survivors has largely focused on determining how social factors and health behaviors among survivors affect their access and use of health services.[58–60] This knowledge has been helpful in characterizing survivors at high risk for morbidity and guiding the development of interventions for populations vulnerable to specific adverse health outcomes. Surprisingly, few studies have addressed the quality and cost-effectiveness of survivorship care delivered within health care systems or its impact on important outcomes such as survivor satisfaction, health-related quality of life, chronic symptoms and disease burden, health care utilization, and survival.[61,62] Correspondingly, despite a plethora of publications describing models of survivorship care, evaluating the use of cancer treatment summaries and survivorship care plans, and promoting risk-based health surveillance recommendations,[63,64] studies are lacking that demonstrate how these resources can be feasibly and effectively implemented in oncology and primary care settings to facilitate care coordination, reduce duplication of services, and improve survivorship outcomes.

Progress in survivorship care and enhancement of the health span of the growing population of childhood cancer survivors requires methodologically rigorous research guided by an analytical framework of established health care quality measures, particularly timeliness, patient-centeredness, efficiency, and equity of care. **Table 2** summarizes the common domains of health care quality measures and potential survivorship topics relevant to these measures advocated by the National Academy of Medicine (formerly the Institute of Medicine).[65] To address knowledge deficits related to survivorship care, careful conceptualization of research aims within the context of survivor, health care provider, community, and health care system factors influencing access to services and survivorship outcomes is essential. In the absence of an integrated health services system, robust infrastructure will need to be

Table 2
Institute of Medicine domains of health care quality

Domain	Aim for Health Care Quality	Relevance to Childhood Cancer
Safe	Avoiding harm to patients from the care that is intended to help them.	Are there efforts and systems in place to monitor late effects of childhood cancer and its treatment?
Effective	Providing services based on scientific knowledge to all who could benefit and refraining from providing services to those not likely to benefit (avoiding underuse and misuse, respectively).	Do survivors have access to surveillance, treatment, and interventions known to impact late effects?
Patient-centered	Providing care that is respectful of and responsive to individual patient preferences, needs, and values and ensuring that patient values guide all clinical decisions.	Is survivorship care designed around the preferences and needs of and resources available to survivors? Is financial toxicity and survivor engagement considered in care planning?
Timely	Reducing waits and sometimes harmful delays for both those who receive and those who give care.	Are diagnoses of posttreatment health problems made quickly and without delay?
Efficient	Avoiding waste, including waste of equipment, supplies, ideas, and energy.	Are resources used efficiently? Is there communication between survivors and providers over time and across settings of care?
Equitable	Providing care that does not vary in quality because of personal characteristics, such as gender, ethnicity, geographic location, and socioeconomic status.	Are there disparities in care and outcomes based on social risk? Are survivors able to receive care in a nearby and convenient location?

developed to support longitudinal investigations of factors influencing access and utilization of health services across the survivorship spectrum from diagnosis, to after completion of therapy, and into long-term follow-up. Improving care coordination should focus on investigation of scalable methods of communication and education at transition milestones, particularly during the transition from oncology to primary care. Historically, survivorship care plans aimed to serve this purpose but, considering the lack of uniform evidence to demonstrate benefit,[66] evaluation of stakeholder perspective (both survivors and providers) is critical to advance understanding about barriers to coordination and implementation of quality, patient-centered survivorship care.

DISSEMINATION AND IMPLEMENTATION SCIENCE TO IMPROVE SURVIVORSHIP CARE

In 2001, the National Academy of Medicine brought to light the major gap between the quality and efficiency of care that could be delivered when health care was informed by scientific evidence and the care that was delivered in routine practice, termed the *quality chasm*.[65] Dissemination and implementation (D&I) science is designed to bridge that chasm and translate research findings into clinical practice. D&I research in survivors is needed to fill the identified gap between what survivorship care could be with improved care coordination, seamless transition from oncology to primary care, and uniform access to evidence-based screening or intervention strategies outlined previously, and what is the reality of often fractured and inconsistent, if any, survivorship care today. Given the emphasis on guideline development and intervention, collaboration with experts in dissemination and implementation will be essential to translate these findings to the almost half million survivors in the United States and many more around the world.[67]

THE FUTURE OF EVIDENCE-BASED GUIDELINE DEVELOPMENT

In Joshua D. Palmer and colleagues' article, "Radiotherapy and Late Effects," in this issue, the international collaboration for guideline development (IGHG) has been described. International collaboration is needed to keep up-to-date with the increasing number of new papers on (interventions for) health problems in childhood cancer survivors, to avoid duplication of work, and to make the process of translating evidence to recommendation transparent. As new knowledge is always emerging, it is essential that a process is in place to update guidelines regularly or perform continuous review of new evidence. Unfortunately, development of guidelines and updating them is a time consuming process. New methods for development and timely updating of these guidelines is essential to bridge the gap between knowledge and practice. The IGHG is developing a living guidelines ICT (Information and Communication Technology) tool in collaboration with a European project (PanCareFollowUp). This ICT tool "the living guideline" will be able to regularly search the literature and to provide guideline groups with new evidence. It will also support the guideline groups to grade new evidence and, if needed, adjust current recommendations. This will help to translate new knowledge into guidelines in an efficient way.

Keeping guidelines up-to-date is important, but simply having guidelines in place does not mean that clinicians are using them for survivorship care in their clinical practice. The complexity of survivorship care may contribute to difficulties with implementation. Many health problems can occur, and the recommendations are based on many different types of cancer treatment. Future solution could include implementation of a digital decisions support tool, based on previous treatment, that could generate a treatment summary and an individual care plan for survivors. Such a tool can help to implement all recommendations in survivorship care.[68] Moreover, risk prediction tools, such as those discussed previously for cardiac risk, may help to refine future recommendations for an individual survivor.

Guidelines are also important to inform survivors and encourage survivorship care. Every survivor of childhood cancer should be aware of their specific treatment-related risks for health problems and suggested risk-based care recommendations from current guidelines. Every survivor of childhood cancer should be aware of their specific treatment-related risks for health problems and suggested risk-based care recommendations from current guidelines. A nice example is the Survivorship Passport initiative of the European Network for Cancer research in Children and Adolescents (ENCCA) in collaboration with other key stakeholders across Europe to develop individualized, Web-based, survivorship care plans using follow-up and screening recommendations from the International Guidelines Harmonization Group (IGHG) and PanCare Childhood and Adolescent Cancer Survivor Care and Follow-Up Studies (www.PanCareFollowUp.eu and www.survivorshippassport.org).[68]

In addition to having an individualized survivorship care plan, ensuring availability of cancer survivorship guidelines in lay language and translation of cancer survivorship guidelines into multiple languages, using nonmedical terminology, will enable survivors to manage their own care. Nice examples are the lay language summaries for guideline recommendations described in the Survivorship Passport (www.survivorshippassport.org) and at the *Together* Web site from St. Jude Children's Research Hospital (together.stjude.org/en-us).

SUMMARY

As survival continues to improve for children diagnosed with cancer and the growing population of childhood cancer survivors in the United States alone now approaches 500,000,[67] we must focus on how to improve not just the duration but also the quality of life after childhood cancer. The future of survivorship research must prioritize expansion of knowledge of late health and psychosocial outcomes, including toxicity of novel therapies and genetic contribution to risk, by leveraging large-scale, collaborative research, and efforts toward prediction and prevention of late effects at the individual survivor level. Further, for these findings to translate into improved outcomes among survivors, they must be adopted by providers and health systems outside of pediatric oncology, which will require coordinated, national, and international efforts to overcome barriers to successful implementation of high-quality, patient-centered survivorship care.

DISCLOSURE

The authors have nothing to disclose.

REFERENCES

1. D'Angio GJ. Pediatric cancer in perspective: cure is not enough. Cancer 1975; 35(3 suppl):866–70.

2. Armstrong GT, Kawashima T, Leisenring W, et al. Aging and risk of severe, disabling, life-threatening, and fatal events in the Childhood Cancer Survivor Study. J Clin Oncol 2014;32(12):1218–27.

3. Bhakta N, Liu Q, Ness KK, et al. The cumulative burden of surviving childhood cancer: an initial report from the St Jude Lifetime Cohort Study (SJLIFE). Lancet 2017;390(10112):2569–82.

4. Teepen JC, van Leeuwen FE, Tissing WJ, et al. Long-term risk of subsequent malignant neoplasms after treatment of childhood cancer in the DCOG LATER Study Cohort: role of chemotherapy. J Clin Oncol 2017;35(20):2288–98.

5. Hudson MM, Ness KK, Gurney JG, et al. Clinical ascertainment of health outcomes among adults treated for childhood cancer. JAMA 2013;309(22):2371–81.

6. Dixon SB, Bjornard KL, Alberts NM, et al. Factors influencing risk-based care of the childhood cancer survivor in the 21st century. CA Cancer J Clin 2018;68(2): 133–52.

7. Hudson MM, Ness KK, Nolan VG, et al. Prospective medical assessment of adults surviving childhood cancer: study design, cohort characteristics, and feasibility of the St. Jude Lifetime Cohort study. Pediatr Blood Cancer 2011; 56(5):825–36.

8. Robison LL, Armstrong GT, Boice JD, et al. The Childhood Cancer Survivor Study: a National Cancer Institute-supported resource for outcome and intervention research. J Clin Oncol 2009;27(14):2308–18.

9. Winther JF, Kenborg L, Byrne J, et al. Childhood cancer survivor cohorts in Europe. Acta Oncol 2015;54(5):655–68.

10. Feijen EA, Leisenring WM, Stratton KL, et al. Equivalence ratio for daunorubicin to doxorubicin in relation to late heart failure in survivors of childhood cancer. J Clin Oncol 2015;33(32):3774–80.

11. Feijen EAM, Leisenring WM, Stratton KL, et al. Derivation of anthracycline and anthraquinone equivalence ratios to doxorubicin for late-onset cardiotoxicity. JAMA Oncol 2019;5(6):864–71.

12. Chow EJ, Chen Y, Hudson MM, et al. Prediction of ischemic heart disease and stroke in survivors of childhood cancer. J Clin Oncol 2018;36(1):44–52.

13. Chen Y, Chow EJ, Oeffinger KC, et al. Traditional cardiovascular risk factors and individual prediction of cardiovascular events in childhood cancer survivors. J Natl Cancer Inst 2019;112(3):256–65.

14. Chow EJ, Chen Y, Kremer LC, et al. Individual prediction of heart failure among childhood cancer survivors. J Clin Oncol 2015;33(5):394–402.

15. Price AL, Spencer CC, Donnelly P. Progress and promise in understanding the genetic basis of common diseases. Proc Biol Sci 2015;282(1821):20151684.

16. Michailidou K, Beesley J, Lindstrom S, et al. Genome-wide association analysis of more than 120,000 individuals identifies 15 new susceptibility loci for breast cancer. Nat Genet 2015;47(4):373–80.

17. Cline MS, Liao RG, Parsons MT, et al. BRCA Challenge: BRCA Exchange as a global resource for variants in BRCA1 and BRCA2. PLoS Genet 2018;14(12): e1007752.

18. Bhatia S. Genetic variation as a modifier of association between therapeutic exposure and subsequent malignant neoplasms in cancer survivors. Cancer 2015;121(5):648–63.

19. Gramatges MM, Bhatia S. Evidence for genetic risk contributing to long-term adverse treatment effects in childhood cancer survivors. Annu Rev Med 2018; 69:247–62.

20. Opstal-van Winden AWJ, de Haan HG, Hauptmann M, et al. Genetic susceptibility to radiation-induced breast cancer after Hodgkin lymphoma. Blood 2019; 133(10):1130–9.

21. Leong SL, Chaiyakunapruk N, Lee SW. Candidate gene association studies of anthracycline-induced cardiotoxicity: a systematic review and meta-analysis. Sci Rep 2017;7(1):39.
22. Wang Z, Wilson CL, Easton J, et al. Genetic risk for subsequent neoplasms among long-term survivors of childhood cancer. J Clin Oncol 2018;36(20): 2078–87.
23. Morton LM, Sampson JN, Armstrong GT, et al. Genome-wide association study to identify susceptibility loci that modify radiation-related risk for breast cancer after childhood cancer. J Natl Cancer Inst 2017;109(11):djx058.
24. Schultz KR, Bowman WP, Aledo A, et al. Improved early event-free survival with imatinib in Philadelphia chromosome-positive acute lymphoblastic leukemia: a children's oncology group study. J Clin Oncol 2009;27(31):5175–81.
25. Rollig C, Serve H, Huttmann A, et al. Addition of sorafenib versus placebo to standard therapy in patients aged 60 years or younger with newly diagnosed acute myeloid leukaemia (SORAML): a multicentre, phase 2, randomised controlled trial. Lancet Oncol 2015;16(16):1691–9.
26. Mosse YP, Voss SD, Lim MS, et al. Targeting ALK with crizotinib in pediatric anaplastic large cell lymphoma and inflammatory myofibroblastic tumor: a Children's Oncology Group study. J Clin Oncol 2017;35(28):3215–21.
27. Laetsch TW, DuBois SG, Nagasubramanian R, et al. A pediatric phase 1 study of larotrectinib, a highly selective inhibitor of the tropomyosin receptor kinase (TRK) family. J Clin Oncol 2017;35(suppl). abstr 10510.
28. Yu AL, Gilman AL, Ozkaynak MF, et al. Anti-GD2 antibody with GM-CSF, interleukin-2, and isotretinoin for neuroblastoma. N Engl J Med 2010;363(14): 1324–34.
29. Younes A, Gopal AK, Smith SE, et al. Results of a pivotal phase II study of brentuximab vedotin for patients with relapsed or refractory Hodgkin's lymphoma. J Clin Oncol 2012;30(18):2183–9.
30. Pollard JA, Loken M, Gerbing RB, et al. CD33 expression and its association with gemtuzumab ozogamicin response: results from the randomized phase III Children's Oncology Group trial AAML0531. J Clin Oncol 2016;34(7):747–55.
31. Minard-Colin V, Auperin A, Pillon M, et al. Results of the randomized Intergroup trial Inter-B-NHL Ritux 2010 for children and adolescents with high-risk B-cell non-Hodgkin lymphoma (B-NHL) and mature acute leukemia (B-AL): Evaluation of rituximab (R) efficacy in addition to standard LMB chemotherapy (CT) regimen. J Clin Oncol 2016;34(15s):10507.
32. von Stackelberg A, Locatelli F, Zugmaier G, et al. Phase I/phase II study of blinatumomab in pediatric patients with relapsed/refractory Acute Lymphoblastic Leukemia. J Clin Oncol 2016;34(36):4381–9.
33. Kantarjian HM, DeAngelo DJ, Stelljes M, et al. Inotuzumab ozogamicin versus standard therapy for acute lymphoblastic leukemia. N Engl J Med 2016;375(8): 740–53.
34. Pinto N, Park JR, Murphy E, et al. Patterns of PD-1, PD-L1, and PD-L2 expression in pediatric solid tumors. Pediatr Blood Cancer 2017;64(11):e26613.
35. Maude SL, Frey N, Shaw PA, et al. Chimeric antigen receptor T cells for sustained remissions in leukemia. N Engl J Med 2014;371(16):1507–17.
36. Chow EJ, Antal Z, Constine LS, et al. New agents, emerging late effects, and the development of precision survivorship. J Clin Oncol 2018;36(21):2231–40.
37. Shima H, Tokuyama M, Tanizawa A, et al. Distinct impact of imatinib on growth at prepubertal and pubertal ages of children with chronic myeloid leukemia. J Pediatr 2011;159(4):676–81.

38. Tauer JT, Hofbauer LC, Jung R, et al. Impact of long-term exposure to the tyrosine kinase inhibitor imatinib on the skeleton of growing rats. PLoS One 2015;10(6): e0131192.

39. Moslehi JJ, Salem JE, Sosman JA, et al. Increased reporting of fatal immune checkpoint inhibitor-associated myocarditis. Lancet 2018;391(10124):933.

40. DuBois SG, Corson LB, Stegmaier K, et al. Ushering in the next generation of precision trials for pediatric cancer. Science 2019;363(6432):1175–81.

41. Turcotte LM, Liu Q, Yasui Y, et al. Temporal trends in treatment and subsequent neoplasm risk among 5-year survivors of childhood cancer, 1970-2015. JAMA 2017;317(8):814–24.

42. Gibson TM, Mostoufi-Moab S, Stratton KL, et al. Temporal patterns in the risk of chronic health conditions in survivors of childhood cancer diagnosed 1970-99: a report from the Childhood Cancer Survivor Study cohort. Lancet Oncol 2018; 19(12):1590–601.

43. Fried LP, Tangen CM, Walston J, et al. Frailty in older adults: evidence for a phenotype. J Gerontol A Biol Sci Med Sci 2001;56(3):M146–56.

44. Ness KK, Krull KR, Jones KE, et al. Physiologic frailty as a sign of accelerated aging among adult survivors of childhood cancer: a report from the St Jude Lifetime Cohort Study. J Clin Oncol 2013;31(36):4496–503.

45. Lopez-Otin C, Blasco MA, Partridge L, et al. The hallmarks of aging. Cell 2013; 153(6):1194–217.

46. Ness KK, Kirkland JL, Gramatges MM, et al. Premature physiologic aging as a paradigm for understanding increased risk of adverse health across the lifespan of survivors of childhood cancer. J Clin Oncol 2018;36(21):2206–15.

47. Braam KI, van der Torre P, Takken T, et al. Physical exercise training interventions for children and young adults during and after treatment for childhood cancer. Cochrane Database Syst Rev 2016;(3):CD008796.

48. Kirkland JL, Tchkonia T. Cellular senescence: a translational perspective. EBioMedicine 2017;21:21–8.

49. Zhu Y, Tchkonia T, Pirtskhalava T, et al. The Achilles' heel of senescent cells: from transcriptome to senolytic drugs. Aging Cell 2015;14(4):644–58.

50. Aminkeng F, Ross CJ, Rassekh SR, et al. Recommendations for genetic testing to reduce the incidence of anthracycline-induced cardiotoxicity. Br J Clin Pharmacol 2016;82(3):683–95.

51. Biro K, Dombradi V, Jani A, et al. Creating a common language: defining individualized, personalized and precision prevention in public health. J Public Health (Oxf) 2018;40(4):e552–9.

52. Oeffinger KC, Ford JS, Moskowitz CS, et al. Promoting breast cancer surveillance: the EMPOWER study, a randomized clinical trial in the Childhood Cancer Survivor Study. J Clin Oncol 2019;37(24):2131–40.

53. Hudson MM, Leisenring W, Stratton KK, et al. Increasing cardiomyopathy screening in at-risk adult survivors of pediatric malignancies: a randomized controlled trial. J Clin Oncol 2014;32(35):3974–81.

54. Zabih V, Kahane A, O'Neill NE, et al. Interventions to improve adherence to surveillance guidelines in survivors of childhood cancer: a systematic review. J Cancer Surviv 2019;13(5):713–29.

55. Nathan PC, Ness KK, Mahoney MC, et al. Screening and surveillance for second malignant neoplasms in adult survivors of childhood cancer: a report from the childhood cancer survivor study. Ann Intern Med 2010;153(7):442–51.

56. Ness KK, Plana JC, Joshi VM, et al. Exercise intolerance, mortality, and organ system impairment in adult survivors of childhood cancer. J Clin Oncol 2020; 38(1):29–42.
57. Daniel CL, Armstrong GT, Keske RR, et al. Advancing Survivors' Knowledge (ASK) about skin cancer study: study protocol for a randomized controlled trial. Trials 2015;16:109.
58. Caplin DA, Smith KR, Ness KK, et al. Effect of population socioeconomic and health system factors on medical care of childhood cancer survivors: a report from the Childhood Cancer Survivor Study. J Adolesc Young Adult Oncol 2017; 6(1):74–82.
59. Casillas J, Oeffinger KC, Hudson MM, et al. Identifying predictors of longitudinal decline in the level of medical care received by adult survivors of childhood cancer: a report from the Childhood Cancer Survivor Study. Health Serv Res 2015; 50(4):1021–42.
60. Mueller EL, Park ER, Kirchhoff AC, et al. Insurance, chronic health conditions, and utilization of primary and specialty outpatient services: a Childhood Cancer Survivor Study report. J Cancer Surviv 2018;12(5):639–46.
61. Siembida EJ, Kadan-Lottick NS, Moss K, et al. Adolescent cancer patients' perceived quality of cancer care: The roles of patient engagement and supporting independence. Patient Educ Couns 2018;101(9):1683–9.
62. Sutradhar R, Agha M, Pole JD, et al. Specialized survivor clinic attendance is associated with decreased rates of emergency department visits in adult survivors of childhood cancer. Cancer 2015;121(24):4389–97.
63. Kadan-Lottick NS, Ross WL, Mitchell HR, et al. Randomized trial of the impact of empowering childhood cancer survivors with survivorship care plans. J Natl Cancer Inst 2018;110(12):1352–9.
64. Landier W, Chen Y, Namdar G, et al. Impact of tailored education on awareness of personal risk for therapy-related complications among childhood cancer survivors. J Clin Oncol 2015;33(33):3887–93.
65. Institute of Medicine Crossing the Quality Chasm. A new health system for the 21st century. Washington, DC: National Academy Press; 2001.
66. Jacobsen PB, DeRosa AP, Henderson TO, et al. Systematic review of the impact of cancer survivorship care plans on health outcomes and health care delivery. J Clin Oncol 2018;36(20):2088–100.
67. Robison LL, Hudson MM. Survivors of childhood and adolescent cancer: life-long risks and responsibilities. Nat Rev Cancer 2014;14(1):61–70.
68. Haupt R, Essiaf S, Dellacasa C, et al. The 'Survivorship Passport' for childhood cancer survivors. Eur J Cancer 2018;102:69–81.

Printed and bound by CPI Group (UK) Ltd, Croydon, CR0 4YY

03/10/2024

01040479-0010